ELECTRON SPIN RESONANCE IN CHEMISTRY

MONOGRAPHS ON ELECTRON SPIN RESONANCE

Editor: H. M. Assenheim, Israel Atomic Energy Commission

INTRODUCTION TO ELECTRON SPIN RESONANCE, H. M. Assenheim
ELECTRON SPIN RESONANCE IN SEMICONDUCTORS, G. Lancaster
ELECTRON SPIN RESONANCE SPECTROMETERS, T. H. Wilmshurst
BIOLOGICAL AND BIOCHEMICAL APPLICATIONS OF ELECTRON SPIN
    RESONANCE, D. J. E. Ingram
ELECTRON SPIN RELAXATION PHENOMENA IN SOLIDS, K. J. Standley and
    R. A. Vaughan
ELECTRON SPIN RESONANCE IN CHEMISTRY, L. A. Blumenfeld,
    V. V. Voevodski, and A. G. Semenov

Electron Spin Resonance in Chemistry

L. A. BLUMENFELD
V. V. VOEVODSKI
A. G. SEMENOV
Academy of Sciences of the U.S.S.R.

translated by

H. M. ASSENHEIM
M.Sc., Ph.D., M.I.E.E., A.Inst.P., C.Eng.

ADAM HILGER LTD
LONDON

This volume is a translation of the German edition
Die Anwendung der Paramagnetischen Elektronenresonanz in der Chemie
published by Akademische Verlagsgesellschaft Geest & Portig K.-G., Leipzig

© H. M. Assenheim, 1973

ISBN 0 85274 108 1

Published by
ADAM HILGER LTD
29 King Street, London WC2E 8JH

Set in cold type by William Clowes & Sons Ltd, London, Colchester and Beccles
Printed by photolithography by J. W. Arrowsmith Ltd, Bristol, BS3 2NT

PREFACE TO THE RUSSIAN EDITION

For six or seven years, most of the working hours of the authors of this book were devoted to the application of the methods of electron spin resonance (E.S.R.) to important topics in chemistry. In the course of this work, it became clear that, for a successful application of E.S.R. in systematic investigations, it is necessary

1. To possess a good, reliable, working instrument and to understand its operation;

2. To be well acquainted with the theoretical groundwork of the method, as is given in popular articles and reviews;

3. To interpret the resulting spectrum so that the maximum amount of information is obtained; and finally

4. To understand the general problems of modern chemistry and so be able, with the help of E.S.R., to distinguish between resolvable and irresolvable problems.

The authors needed considerable time to come to these simple conclusions. Even more time was spent in overcoming the problems caused by the lack of a reliable instrument and in collating the analytical methods to be used for the various spectra and the systematic application of E.S.R. to chemistry.

The aim of this book, which represents a complete summary of the authors' work, is to instruct those who may wish to use this technique and also to ease their path to success by enabling them to learn from our experiences.

The monograph consists of two parts. In the first part (Chapters 1 to 6), the experimental aspects of the technique, the theory of the method, and the interpretation of experimental results are considered. The second part (Chapters 7 to 12) concerns the solutions of a series of problems in the application of E.S.R. to modern chemistry.

The introduction (Chapter 1) comprises a general review of the method and its theoretical foundations, and of E.S.R. spectrometers. The second chapter describes in more detail the principles of construction of spectrometers, compares the most important features in existing types of spectrometer, and discusses the requirements of instruments designed for chemical applications.

Chapter 3 gives a short account of the theory of E.S.R. The purpose of this chapter is to introduce the reader to some problems in theoretical physics which he is likely to meet during a deeper analysis of E.S.R. results. It is clear that the mathematics of Chapters 2 and 3 will present some considerable difficulties to the unprepared reader. This should not discourage those chemists who wish to use E.S.R. to obtain quick solutions to their particular problems. The Introduction is a sufficient basis for the understanding of the subsequent chapters, and a more detailed study of the more difficult sections of Chapters 2 and 3 can be postponed until such time as the reader considers it worth his while to expend the effort required.

Chapters 4, 5 and 6 contain relatively simple and, in our opinion, extremely useful methods for the primary interpretation of spectra, which allow one to obtain much useful chemical information. The essentials of these methods were developed in the authors' laboratories.

Considering the rapid growth of published literature in chemical applications of E.S.R., it was considered pointless to try to write a critical summary of existing literature. Such a summary would be hopelessly out-dated even by the time of its publication. For this reason, in the second part of the book we have chosen problems in modern chemistry which we consider to be particularly interesting, and have tried to show what results can be achieved by investigating these problems with the help of E.S.R.

Naturally we have tried to choose problems in which the application of E.S.R. throws new light on the subject, and in which results are not obtainable by other techniques. However, it may seem that, of the examples used for demonstration, work carried out in the authors' laboratories plays a disproportionately large part. This is understandable, since we are more familiar with our own work than with other people's, and were thus able to find in it more features of general theoretical interest. This book is unlike other published monographs on E.S.R. largely because of our essentially different selection of material.

At this point, the authors wish to thank our collaborators at the Institute of Chemical Physics of the Academy of Science of the U.S.S.R.* and at the Institute for Chemical Kinetics at the Siberian Department of the Academy of Science of the U.S.S.R.†; J. N. Molin, J. S. Lebedev, W. B. Kasanski and J. D. Zvetkov, for their participation in the discussion of various problems appearing in this book; I. I. Tschcheidse, W. K. Jermolajev,

---

* In this translation, designated as ICP. (Translator)
† In this translation, designated as ICK. (Translator)

A. E. Kalmanson and D. M. Tschernikova, for performing special experiments and calculations; N. N. Tichomirova, N. N. Bubnov, I. W. Nikolajeva, G. B. Pariski, L. I. Schapovalova, M. D. Stschirov, A. A. Semenova and J. M. Shidomirova, for their encouragement in the writing of the monograph.

We take this opportunity of expressing our thanks to the engineers of the Institute for Chemical Physics, J. K. Russian and W. D. Grischin, with whose active co-operation the first spectrometer type E.P.R.-2 was designed and constructed.

                                        L. A. BLUMENFELD
                                        V. V. VOEVODSKI
                                        A. G. SEMENOV

PREFACE TO THE ENGLISH EDITION

As this book was written by the founders of the principles of E.S.R., its inclusion in our series of monographs was considered essential. The subject of the book, the chemical applications of E.S.R., is also one of the most important topics in this field.

The original text was published in Russia and subsequently, some years later, translated into German. For the German edition additional material was added. My translation has been made from the German edition, and I thank the publishers of that edition for granting me permission to translate.* I think that little has been lost in translating via a second language. I have kept as close as possible to the original text, and to the expressions and concepts of the authors. I have retained the use of the original M.K.S. units.

Though the original text was published in the previous decade, it, like many first works on new subjects, is essential reading if a full understanding of E.S.R. is to be obtained. All too often the original thinking of the inventors is forgotten, and one obtains a rather narrow and over-specialized treatment of the subject. This book will help the reader to see E.S.R. in full perspective, as it was seen by its inventors and used in its first applications.

The chemical applications of E.S.R. have long been considered the most important branch of the subject, first, with respect to the use of the technique as a tool in studying all aspects of chemical science, and second, as being the most fruitful field for future research, including such areas as irradiation chemistry, enzyme catalysis, and the study of human tissue. The authors have dwelt at some length on the biological applications, and their approach may well add to Western thought on the subject.

The book is in two parts. The first deals with the general concepts of E.S.R., and introduces some techniques which may be little known in the West. The second part deals with the application of E.S.R. to the solution of chemical problems, and gives many good examples. This section also covers the application to biological systems.

Generally speaking, this book is complementary to many monographs published in the series and, as a model of how the other half of the world does its research, it should find its way onto the bookshelves of most technical libraries, as well as into personal collections.

* Passages and references added by the German translator of the Russian edition are marked with an asterisk.

Finally, I should like to thank Dr Yehuda Suss for his considerable help in the first stages of the translation, and Stella Redwood of Jerusalem for typing the manuscript. Last, but not least, I should like to thank my daughter Julia, who started typing this preface and commented, 'I can type it, but I don't understand it.' I then rewrote the preface and now hope that it is comprehensible.

Tel-Aviv,
April 1973   H. M. ASSENHEIM

CONTENTS

Part 1: General Fundamentals of E.S.R.

1 INTRODUCTION   3

2 CONSTRUCTION PRINCIPLES OF E.S.R. SPECTROMETERS   10

Microwave systems in E.S.R. spectrometers. Magnetic field modulation. Amplifier and recorder systems for E.S.R. signals. Electrical interference and microphone effects. Reasons for distortion of the spectral line shape. Spectrometer sensitivity.

3 THEORY OF E.S.R. SPECTRA   46

The free paramagnetic atom. Fundamentals of the theory of groups and their representation: group theory. Group theory and quantum mechanics. The splitting of levels of the free paramagnetic atom in crystal fields of different symmetry. Calculation of the g-factor of a paramagnetic atom in a crystal. The anisotropy of the g-factor. Anisotropy and shift of the g-factor for organic free radicals. The hyperfine structure of E.S.R. spectra. Width and shape of E.S.R. lines. Summary.

4 ISOLATED, SYMMETRIC LINES IN E.S.R. SPECTRA   107

5 ASYMMETRIC E.S.R. LINES   122

Simple crystals with axial symmetry. Asymmetric E.S.R. lines in polycrystals: methods for the determination of $g_\perp$ and $g_\parallel$. Determination of the true line width from the shape of the asymmetric line. Line shapes of partially orientated polycrystals with axial symmetry.

6 THE HYPERFINE STRUCTURE OF THE E.S.R. SPECTRA   143

Basic characteristics of the H.F.S. formed by interaction with a magnetic nucleus. H.F.S. of several equivalent nuclei. H.F.S. of non-equivalent nuclei. E.S.R. spectra with poorly resolved H.F.S.: analytical treatment. E.S.R. spectra with poorly resolved H.F.S.: analysis using electronic computers. E.S.R. spectra with unresolved H.F.S.

Part 2: The Application of E.S.R. to the Solution of Chemical Problems

7 FREE RADICALS IN CHEMICAL REACTIONS   179

8 THE APPLICATION OF E.S.R. IN THE INVESTIGATION OF ELECTRON DELOCALIZATION PHENOMENA   188

Delocalization of unpaired electrons in stable radicals and radical ions. Spin delocalization in connection with multi-electron bonds. On the possibility of 'blocking' the delocalization. Electron delocalization in high molecular bonds. Chemical processes in complex systems which are connected with electron transfer and delocalization. Electron transfer under the influence of light. Production of free radicals.

xi

9 THE APPLICATION OF E.S.R. TO THE STUDY OF PROCESSES
WHICH TAKE PLACE VIA THE RADIOLYSIS OF SOLIDS 230

The investigation of radicals formed by irradiation of organic materials:
general remarks on the capabilities of E.S.R. in this field. On the
mechanism of the radiolysis of organic solids. Dependence of the
radiation yield on the chemical structure: 'hot' hydrogen atoms. Free
radicals from the radiolysis of biological materials.

10 THE KINETICS OF RADICAL REACTIONS IN THE SOLID PHASE 262

Determination of the reaction rates of free radicals in irradiated
polymers. On some peculiarities of the reaction kinetics of radical
recombination in the solid phase.

11 THE APPLICATION OF E.S.R. IN THE STUDY OF CATALYSTS
AND IN PRIMARY REACTIONS ON SURFACES 278

Free radicals which are absorbed on solid surfaces. The study of
catalytic agents which contain paramagnetic ions. The study of the
processes of enzyme catalysis.

12 THE APPLICATION OF E.S.R. TO THE INVESTIGATION OF
ORGANIC STRUCTURES 301

APPENDIX 1: TABLES OF THE CHARACTERISTICS OF THE
IRREDUCIBLE REPRESENTATIONS OF SOME SYMMETRY
GROUPS 313

APPENDIX 2: SPIN FUNCTIONS AND PAULI MATRICES 317

APPENDIX 3: INTENSITY DISTRIBUTION IN AN H.F.S.
SPECTRUM FOR n EQUIVALENT NUCLEI WITH $I = \frac{1}{2}$, 1, and $\frac{3}{2}$ 318

INDEX 321

PART I

GENERAL FUNDAMENTALS
OF E.S.R.

Chapter 1

Introduction

In 1944 at Kazan University, Zavoisky carried out investigations of paramagnetic relaxation at high frequencies (10^7 to 10^8 Hz), with the high frequency component oriented parallel and perpendicular to the static magnetic field. This was the first time that a systematic investigation of relaxation in crossed fields was performed, and he discovered in paramagnetic salts ($MnCl_2$, $CuSo_4 . 5H_2O$, etc.) an intensive resonance absorption of the high frequency energy, with a well-defined relationship between the magnetic field strength and the frequency. So a new physical phenomenon was discovered, which is now generally known as *electron spin resonance* or E.S.R.†

In the first years after this discovery, E.S.R. was used to solve special problems in fundamental physics. In the late forties came the successful application of the technique to the investigation of the finer details of electronic structure of paramagnetic ions in crystalline lattices of various symmetries. In the early fifties began the widespread use of E.S.R. for the solution of problems in chemistry. The reasons for this application are clear, for in modern chemistry it is extremely important to understand the structure and chemical properties of paramagnetic materials, which are closely involved in many complex chemical processes. On the one hand was the study of the paramagnetic metal ions of the transition groups of the periodic table, which form the active centres of a very large number of heterogeneous catalysts, or which are connected in metallo-organic complexes which determine the activity of complicated organic catalysts, among them the majority of the biological enzymes. On the other hand there were the detailed investigations of a large number of chemical reactions in the gas and liquid phase, among them photochemical, radiation-chemical, and biochemical processes, in which radical formation and chain mechanisms are widespread.

---

† In literature abroad the following abbreviations are used: PER (paramagnetische Elektronenresonanz), RPE (resonance paramagnetique electronique)

Owing to the difficulties of direct detection, concentration determination and structure interpretation of free radicals, the detection of the radical character was in most cases, and especially for fast reactions, carried out indirectly, on the basis of kinetic data. As will be shown later, the E.S.R. solution to both problems, which can be grouped together under the general heading of 'the role of particles with unpaired electrons in chemical processes', created a completely new and far deeper experimental and theoretical basis.

E.S.R. is based on the well-known Zeeman effect, which may be described as follows. If one introduces a paramagnetic particle, characterized by its quantum number S, into a constant magnetic field, then its ground state will be split into $2S + 1$ levels, which are separated in energy from each other by:

$$\Delta E = g\beta B$$

where B is the magnetic induction, β the unit of atomic magnetism, the Bohr magneton, and g the spectroscopic splitting factor, which determines the size of the effective magnetic moment of the particle.†

We will limit ourselves now to the simplest case, which is also the most frequent in chemistry, of $S = \frac{1}{2}$ (one unpaired electron). Here, two Zeeman levels arise in the applied magnetic field, with magnetic quantum numbers $S_z = \pm\frac{1}{2}$ and a separation of $2\beta B$. This corresponds to a magnetic induction of approximately $0\cdot3$ Wb m^{-2} at an energy difference of

$$\Delta E \simeq 0\cdot3 \text{ cm}^{-1} \simeq 4.10^{-5} \text{ eV} \simeq 1 \text{ cal/mol}$$

From this it follows that the magnitude of the splitting, at temperatures which are not too low, is from 10^2 to 10^3 times smaller than the mean thermal energy. The population of the levels in the magnetic field will differ in accordance with the Boltzmann law (for $\Delta E/kT \approx 2.10^{-3}$) by about $0\cdot2$ per cent. Equilibrium will be achieved in this case by transition processes of the magnetic moments between the levels $S_z = +\frac{1}{2}$ and $S_z = -\frac{1}{2}$ (orientation parallel and antiparallel to the field), at the expense of thermal motion, where the probability W_1 of the transitions from lower to higher level is $\exp[\Delta E/RT] \doteq 1\cdot002$ times smaller than the probability W_2 of the downward transition.

† In the simplest case, where the magnetic properties of the particle are caused by spin magnetism only, the equation $g = g_{el} = 2\cdot0023$ is valid, as is usual in atomic physics. In the case where the effective moment also depends on the orbital motion of the electrons, g can be either larger or smaller than g_{el}. In the majority of cases of interest in chemistry, and particularly for all free radicals, the deviation of the g value from the pure spin value is very small.

The essence of Zavoiski's discovery is the following: if a paramagnetic material is placed in a static magnetic field B, and a high frequency magnetic field of frequency

$$\nu = \frac{\Delta E}{h} = \frac{g\beta B}{h} \tag{1.1}$$

is applied perpendicular to the static magnetic field, then transitions between the neighbouring levels are induced with equal probability. During this process population levels will also tend to equalize themselves. The usual formula for the relative populations of both levels,

$$\frac{N_2}{N_1} = \frac{k_1}{k_2} = \frac{k_0 e^{-\Delta E/RT}}{k_0} = e^{-\Delta E/RT} \tag{1.2}$$

must, in accordance with the above, be replaced by the equation

$$\frac{N_2}{N_1} = \frac{k_1 + k_{ind}}{k_2 + k_{ind}}$$

where k_{ind} is the constant part of the transition velocity under the influence of the high frequency field B_1 (moreover $k_{ind} \simeq B_1^2$).

As a result of this, the population of the higher level becomes larger than that indicated by the Boltzmann distribution alone; also, in the stationary state, the number of downward thermal transitions will be larger than the number of upward thermal transitions. This means that a part of the energy of the high frequency field is absorbed in the sample, and heats it up. It can be easily shown that the rate of energy absorption in a system of N_0 paramagnetic particles is equal to

$$W \approx \frac{N_0 k_0}{2} \cdot \frac{\Delta E}{RT} \cdot \frac{k_{ind}}{k_0 + k_{ind}} \tag{1.3}$$

The experimental problem in observing the effect of E.S.R. is the accurate measurement of the absorbed high frequency energy. From the basic equation of E.S.R. (1.1) we can see that observation of spectra can be carried out in one of two ways:

(a) by changing the frequency and keeping a constant value of B, and
(b) by changing the magnetic induction and keeping a constant value of ν.

For technical reasons (see Chapter 6), the second method is used in all E.S.R. spectrometers, and so the presentation of the spectrum is in coordinates of $I_{abs} = f(B)$ with ν = constant, where I_{abs} is the intensity of the absorbed high frequency energy.

E.S.R. in Chemistry

The main components of an E.S.R. spectrometer are:
1. A high frequency or microwave generator.
2. A resonant circuit, in the magnetic field of which is placed the sample to be investigated. (For the high frequency region the sample is placed in the coil of an oscillator, and for the microwave region, in a cavity resonator.)
3. A detector with suitable amplification.
4. A pen recorder or similar device for displaying the signal.
5. A magnet.

The majority of standard E.S.R. spectrometers work at a wavelength of 3 cm, which for $g = 2$ corresponds to a magnetic induction $B \simeq 0.3$ Wb m^{-2}. This is done for several reasons: the samples have convenient dimensions, the magnetic fields may easily be generated, and microwave components readily available from radar systems may be used. For detailed structure investigations, it is frequently necessary to measure E.S.R. spectra at other frequencies as well. Such measurements are made at shorter as well as longer wavelengths, from 8 mm to 100 cm (in fields ranging from 1·2 to 0·01 Wb m^{-2}).

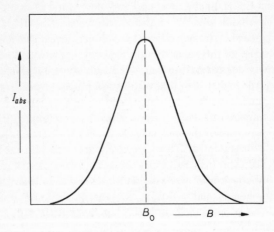

Fig. 1.1. E.S.R. absorption line.

Figure 1.1 shows a typical absorption line. The peak of the line corresponds to the value $B = B_0$, at which equation (1.1) is exactly fulfilled. In other words, from equation (1.1), at known ν and with a measured value of B_0, one can calculate the value of g, i.e. the effective magnetic moment of the paramagnetic centres. Since g is a specific value, measurements made at different frequencies will give resonance lines at different field strengths. The area under the absorption curve is proportional to the number of paramagnetic particles in the sample, assuming of course that measurements are made under otherwise equal conditions. The width and slope of the line can yield structural information about the paramagnetic particles, and information about the exchange interaction between the particles themselves and also with their surroundings. This will be shown in later chapters. The E.S.R. spectrum can give particularly valuable information in the case where the paramagnetic particle contains atoms with nuclear magnetic moments. In this case, the so-called hyperfine structure (H.F.S.) of the E.S.R. line is produced (the line being split into several components). From the number of components, their relative intensity and the magnitude of the splitting, one can obtain extremely important information about the structure and electron distribution of radicals which is not accessible by other methods. Electron displacement in complex organic structures was detected in this way for the first time.

Modern E.S.R. spectrometers are characterized in the following manner. For a very good instrument, the detection sensitivity for paramagnetic materials with an E.S.R. line width of 10^{-4} Wb m^{-2}, and a sample volume of 0·5 cm^3, is approximately 10^{12} unpaired electrons or $2 . 10^{-12}$ mol. The sensitivity of standard instruments used for chemical investigations usually reaches only $\frac{1}{5}$ or $\frac{1}{10}$ of this value. For particles with very wide lines the absolute sensitivity decreases. However, the sensitivity still remains several orders of magnitude higher than that of other techniques used for the detection of paramagnetic centres arising in chemical reactions. The advantage of E.S.R. compared to classical static magnetic measurements, is that in E.S.R. the diamagnetism of the molecules in the system has no influence on the results of the measurement. This is precisely the reason for the high sensitivity of E.S.R. This high sensitivity, however, is generally not sufficient for the investigation of free radicals formed by chemical reactions and during photochemical and radiation reactions in the liquid or gaseous phase. The concentration of radicals under these conditions does not usually exceed 10^{12} to 10^{13} cm^{-3}, and may be considerably smaller. It would appear possible that the sensitivity could be considerably increased by increasing the power of the microwave source, but this, from the foregoing treatment, gives rise to an increase in k_{ind} and does not permit an unlimited increase in sensitivity. In fact, (1.3) shows that for $k_{ind} \gg k_0$

$$W \approx \frac{k_0 N_0}{2} \cdot \frac{\Delta E}{RT} \tag{1.4}$$

which is independent of k_{ind}. This effect, called *saturation*, follows from the fact that at high microwave powers, the ratio of the population of both levels tends asymptotically to unity, and the rate of the change of microwave energy into heat (at a given k_0) is determined only by the thermal transition probability. On the one hand, saturation may be observed in many samples at relatively low powers; whilst on the other hand, with organic radicals, for which k_0 is usually very large, the sensitivity of standard spectrometers may be considerably increased by using more microwave power, provided that the temperature is not too low.

An important characteristic of E.S.R. spectrometers is their resolution, i.e. the ability to resolve finely spaced lines into separate components, and the accurate determination of line shape in a narrow field range. As the width of individual lines is usually larger than 10^{-5} Wb m^{-2}, one requires a homogeneity of approximately 10^{-5} over the sample volume at fields of 0·3 Wb m^{-2} (i.e. in the 3 cm wavelength region). This does not present much technical difficulty.† Similar requirements are also set for the frequency stability and other parameters of the electronic components (see Chapter 2).

The use of E.S.R. in chemistry requires particular attention to the stability and reproducibility of the spectrometer, as solutions to such problems require many series of experimental measurements carried out under identical conditions. The measurements of most importance are those concerned with the property changes of a system, which depend on such factors as time (kinetic measurements), the effect of added or substituted components, temperature, the nature of the solvent, and many other experimental conditions. With modern spectrometers, continuous measurements may be carried out over several hours, and at sample temperatures varying from below that of liquid helium to about 500°C.

The limitation of the use of E.S.R. in chemistry is usually insufficient sensitivity, which is particularly important in investigations of free radicals produced only in very small quantities. One must also take into account that some paramagnetic particles (some transition metal ions, complex molecules in the triplet state, etc.) do not normally give an E.S.R. signal, for reasons which will be dealt with in detail in Chapter 3; either because of strong line broadening or because the corresponding transitions fall well outside the usual frequency range. In many such cases, the E.S.R. spectra could be observed if measurements were performed at very low temperatures. On the other hand, components with measurable E.S.R. spectra could

† The homogeneity of the magnetic field in high resolution nuclear resonance spectrometers must not be less than 10^{-8}.

be obtained by bonding the magnetic ions to organic ligands, i.e. by changes of the electronic structure.

The sensitivity of the E.S.R. method deteriorates noticeably in cases where the sample exhibits a large dielectric loss or a large electric conductivity. The decrease in sensitivity follows from a reduction in the usable microwave power, a significant part of which now goes to the lossy dielectric. This effect is particularly troublesome in the study of aqueous solutions and biological samples, and in these cases one generally has to accept a reduced sensitivity.

With high electric conductivity, the microwave power is absorbed in the surface layer only, and will not penetrate further into the body of the sample. This will also make for a noticeable reduction in the sensitivity. Because of this, some measurements are made on specially prepared samples (e.g. alkali metals) consisting of finely dispersed particles of diameters from 1 to 10 μm. In the case of aqueous electrolytic solutions, very fine capillaries or thin films are used, giving a very high ratio of sample surface area to volume.

As can be seen from the above, E.S.R. offers unique facilities for the detection and measurement of active paramagnetic centres like free radicals and complexes, and also for the investigation of the electronic structure of paramagnetic ions in widely different compounds. In contrast to all other methods of investigation, E.S.R. not only detects free radicals, measures their concentration, identifies them and determines their structure, but may also give answers to questions which were unanswerable prior to direct experimental measurement, concerning the degree and character of the displacement of the unpaired electrons in the paramagnetic centre, or their exchange interaction with other nuclei in the molecule and with other unpaired electrons of the system. In addition to this, through the application of E.S.R. measurement to different materials, together with theoretical analysis of the results, many discoveries of prime importance in chemistry have been made; in particular, in the investigation of the structure of chemical bonds and the mechanisms of chemical processes. It is evident that the reactions and physico-chemical properties of condensed phases (among which are many molecules of high molecular weight) depend to a much greater extent than was previously assumed on very weak inter- and intramolecular exchange interactions. These interactions, being so weak, have such a small effect on the energy levels that they could not be identified using the usual methods.

In this book, the applications of E.S.R. in classical chemistry will be considered in detail, as well as completely new applications which stem from the technique.

Chapter 2

Construction Principles of E.S.R. Spectrometers

MICROWAVE SYSTEMS IN E.S.R. SPECTROMETERS

As we have already said, most of the present-day spectrometers are used in the centimetre wavelength region. In this type of spectrometer the sample to be investigated is located in the magnetic field of a cavity resonator. The cavity is placed between the pole pieces of an electromagnet so that, at the sample, the microwave magnetic field is perpendicular to the static magnetic field. If the magnetic field is slowly swept through the region which satisfies the condition for paramagnetic resonance (1.1), the damping in the cavity changes as a result of the absorption of microwave energy by the sample. At the same time, the resonant frequency of the cavity also changes. This second effect is induced by the change in the real part of the magnetic susceptibility χ' in the vicinity of the resonance, and produces a dispersion signal.

The power absorbed by the sample is calculated from the following equation:

$$P_{\text{sam}} = \frac{1}{2\mu_0}\omega \int\limits_{V_{\text{sam}}} \chi_0'' B_1^2 \mathrm{d}V \tag{2.1}$$

Here, ω is the angular frequency of the microwave oscillations, χ_0'' the imaginary part of the magnetic susceptibility, B_1 the amplitude of the microwave induction field, and V_{sam} the sample volume.

If the sample is physically very small, i.e. when it can be placed entirely in the region of maximum microwave field B_{1M}, one may write instead of (2.1),

$$P_{\text{sam}} = \frac{1}{2\mu_0}\omega\chi'' B_{1M}^2 \tag{2.2}$$

Here $\chi'' = \chi_0''$. V_{sam} is the susceptibility of the whole sample. The damping of the cavity is defined by the following equation:

$$d_0 = \frac{1}{Q_0} = \frac{1}{\omega_0} \cdot \frac{P_{cav}}{W_{cav}} = \frac{1}{\omega_0} \cdot \frac{P_{cav}}{\dfrac{1}{2\mu_0} \displaystyle\int_{V_{cav}} B_1^2 \mathrm{d}V} \tag{2.3}$$

where Q_0 is the unloaded Q of the cavity, P_{cav} the power converted to heat in the cavity, W_{cav} the energy stored in it, V_{cav} its volume, and ω_0 the angular resonance frequency.

Taking into account the E.S.R. absorption in the sample, for $\omega = \omega_0$ the damping of the cavity will be

$$d = \frac{P_{cav} + \dfrac{1}{2\mu_0} \omega_0 \chi'' B_{1M}^2}{\dfrac{\omega_0}{2\mu_0} \displaystyle\int_{V_{cav}} B_1^2 \mathrm{d}V} = d_0 + \frac{\chi''}{V_{eff}} \tag{2.4}$$

where

$$V_{eff} = \frac{\displaystyle\int_{V_{cav}} B_1^2 \mathrm{d}V}{B_{1M}^2} \tag{2.4a}$$

is usually called the effective cavity volume. From equation (2.4), we find that the change in damping of the cavity as a result of the E.S.R. absorption is

$$\Delta d = \frac{\chi''}{V_{eff}} \tag{2.5}$$

From the viewpoint of experimental technique, the problem of detecting E.S.R. spectra reduces to detecting changes in the damping of the cavity as a function of the field of the electromagnet.

Figures 2.1 and 2.2 show the two basic arrangements of the microwave part of centimetre-wave spectrometers. The spectrometer in Fig. 2.1 includes a transmission cavity. A change in damping of the cavity produces a change in the power passing through the cavity. The power incident on the detector in this arrangement is

$$P_D = P_0 \left| \frac{2\sqrt{(\beta_1 \beta_2)}}{1 + \beta_1 + \beta_2 + iQ_0 \left(\dfrac{\omega}{\omega_0} - \dfrac{\omega_0}{\omega}\right)} \right|^2 \tag{2.6}[1]$$

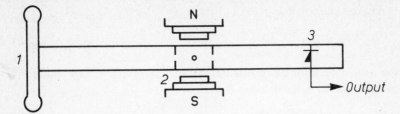

Fig. 2.1 Arrangement with transmission cavity.
1. microwave generator. 2. cavity with sample. 3. microwave detector.

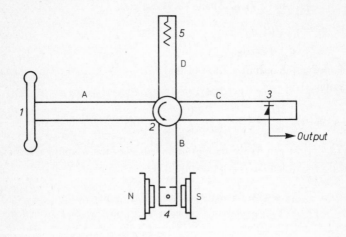

Fig. 2.2. Arrangement with reflection cavity.

1. microwave generator	4. cavity with sample
2. microwave bridge	5. matched load
3. microwave detector	

where P_0 is the power supplied by the microwave generator, and β_1 and β_2 the coupling coefficients of the cavity with the waveguide.

The coupling coefficients are determined from the following relationships:

$$\beta_1 = \frac{d_1}{d} \quad \text{and} \quad \beta_2 = \frac{d_2}{d} \tag{2.7}$$

where d_1 and d_2 are the damping factors due to the radiation through the coupling holes.

For $\omega = \omega_0$ we find

$$P_D = \frac{4\beta_1\beta_2}{(1 + \beta_1 + \beta_2)^2} P_0 \tag{2.8}$$

For a linear detector the relationship between its output voltage and the power absorbed in the detector is given by

$$U_D = \sqrt{(GP_DR_D)} \tag{2.9}$$

where G is the conversion factor of the detector and R_D its output resistance.

From equations (2.7), (2.8) and (2.9), we get

$$U_D = \frac{2\sqrt{(d_1d_2)}}{d + d_1 + d_2} \sqrt{(GP_0R_D)} \tag{2.10}$$

The change in the output voltage of the detector as a result of the change in the damping is

$$\Delta U_D = \frac{\partial U_0}{\partial d} \Delta d = -\frac{2\sqrt{(d_1d_2)}}{(d + d_1 + d_2)^2} \sqrt{(GP_0R_D)}\Delta d \tag{2.11}$$

From (2.11), we can derive the optimum values of the coupling coefficients β_1 and β_2 for which ΔU_D is a maximum. These values are

$$\beta_1 = \frac{d_1}{d} = \beta_2 = \frac{d_2}{d} = \beta_{\text{opt}} = \frac{1}{2} \tag{2.12}$$

Using (2.5) and (2.12) we can derive from (2.11) the optimum value of the usable signal at the detector output:

$$\Delta(U_D)_{\text{opt}} = -\frac{\chi''}{4dV_{\text{eff}}}\sqrt{(GP_0R_D)} = -\frac{1}{4}\chi''\frac{Q_0}{V_{\text{eff}}}\sqrt{(GP_0R_D)} \tag{2.13}$$

In the arrangement of Fig. 2.2, one uses the dependence of the reflection coefficient of a cavity on its damping. The cavity is connected to one arm of a microwave bridge. Either a Hybrid tee or a Hybrid ring[2] may be used as the bridge element. The microwave signal from the generator passes along arm A, and is incident on the bridge, where it is split equally between the two arms B and D. The wave along arm D is absorbed in a reflectionless termination (matched load). The wave travelling along arm B is partly reflected by the cavity, and returns to the junction, where it is again divided between arms A and C. In arm A the wave is absorbed by the generator, which should be matched to the waveguide. In arm C the wave reaches the microwave detector, which is also matched to the waveguide. Thus the power incident on the detector is

$$P_D = \frac{1}{4}P_0 \, |\Gamma_{cav}|^2 \tag{2.14}$$

where $|\Gamma_{cav}|$ is the reflection coefficient of the cavity.

If one considers the equivalent circuit of the cavity,[1] the equivalent input resistance may be taken as the resistance of a conventional parallel resonant circuit consisting of a capacitance, inductance and resistance. For slight mistuning, i.e. for $|\omega - \omega_0| = \Delta\omega \ll \omega_0$, the input resistance of such a circuit is approximately equal to

$$Z_{in} = R\left(1 + i \cdot 2Q_0 \frac{\Delta\omega}{\omega_0}\right)$$

where R is the resistance.

The reflection coefficient[2] is defined by

$$\Gamma = \frac{Z_{in} - Z_0}{Z_{in} + Z_0}$$

where Z_0 is the characteristic impedance of the waveguide.

$$\Gamma_{cav} = \frac{1 - \beta + i \cdot 2Q_0 \dfrac{\Delta\omega}{\omega_0}}{1 + \beta + 1 \cdot 2Q_0 \dfrac{\Delta\omega}{\omega_0}} \tag{2.15}$$

where $\beta = Z_0/R = d_1/d$, and d_1 is the damping produced by connection to the waveguide.

If we put $\Delta\omega = 0$ in (2.15) and use (2.9) and (2.14), we obtain a detector output voltage of

$$U_D = \frac{1}{2}\sqrt{(GP_0R_D)}\frac{d - d_1}{d + d_1} \tag{2.16}$$

The voltage change induced by the change in damping is equal to

$$\Delta U_D = \frac{\partial U_D}{\partial d}\Delta d = \frac{d_1}{(d_1 + d)^2}\sqrt{(GP_0R_D)}\Delta d \tag{2.17}$$

This value reaches a maximum under the condition

$$d_1 = d \quad \text{or} \quad \beta = \beta_{opt} = 1 \tag{2.18}$$

From (2.17) and using (2.5) and (2.18) we get

$$\Delta(U_D)_{\text{opt}} = - \frac{\chi''}{4dV_{\text{eff}}} \sqrt{(GP_0 R_D)} \qquad (2.17a)$$

Comparing this expression with equation (2.13), we can see that the arrangements of Figs. 2.1 and 2.2 are completely equivalent so far as the size of the usable signal at the output of the microwave detectors is concerned, provided that the detector characteristics are equal in both cases, and that the coupling coefficients assume their respective optimum values.

It should be noted that some workers[3,4] incorrectly assign a somewhat larger value to the usable signal from a reflection cavity system than to that from a transmission cavity system.

In both systems a semiconductor diode or a metal wire bolometer can be used as the microwave detector. Although a satisfactory high sensitivity can be achieved with bolometers,[4,5] they are used much less frequently than semiconductor diodes. This arises from the relatively long response time of the bolometer,[6] which considerably reduces the versatility of the spectrometer. Spectrometers using bolometers cannot be used to investigate fast processes (of duration less than about 0.1 s). The long response time of the bolometer also prohibits the use of high frequency magnetic field modulation. As a result of this, such spectrometers are very sensitive to mechanical vibration. Consequently spectrometers with bolometer detection will not be considered here.

The parameters of semiconductor diodes depend to a large extent on the microwave power P_D.[7,3] At power levels below 10^{-4} W, the conversion factor G increases rapidly with increase in power, and for $P_D \leqslant 10^{-5}$ W there exists a linear relationship between the output voltage and the input power:

$$U_D = \beta P_D \qquad (2.19)$$

with β = const. This range of the diode characteristic is generally known as the square-law region.† When the power is raised above 10^{-4} W, G increases

---

† If we put $P_D = U_{\text{in}}^2 / R_{\text{in}}$ in equation (2.19), where U_{in} is the microwave voltage at the input to the detector and R_{in} the input resistance of the detector, we get the following relationship between the output and input voltages of the detector:

$$U_D = (\beta/R_{\text{in}}) U_{\text{in}}^2$$

Hence, for the region we are considering, the output voltage is proportional to the square of the input voltage, and so this part of the characteristic is called the square-law region.

less rapidly and approaches a limiting value. For this part of the characteristic (the linear region), equation (2.9) may be considered sufficiently accurate with $G \approx$ const.

The noise produced in the diode will depend also to a large extent on P_D. It is known that the noise from a semiconductor diode arises largely from two contributions,[7,8] the thermal noise and the excess noise. The spectral density of the thermal noise is frequency-independent. The thermal noise power delivered by a diode into a matched resistance load is

$$P_{th,R} = kT\Delta f \tag{2.20}$$

where k is Boltzmann's constant, T the absolute temperature, and Δf the bandwidth of the amplifier.

The spectral density of the excess noise increases with decreasing frequency and with increasing power at the detector. The causes of the excess noise are considered to be the relatively small statistical oscillations of the detector resistance. If a resistance load, matched over a wide frequency range, is connected to the output of the detector, and microwave power supplied to the input, then the rectified voltage produced in the resistor is noise-modulated as a result of the statistical oscillations in the resistor. The noise power delivered by this resistor is approximately given by the following equation:[8,3]

$$P_{exc,R} = \frac{\alpha P_D}{f_M} kT\Delta f \tag{2.21}$$

Here, f_M is the centre frequency in the transmission range, $\alpha \approx 10^{11}$ W^{-1} s^{-1} for the linear part of the characteristic;[3] for the square-law region, α is dependent on P_D. The total detector noise power delivered into the load is

$$P_R = P_{th,R} + P_{exc,R} = \left(\frac{\alpha P_D}{f_M} + 1\right) kT\Delta f \tag{2.22}$$

If the amplifier used to increase the rectified signals is suitably constructed, the spectrometer sensitivity is limited mainly by imperfections of the microwave detector. The conversion factor of an ideal detector is $G_0 = 1$. If an ideal detector is working into a matched load, i.e. for $R_D = R_L$, we may determine the effective noise voltage at the load resistor from the thermal noise of the resistors R_D and R_L:

$$(U_R)_{opt} = \sqrt{(2kT\Delta f R_D)} \tag{2.23}$$

If it is assumed that the amplitude of the smallest detectable signal is equal to the effective noise voltage, we obtain from equations (2.13) and (2.23) the smallest value $\chi''_{min,opt}$ which can in principle be detected by the spectrometer:

$$\chi''_{min,opt} = \frac{4V_{eff}}{Q_0} \sqrt{\frac{2kT\Delta f}{P_0}} . \tag{2.24}$$

The noise power in the load resistor of a real detector, including the thermal noise of the load, is given by

$$P_{R,L} = kTt\Delta f \tag{2.25}$$

with

$$t = \frac{\alpha P_D}{f_M} + 2 \tag{2.25a}$$

The effective noise voltage in the load resistance of a real detector will be

$$U_{R,L} = \sqrt{(P_R R_D)} = \sqrt{(kTt\Delta f R_D)} \tag{2.26}$$

If we compare equations (2.13) and (2.26), we find the minimum value χ''_{min} which can be detected by a practical spectrometer:

$$\chi''_{min} = \frac{4V_{eff}}{Q_0} \sqrt{\frac{kTt\Delta f}{P_0 G}} \tag{2.27}$$

From equations (2.27) and (2.24) we obtain the noise figure of such a spectrometer:

$$k_R = 20 \log\left(\frac{\chi''_{min}}{\chi''_{min,opt}}\right) = 10 \log\left(\frac{t}{2G}\right) \text{ in dB} \tag{2.28}$$

One sees that G must be increased to improve spectrometer sensitivity. This means that, in accordance with the above, P_D must be increased until the linear range of the characteristic is reached. On the other hand, t should be as small as possible. From equation (2.25a), this can be achieved by making f_M larger and P_D smaller. It is desirable to amplify the signal from the detector at as high a frequency f_M as is possible. Also in the setting up of the spectrometer one has to set the optimum value P_D, at which t/G becomes a minimum. In the spectrometer ESR-2 a modulation frequency $f_M \approx 10^6$ Hz was used. Experience with this spectrometer shows that with a modulation frequency of 1 MHz, the optimum value of the microwave power P_D which reaches the diode is approximately between 0·2 and 0·5 mW (for semiconductor diodes types DK-S4 and D405). For $f_M < 1$ MHz the optimum power is less, as a result of the increase in excess noise.

The arrangement of Fig. 2.1 is not satisfactory so far as the choice of optimum power P_D goes. With this arrangement the optimum noise figure can only be achieved with one particular value of power from the micro-wave generator; e.g., for the spectrometer ESR-2, as we have already mentioned, $(P_D)_{opt} \approx 0.5$ mW. With optimum coupling coefficients, i.e. with $\beta_1 = \beta_2 = \frac{1}{2}$, from this spectrometer, one obtains, according to equation (2.8), $(P_0)_{opt} = 4P_D = 2$ mW. However, the experimental conditions often require a change in the power P_0; for example in relaxation measurements using the saturation technique, where P_0 must be varied over a very wide range. Also, as can be seen from equation (2.13), the usable signal at the output of the microwave detector, i.e. the spectrometer sensitivity, can be increased by an increase in P_0. In this case, whilst P_0 is increased above $(P_0)_{opt}$, the coupling coefficients β_1 and β_2 would have to be made smaller compared to their optimum value $\beta_1 = \beta_2 = \frac{1}{2}$, in order to retain favourable conditions at the detector. Also, in this arrangement, the increase in the noise figure does not allow a noticeable improvement in the sensitivity when P_0 is increased. In some cases, P_0 has to be made smaller than $(P_0)_{opt}$, to prevent saturation effects. This will increase the noise figure of the spectrometer.

In order to enable P_0 and P_D to be adjusted independently of each other, the arrangement of Fig. 2.1 may be extended by placing a microwave shunt in parallel with the cavity (Fig. 2.3).[3] The shunt includes a variable attenuator and a variable phase shifter, so that the amplitude and phase of the microwave signal which reaches the detector through the shunt may be adjusted.

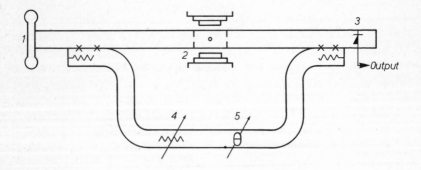

Fig. 2.3. Arrangement with microwave shunt.

1. microwave generator   4. variable attenuator
2. cavity with sample   5. phase shifter
3. microwave detector

The arrangement in Fig. 2.2 is more adaptable than the one in Fig. 2.1. In this arrangement arm D of the microwave bridge is terminated by a load in which amplitude and phase can be altered, so controlling the value of P_D. For example, for the phase adjustment a variable short-circuit may be used, and for the amplitude adjustment, a variable attenuator (Fig. 2.4a).[9] It is assumed here that the microwave generator and detector are matched to the waveguide, so that in this particular case the wave reflected from arm D is completely absorbed by the generator and detector. The wave reflected from arm B is similarly absorbed. Thus the two arms of the microwave bridge in Fig. 2.4 work completely independently of each other. Consequently, the power incident on arm B (and absorbed in the cavity), and the amplitude of the E.S.R. signal at the input of the detector, are independent of the reflection coefficient in arm D, which may be adjusted to

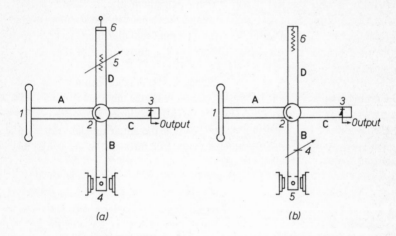

(a)   *(b)*

Fig. 2.4. Variations of the arrangements with reflection cavities.

(a) Arrangement with adjustable reflection coefficient in arm D

    1. microwave generator   4. cavity with sample
    2. waveguide bridge   5. variable attenuator
    3. microwave detector   6. movable short

(b) Arrangement with adjustable reflection coefficient in arm B

    1. microwave generator   4. matching unit
    2. waveguide bridge   5. cavity with sample
    3. microwave detector   6. matched load

give the optimum value of P_D. P_D is determined from the sum of the reflection coefficients in arms D and B; i.e.

$$P_D = \tfrac{1}{4}P_0|\Gamma_1 + \Gamma_{\text{cav}}|^2 \qquad (2.29)$$

where $\Gamma_1 = \Gamma' + i\Gamma''$ is the reflection coefficient of arm D. However, even the arrangement of Fig. 2.4a does not give an optimum value of P_D if the generator power P_0 is small. Since the coupling coefficient of the cavity is chosen, for sensitivity considerations, to be close to the optimum value, i.e. $\beta \to 1$, it follows from equation (2.15) that the reflection coefficient of arm B may be neglected ($\Gamma_B \to 0$). As a result of this, the amount of power absorbed by the detector is determined primarily by the reflection coefficient of arm D. P_D reaches its maximum value on total reflection in arm D, i.e. for $\Gamma_1 = 1$. For $\Gamma_1 = (\Gamma_1)_{\text{max}} = 1$, from equation (2.29) we get $(P_0)_{\text{min}} = 4(P_D)_{\text{opt}}$. We can also see that the arrangement of Fig. 2.4a allows optimum performance of the detector only if $P_0 \gg (P_D)_{\text{opt}}$. Putting $(P_D)_{\text{opt}} = 0.5$ mW in the arrangement of Fig. 2.1, we arrive at the following limiting condition:

$$P_0 \geqslant 2 \text{ mW}$$

Figure 2.4b shows another variation of the arrangement of Fig. 2.2. Here, another component is placed before the cavity in arm B, which reflects back to the bridge a part of the power passing through this arm. This may be achieved by means of a three-stub tuner, or a variable probe matching unit. Altering the depth and position of the probe in the waveguide will change the amplitude and phase of the reflected wave (which falls on the detector). However, it should be pointed out that in the arrangement of Fig. 2.4b, the power entering the cavity alters when P_D is adjusted, and this also affects the amplitude of the E.S.R. signal at the detector input. This mutual dependance makes the setting-up of the spectrometer more difficult, and is an inherent disadvantage of this arrangement, although in other ways it does allow more possibilities than that of Fig. 2.4a of adjustment for the optimum value of P_D.

E.S.R. spectrometers are also used with intermediate frequency (superheterodyne mixer) detectors. In this case there is an additional component in the microwave detector arm, and an additional microwave generator, the local oscillator. The signal voltage and the heterodyne voltage reach the detector diode simultaneously. As a result of the mixing of these two oscillations, one gets at the output of the mixer an intermediate frequency (I.F.) signal, with a frequency f_{IF}, which is equal to the difference between the frequencies of the local oscillator and signal oscillator. Further signal amplification is achieved with an I.F. amplifier tuned to f_{IF}. The signal voltage at the output of the mixer is calculated from equation (2.9), i.e. the mixer acts as a linear detector. The optimum working point of the mixer diodes is found by adjusting the power level of the local oscillator frequency reaching them.

The I.F. amplifiers of superheterodyne spectrometers usually have a bandwidth (of several MHz) which is considerably greater than would normally be allowed for the detection of distortion-free spectral lines. This is the price one pays for the relatively good frequency stability of the I.F., which is a function of the fluctuations of the local and signal oscillators. If a narrow-band I.F. amplifier were to be used, the frequency modulation of the I.F. signal would be changed into amplitude modulation by the response curve characteristic of the I.F. amplifier, and this would give rise to additional noise. With increasing bandwidth of the I.F. amplifiers, the requirement of tuning stability of both microwave sources is lessened. The stability of the frequency f_{IF} can be considerably increased if one uses the arrangement of the local oscillator shown in Fig. 2.5. Here, a part of the power from the main generator is fed to a bridge modulator, the input diodes of which also receive a signal of frequency f_{IF} from a high frequency generator. The output of the modulator contains, apart from a very weak component of frequency ν, two sidebands with frequencies $\nu + f_{IF}$ and $\nu - f_{IF}$. One of these sidebands is filtered out through a cavity-filter, and is used as the heterodyne frequency. The advantage of such an arrangement is that the stability of the intermediate frequency depends solely on the stability of the high frequency generator, which can be made very great. Thus a very narrow bandwidth of the I.F. amplifier may be used. However, this particular arrangement also has its disadvantages. Statistical fluctuations in the crystal diodes will modulate the microwave signal at the output of the modulator with low frequency noise. If the heterodyne voltage $U_{\nu \pm f_{IF}}$ at the input to the mixer is modulated with low frequency noise, then the I.F. voltage at its output,

$$U_{IF} = A \cdot U_\nu \cdot U_{\nu \pm f_{IF}} \qquad (2.30)$$

will also be modulated with the same noise. Here A is a constant and U_ν the output voltage from the waveguide bridge in the absence of an E.S.R. signal.

From equation (2.30), we see that the above-mentioned noise will disappear for $U_\nu = 0$. This condition may be achieved by complete balance of the microwave bridge. Under these conditions, an I.F. signal will appear only when an E.S.R. absorption unbalances the bridge. Even under these conditions there will still be some noise, as the modulator and the cavity con-

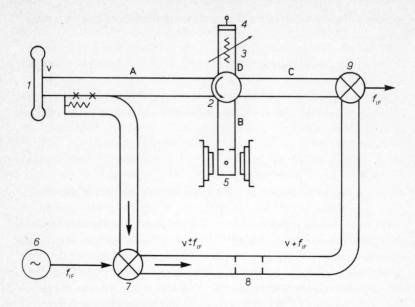

Fig. 2.5. Superheterodyne spectrometer with only one microwave source

1. microwave generator	6. high frequency generator
2. waveguide bridge	7. push-pull modulator
3. variable attenuator	8. cavity
4. movable short	9. mixer
5. cavity with sample	

nected to it generally let through a small component of noise oscillations at a frequency ν. Complete suppression of this noise appears impossible because of the relatively small difference in frequency between the sidebands and the main frequency ν.

The main advantage of the microwave superheterodyne receiver is that the intermediate frequency can be chosen to be very high (30 MHz or higher). Consequently the excess noise is very small. For example, radar superheterodyne receivers have noise figures of 12 to 14 dB, i.e. the sensitivity is lower than the best theoretically possible by a factor of only 4 or 5.

In practice, we assume that only the voltage from the local oscillator reaches the mixer diode; thus the operation of the mixers, so far as the signal from the local oscillator is concerned, is virtually the same as the operation of a normal detector. The diode output contains an excess-noise power

$$P_{\text{exc},R} = \frac{\alpha P_{\text{loc}}}{f_M} kT\Delta f \tag{2.31}$$

where P_{loc} is the local oscillator power which is absorbed by the mixer. If we take into account only the noise component which the I.F. amplifier lets through, we get

$$P_{\text{exc},R} = \frac{\alpha P_{\text{loc}}}{f_{\text{IF}}} kT\Delta f_{\text{IF}} \tag{2.31a}$$

where Δf_{IF} is the bandwidth of the I.F. amplifier. If we choose a sufficiently large value of f_{IF}, then the effect of this noise may be neglected.

Superheterodyne spectrometers do have, however, considerably larger noise figures than radar receivers.[3,11] The noise figure increases very rapidly with the power P_0. This may be explained by taking into account that the excess noise is produced by statistical fluctuations in the resistance of the semiconductor diodes. The magnitude of these fluctuations may be calculated from equation (2.31). The normalized fluctuations are given by

$$\frac{\Delta R_D}{R_D} = 2\sqrt{\frac{\alpha kT\Delta f}{G f_M}}$$

If an I.F. voltage appears at the output of the mixer, then it is amplitude-modulated with noise, as a result of the fluctuations of R_D. The depth of noise modulation is

$$m = \sqrt{\frac{\alpha kT\Delta f}{G f_M}} \tag{2.32}$$

and the effective noise voltage at the output of the mixer becomes

$$U'_{\text{IF},R} = mU_{\text{IF}} \tag{2.33}$$

From equation (2.33) it follows that the 'optimum working point' of the mixer is $P_D = 0$. As (2.32) shows, the depth of modulation m increases with decreasing f_M, i.e. this type of noise is dominated by low frequency components.

The radar signal consists of pulses, and between these pulses the microwave power is equal to zero. From (2.33), this type of noise in a radar receiver will lead to a meaningless distortion of the pulses. In principle, one can balance the bridge in the arrangements of Figs. 2.2 and 2.3 in a similar way, the microwave energy falling on the mixer only if an E.S.R. absorption occurs. Thus the noise of (2.33) would disappear, as in the case of a radar receiver. However, the following will show that a complete balance of the waveguide bridge cannot generally be used, and the E.S.R. signal presents itself as a relatively small modulation of a high power microwave signal. If the low frequency noise modulation is not to influence the sensitivity of the spectrometer, then the statistical fluctuations of the I.F. voltage should not be larger than the thermal noise at the output of the mixer; i.e.

$$m(U_{IF})_0 < \sqrt{(2kT\Delta f R_D)} \tag{2.34}$$

Considering (2.32), this leads to the condition

$$(U_{IF})_0 < \sqrt{\frac{2GR_D f_M}{\alpha}} \tag{2.34a}$$

If we put in the numerical values $G = 0.25, f_M = 10^3$ Hz, $\alpha = 10^{11}$ W^{-1} s^{-1}, R_D (for push-pull mixer) = 150 Ω, we get $(U_{IF})_0 < 1$ mV, which corresponds to a microwave power $P_D < 2.10^{-8}$ W at the input of the mixer. As one can see from this example, the advantages of a superheterodyne spectrometer can be fully utilized only at a sufficiently small P_D. At $P_0 > 10^{-7}$ W a corresponding decrease of P_D can only be achieved with microwave balancing. As the power from the microwave source increases, so the required degree of balance is increased.

More recently, some superheterodyne spectrometers have appeared which do not exhibit the above disadvantages; with high klystron powers these reach sensitivities which correspond to those of heterodyne receivers with low noise figures. Some improvements in experimental technique have been evolved in this connection, and these will now briefly be discussed.

The principle of phase-sensitive detection, until recently used only in connection with magnetic field modulation, has been used for the demodulation of microwave signals. As a result of this, one can work with completely balanced measuring bridges, which simplifies the operation of the spectrometer (particularly when there are changes in the amplitude of the microwave field at the sample position). Besides this, klystron noise may be eliminated. A typical spectrometer with phase-sensitive detection is described by Henning.[26*] As a frequency modulation of 30 Hz was used, the sensitivity obtained was only 10^{13} spins. Phase-sensitive detection in microwave systems using heterodyne detection was realized in the spectrometer of Laffon *et al.*[27*] In this spectrometer part of the signal klystron power was coupled through a phase shifter into the heterodyne arm. A sensitivity of 10^{12} spins was achieved for a sample volume of 300 mm^3.

In a spectrometer with phase-sensitive microwave detection, both the signal and the reference voltage have to undergo a frequency change. In the system of Laffon *et al.*, this is achieved for both the signal and the reference using only one pair of mixer diodes. As a result of this, the noise, which originates from the modulation of the reference voltage by statistical resistance fluctuations (see p. 23), cannot be separated from the signal, and the noise figure of the spectrometer deteriorates. This deterioration may be prevented if separate mixer diodes are used for frequency changing the signal and the reference. The diodes in the signal input arm are then in fact only loaded by the signal, and the noise figure is the same as for a radar receiver. The amplitude noise of the reference voltage can be prevented in the usual way by the use of a limiter circuit, since the signal and the reference are being amplified in separate I.F. amplifiers. Naturally such a system requires a large amount of electronic equipment, but this can be housed in a relatively small space by the use of modern miniaturized components. Spectrometers in which this type of phase-sensitive detection is used have been described by Teaney, Klein and Portis,[24*] and by Holton and Blum.[28*]

If the local oscillator is used in an arrangement such as is shown in Fig. 2.5, then the reference voltage for the phase sensitive I.F. detector can be taken directly from the high frequency oscillator. Fig. 2.6* shows some more possible arrangements for phase sensitive microwave detection.

A second improvement in experimental technique involves the balancing of the microwave bridge. The arrangements in Fig. 2.3 (transmission cavity) and Fig. 2.4 (reflection cavity) allow a complete bridge balance to be obtained (which is necessary if we are to take advantage of phase-sensitive detection) only for one single frequency. This puts very stringent requirements on the tuning of the klystron and the cavity resonator (see also Fig. 2.7). If a resistive termination is used which has the same frequency response as the resonant cavity, in the arrangements of Figs. 2.3 and 2.4*a*, then the bridge may be balanced over a wide band. Such a termination can be another tuned cavity, and so allows a variation of the three parameters, resonant frequency, Q factor and coupling coefficient. In addition to this, the E.S.R. cavity and balance arms of the bridge have to be the same electrical length. Thus for a complete balance, four operating elements are necessary. Arrangements of this type have been built for use with transmission cavities[29*] as well as reflection cavities.[23,30*] The sensitivities of detection which have been achieved are approximately ten times better than with the more simple systems. Calculations carried out by Redhardt[30*] show that if a spectrometer of the type shown in Figs. 2.3 and 2.4 is balanced to detect

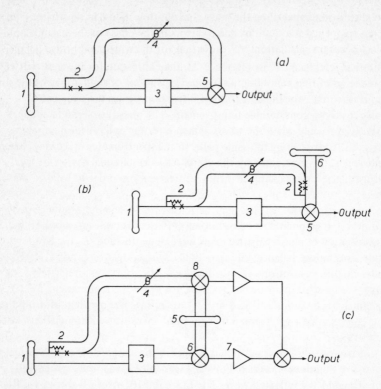

Fig. 2.6.* Spectrometer arrangements with phase-sensitive detection of the micro-wave signals.

(*a*) Homodyne spectrometer

1. microwave generator	4. phase shifter
2. directional coupler	5. push-pull homodyne detector
3. microwave bridge	

(*b*) Superheterodyne spectrometer with phase-sensitive detection

1. microwave generator	4. phase shifter
2. directional coupler	5. push-pull mixer
3 microwave bridge	6. heterodyne oscillator

(*c*) Superheterodyne spectrometer with phase-sensitive detection of the I.F.

1. microwave generator	5. heterodyne oscillator
2. directional coupler	6. signal mixer
3. microwave bridge	7. signal I.F. amplifier
4. phase shifter	8. phase sensitive I.F. detector

an absorption signal, then the main contribution to loss in sensitivity comes from frequency fluctuations due to errors in the phase of the balance arm. More accurate calculations[31]* show that for the wide-band bridge balance of either reference 29* or reference 23, the expression for the sensitivity as a function of frequency fluctuation contains terms of similar magnitude. In contrast to this, for the detection of dispersion signals the wide-band balance gives a considerable improvement. The phase error can be made exactly zero only when the waves, which interfere and cancel themselves, are made to pass along the same path. In the spectrometer of Teaney, Klein and Portis, this is effected by the use of a special bimodal cavity. In fact, altogether seven balancing elements are necessary in order to balance the cavity.

Summarizing, we can say that the sensitivity of superheterodyne spectrometers as compared to conventional systems has been increased by the introduction of phase-sensitive microwave detection and the use of the wide-band bridge balance, and also by using high klystron powers. However, balancing these spectrometers for highest sensitivity takes a relatively long time, so this type of spectrometer does not fulfill the requirement for chemical applications as stated in §2.7 under (a). The problem of using the highest sensitivity spectrometers for routine investigations is a difficult one to solve.

As has already been mentioned, arm D in the circuit of Fig. 2.4a contains balancing components which allow changes to be made in the phase and amplitude of the reflected wave. The E.S.R. cavity in arm B acts as a reflection component. Since the reflection coefficient of the cavity is strongly frequency-dependent, as equation (2.15) shows, we can expect that the waveguide bridge output voltage is extremely sensitive to mistuning of the cavity $\Delta\omega/\omega$ with respect to the microwave generator. For $2Q_0\,\Delta\omega/\omega \ll 1$ we find, from equation (2.15),

$$\Gamma_{cav} \approx \frac{1-\beta}{1+\beta} + \frac{8\beta Q_0^2}{(\beta+1)^3}\left(\frac{\Delta\omega}{\omega}\right)^2 + i\,\frac{4\beta Q_0}{(\beta+1)^2}\left(\frac{\Delta\omega}{\omega}\right) \qquad (2.35)$$

From (2.9) and (2.29), the voltage at the output of the mixer is

$$U_{IF} = \tfrac{1}{2}\sqrt{(GP_0R_D)}\left[\Gamma_0 + \frac{8\beta Q_0^2}{(\beta+1)^3}\left(\frac{\Delta\omega}{\omega}\right)^2 + i\left(\Gamma'' + \frac{4\beta Q_0}{(\beta+1)^2}\frac{\Delta\omega}{\omega}\right)\right]$$

where $\qquad\qquad\qquad\qquad\qquad\qquad\qquad\qquad\qquad\qquad\qquad\qquad$ (2.36)

$$\Gamma_0 = \Gamma' + \frac{1-\beta}{1+\beta}$$

If an amplitude detector is placed at the output of the I.F. amplifier, which is usually the case, then its output voltage is proportional to the contribution of U_{IF}, i.e. proportional to the magnitude

$$
| U_{IF} | = \tfrac{1}{2}\sqrt{(GP_0 R_D)}\left[\Gamma_0 + \frac{8\beta Q_0^2}{(1 + \beta)^3}\left(\frac{\Delta\omega}{\omega} \right)^2 \right.
$$

$$
\left. + i \left(\Gamma'' + \frac{4\beta Q_0}{(1 + \beta)^2}\frac{\Delta\omega}{\omega} \right) \right] \tag{2.37}
$$

The E.S.R. absorption signal represents a change in the real part of the reflection coefficient, i.e. a change in the magnitude of Γ_0. The dispersion signal causes a mistuning of the cavity and can therefore be represented as a change in the value of $\Delta\omega/\omega$. To prevent distortion of the absorption signal by dispersion, the waveguide bridge must be so balanced that the total reflection coefficient depends as little as possible on $\Delta\omega/\omega$. This can be achieved by the condition

$$
\Gamma'' = 0 \quad \text{and} \quad \Gamma_0 \gg \frac{4\beta Q_0}{(1 + \beta)^2}\frac{\Delta\omega}{\omega} \tag{2.38}
$$

If the quantity $\Delta\omega/\omega$ is rapidly changing as a result of statistical fluctuations of the generator frequency or as a result of mechanical vibration of the components, then this, according to (2.37), constitutes a noise source for the spectrometer. If condition (2.38) is also satisfied, then this noise becomes very small. This would imply that the waveguide bridge should not be completely balanced, since then $\Gamma_0 = 0$. If we consider (2.38) and put $\beta = 1$ in (2.37) (optimum coupling of the cavity), then we obtain

$$
U_{IF} \approx \tfrac{1}{2}\sqrt{(GP_0 R_D)}\left[\Gamma_0 + \frac{1 + 2\Gamma_0}{2\Gamma_0}Q_0^2\left(\frac{\Delta\omega}{\omega} \right)^2 \right] \tag{2.39}
$$

From this equation, it follows that the mean I.F. voltage at the output of the mixer is

$$
(U_{IF})_0 = \tfrac{1}{2}\Gamma_0\sqrt{(GP_0 R_D)} \tag{2.40}
$$

The noise voltage caused by the fluctuations of $\Delta\omega$ will be

$$
U_{IF, R}'' = \frac{1 + 2\Gamma_0}{4\Gamma_0}Q_0^2\left(\frac{\Delta\omega}{\omega} \right)_{eff}^2 \sqrt{(GP_0 R_D)} \tag{2.41}
$$

where $\Delta\omega/\omega_{\text{eff}}$ is the effective value of the fluctuations of the relative mistuning in a given frequency band Δf.

From the requirement that this noise voltage should be smaller than the thermal noise, we find, with the help of (2.41) and (2.23), that the required stability is achieved only by successive adjustment of both sides of the bridge† :

$$\left(\frac{\Delta\omega}{\omega}\right)_{\text{eff}} < \frac{2}{Q_0} \sqrt{\frac{\Gamma_0}{1+2\Gamma_0}} \sqrt[4]{\frac{2kT\Delta f}{GP_0}} \tag{2.42}$$

As we can see, the stability requirements for $\Gamma_0 \to 0$ are increasing quite rapidly. Therefore, if we consider the factors which influence the mistuning of the cavity with respect to the microwave source, Γ_0 must be made as large as possible in order to improve the stability of the spectrometer. On the other hand, for sensitivity considerations, using equations (2.34a) and (2.40), we get

$$\Gamma_0 < 2 \sqrt{\frac{2f_M}{\alpha P_0}} \tag{2.43}$$

With the maximum value of the reflection coefficient,

$$\Gamma_0 = (\Gamma_0)_{\text{max}} = 2 \sqrt{\frac{2f_M}{\alpha P_0}} \tag{2.44}$$

we can find from (2.42) the permissible value of the mistuning on one side with respect to the other, $(\Delta\omega/\omega)_{\text{eff}}$.

If in the arrangement of Fig. 2.4a direct rectification is used, then the optimum value $(\Gamma_0)_{\text{opt}}$ of the reflection coefficient follows from the optimum working point of the microwave detectors. From equation (2.29) it follows that

$$(\Gamma_0)_{\text{opt}} = 2 \sqrt{\frac{(P_D)_{\text{opt}}}{P_0}} \tag{2.45}$$

This is illustrated by Fig. 2.7, showing the curves, calculated from equations (2.44) and (2.45), of $(\Gamma_0)_{\text{max}}$ and $(\Gamma_0)_{\text{opt}}$ as functions of the power P_0. Fig. 2.8 shows the dependence of the mistuning $(\Delta\omega/\omega)_{\text{eff}}$ on P_0, calculated from equation (2.42). From these figures, it is clear that the requirements of frequency stability from a superheterodyne spectrometer are considerably higher than for a conventional spectrometer. In addition, these stability requirements increase as the power P_0 increases. Experiment[10] shows that for powers $P_0 > 1$ mW the reflex klystrons now

† It should not be forgotten that the derived formulae are only approximate.

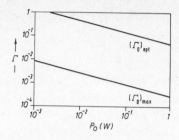

Fig. 2.7. Dependence of the optimum reflection coefficient on microwave power for reflection-cavity system

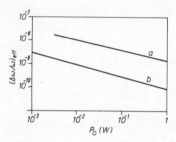

Fig. 2.8 Permissible frequency instability $(\Delta\omega/\omega)_{eff}$ for a reflection-cavity system:

(a) for direct rectification
(b) for superheterodyne operation

used as microwave sources no longer fulfil the requirements set on frequency stability for superheterodyne spectrometers. If $P_0 > 1$ mW, the noise figure of the spectrometer becomes considerably larger than that of a radar receiver.[11] It is clear from this that superheterodyne spectrometers are very prone to microphonic effects and temperature changes in the components.

The above arguments are also valid for transmission-cavity systems with a waveguide shunt (see Fig. 4), as this arrangement is basically only a modification of the waveguide bridge. For systems with a transmission cavity but without the shunt (see Fig. 2.1), from (2.6) and (2.9) we get the approximation

$$U_D \approx \tfrac{1}{2}\sqrt{(GP_0R_D)}\left[1 - \tfrac{1}{2}Q_0^2\left(\frac{\Delta\omega}{\omega}\right)^2\right] \tag{2.46}$$

where we have put $\beta_1 = \beta_2 = \beta_{opt} = \tfrac{1}{2}$.

With analogous conditions in equation (2.42), we find for the permissible mistuning

$$\left(\frac{\Delta\omega}{\omega}\right)_{\text{eff}} < \frac{2}{Q_0}\sqrt[4]{\frac{2kT\Delta f}{Q \cdot P_0}} \tag{2.47}$$

Comparing this equation with (2.42), we see that in this case the restrictions on the amount of mistuning are less stringent than in the system with microwave balance. The foregoing arguments lead us to the following conclusions.

1. All microwave arrangements of spectrometers are similar, so far as the size of the E.S.R. signal at the input to the microwave detector goes (conditional on the coupling coefficients of the cavities being optimum).

2. The transmission-cavity system of Fig. 2.1 is considered to be the simplest one. It is least sensitive to all types of instabilities which result from the mistuning of the cavity with respect to the microwave source. The disadvantage of this arrangement is that it does not allow independent adjustment of P_D and P_0, so the noise figure will be optimum only for a particular value of power P_0. This arrangement is to be recommended if the major requirements of the spectrometer are maximum reliability and simple operation.

3. If the microwave power reaching the cavity is required to be varied over a wide range, and if very high sensitivity is required, then one should use a system with microwave balance. In this case, the higher the power P_0, the more care has to be taken in balancing the waveguide bridge (particularly if a superheterodyne receiver is used). The construction of such a spectrometer usually presents many problems with regard to the high stability requirements of the relative tuning between the microwave source and the E.S.R. cavity.

4. Since their requirements as to the stability of the tuning are very high, superheterodyne spectrometers may be used to advantage only if P_0 is not larger than 1 mW (e.g. in the investigation of very narrow lines, and at very low sample temperatures[3]).

§2.2

MAGNETIC FIELD MODULATION

In Chapter 1 we showed that spectra may be plotted in two ways. In the first, one changes the frequency of the microwave source whilst the magnetic induction B is held constant. In the second, the magnetic induction is changed, and the frequency remains constant. If the operating frequency of the spectrometer is changed, then at least two operating elements of the spectrometer (klystron and cavity) also have to be changed. As we have seen from the preceding section, the relative tuning of these elements imposes severe restrictions on the performance, so it is clear that the former method is virtually unusable. Thus in the spectrometers used today, the latter method is used.

We have already mentioned that the spectral density of the excess noise of a microwave detector increases very rapidly with decreasing frequency. For this reason, direct measurement of the E.S.R. signal at the output of the detector, for example with a high sensitivity galvanometer or a d.c. amplifier, is not used in high frequency spectrometers. In its place, we use the principle of magnetic field modulation.

If one succeeds in holding a very good balance of the measuring bridge during a measurement, and if a phase-sensitive heterodyne receiver is used (see p. 24), then magnetic field modulation may be completely dispensed with, without reducing the sensitivity. This type of spectrometer was described by Teaney, Klein and Portis.[24] Here a bimodal cavity was used as the bridge element, its method of operation being analogous to that of Bloch's two-coil system in nuclear magnetic resonance. By dispensing with magnetic field modulation, one also prevents all kinds of undesirable modulation distortion of the line shape, for example in resolving closely spaced lines of different widths. Also for very wide lines there is no loss in sensitivity through insufficient modulation amplitude.*

At the present time, two methods of magnetic field modulation are used. In the first method, the so-called crystal-video spectrometer, a sinusoidal magnetic field (the magnetic 'sweep' field), the amplitude of which is greater than that of the spectral lines, is superimposed on the static field on the electromagnet. This field is usually produced by modulation coils mounted on the pole pieces of the magnet. The modulation coils are very often fed from an a.c. network through a variable transformer. The magnet goes through the resonance value of the magnetic induction B_0 twice in one cycle, so the E.S.R. signal appears twice at the output of the microwave detector during each cycle of the modulation voltage. This signal is amplified in an electronic amplifier and fed to the vertical plates of a cathode ray oscilloscope. The horizontal plates receive the a.c. voltage via a phase shifter. Thus a picture of the spectral line appears on the screen of the oscilloscope. For a distortionless representation of the line shape, the amplifier must have a bandwidth from 50 Hz to 10 kHz. This is the audio-frequency range. For this reason, such spectrometers are very sensitive to mechanical shock and vibration, despite the use of modulation, and the signal strength is very high. In addition, the detection sensitivity of this type of spectrometer is very low, as the excess noise of the microwave detectors is very large. To increase the modulation frequency in a crystal-video spectrometer is pointless, since this also requires a considerable increase in the bandwidth of the signal amplifier if distortion of the line shape is to be avoided.

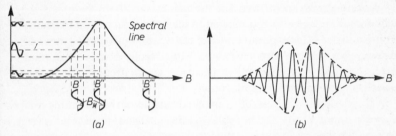

Fig. 2.9 (*a*) Example of high frequency modulation. B', B'' and B''' are arbitrarily chosen, and are the instantaneous values of the magnetic induction during the tracing of the spectral line. (*b*) The resulting signal at the output of the microwave detector (a.c. component). The envelope of the signal represents the first derivative of the spectral line.

∗If one assumes that the noise temperature of the receiver is inversely proportional to the frequency, which is the case for crystal diodes in the low frequency range, then a spectrometer noise figure which is independent of modulation frequency is obtained. An improvement of the noise figure is here possible only through repeated recordings of the spectrum and a subsequent correlation analysis.∗

In the second method (the double modulation method), a sinusoidal high frequency magnetic field, the amplitude of which is smaller than half the line width, is superimposed on the slowly varying magnetic field which passes through the entire spectral line (such a field change is usually called a *sweep*). At the output of the microwave detector, a signal appears with the modulation frequency. The envelope of this signal is the first derivative of the spectral line (Fig.2.9). From the output of the detector, the signal is passed to a high frequency amplifier, then to a phase-sensitive detector, and thereafter to a recorder. In a spectrometer with double modulation, the signal amplifier only lets through the high frequency components of the noise, which appear at the output of the microwave detector. Since the intensity of these components is considerably smaller than those of low frequency, the detection sensitivity and the insensitivity to disturbances in such a spectrometer are considerably better than in a crystal-video system.

As the amplitude of the high frequency modulation field B_M increases, the useful signal from the output of the amplifier rises until a certain level is reached, after which it falls. The distortion of the line shape increases with an increase in B_M. This line distortion can only be neglected if the spectrometer is set suitably.

The double modulation technique is also known as the *method of differential tracing*. However, this description is correct only for modulation amplitudes which are small compared to the line width. To achieve an optimum signal-to-noise ratio it is necessary to use a modulation amplitude for which the tracing is not 'differential'. One can, however, calculate the real line shape from the plotted curve for any modulation amplitude. Such a technique, using an integral transformation, has been described by Spry.[25]* This is almost identical to another mathematical technique using the Fourier series expansion of the signal. If the signal can be expanded into a Fourier series in the interval from $B_0 - B_b/2$ to $B_0 + B_b/2$,

$$U_S = A \sum_{n=1}^{\infty} (a_n \cos nx + b_n \sin nx) \qquad x = 2\pi \frac{B - B_0}{B_b}$$

then the following expression is obtained for the plotted curve:

$$U_S^{(1)} = 2A \sum_{n=1}^{\infty} J_1\left(2\pi n \frac{B_M}{B_b}\right) (b_n \cos nx - a_n \sin nx)$$

One can see that only those Fourier components of the signal with an optimum signal-to-noise ratio are employed, for which the Bessel function assumes its maximum value. This is the case for $2\pi n B_n/B_b = 1.84$. If the signal contains lines of different widths, i.e. if the essential Fourier components of the signal lie in different n-regions, then the simultaneous optimization of the modulation amplitude for all lines is no longer possible.*

For a line with Lorentzian shape, the modulation amplitude for which the E.S.R. signal is maximum, is given by $B_M = \Delta B_{1/2}$, where $\Delta B_{1/2}$ is the line width measured at half height.[4] In this case, the recorded line is broadened by a factor $\sqrt{3}$, and the signal amplitude at the detector output is smaller by a factor 0.354, as compared to a crystal-video system. In a spectrometer using double modulation of the magnetic field, the bandwidth of the signal amplifier is independent of the modulation frequency, since the time taken to record the spectrum line is determined only by the sweep rate of the magnetic field. For this reason, the noise figure of the spectrometer may be reduced by increasing the modulation frequency. However, there is a limit to how much the modulation frequency may be increased, and this is imposed by the distortions of the line shape which are produced. It is known that the stationary value of the absorption line appears in a time which is determined by the relaxation time of the sample (see Chapter 3). Therefore, for an undistorted reproduction of the line, it is necessary that the sweep rate of the polarizing magnetic field satisfies the following condition:

$$\frac{dB}{dt} \ll \gamma(\Delta B_{1/2})^2 \tag{2.48}$$

where γ is the gyromagnetic ratio.

For a sinusoidal modulation, we get

$$\frac{dB}{dt} = \omega_M B_M \tag{2.49}$$

and equation (2.48) can be written in the form

$$\omega_M B_M \ll \gamma(\Delta B_{1/2})^2 \tag{2.50}$$

As we have already mentioned, for maximum spectrometer sensitivity, the modulation amplitude must have the value $B_M = \Delta B_{1/2}$. From (2.50) we then obtain the following expression for the limiting value of the modulation frequency:

$$f_M \ll \gamma \frac{\Delta B_{1/2}}{2\pi} \tag{2.51}$$

There are many problems associated with the production of a high frequency magnetic field inside the resonant cavity, as the cavity walls usually present an effective shield against such fields and prevent them from entering the cavity. In some cases[13,14] these difficulties have been overcome by having a slit in the cavity and feeding the high frequency current directly to the metal parts of the cavity. The current flowing around the slit then produces high frequency magnetic field inside the cavity. The location of the slit is such that it does not cut any of the microwave current lines in the walls of the cavity. In some cases the current is allowed to flow through a wire loop[15,16] or a pair of copper rods[17] inserted into the cavity.

The literature[18] also describes cavities made of quartz which have a thin layer of silver plating on the inside. The high frequency magnetic field inside such cavities is produced by modulation coils placed outside the cavity walls.

§2.3

AMPLIFIER AND RECORDER SYSTEMS FOR E.S.R. SIGNALS

The block diagram of the electronic part of the spectrometer must be designed in accordance with the modulation system chosen and the type of microwave receiver used (direct rectification or frequency conversion). If the modulation system of the crystal-video spectrometer is used, with direct rectification, as we have already mentioned, a low frequency amplifier with a sufficiently wide bandwidth must be connected to the detector output, and the output voltage of the amplifier passed to the vertical plates of an oscilloscope. Since the magnetic field is usually sinusoidal, for an undistorted representation of the line shape on the screen, the horizontal deflection voltage must also be made sinusoidal. To do this, the voltage which is put on the horizontal plates of the oscilloscope tube (via a phase shifter) is taken from the same source that feeds the modulation coils of the electromagnet. If a mixer stage is used as the microwave detector, then the amplifier circuit becomes more complicated. In this case, the mixer stage is followed by an I.F. amplifier, on the output of which a second detector is located. The output from the second detector carries the E.S.R. signal to an L.F. amplifier, and then to the deflection plates of the cathode ray tube. As a second detector, a peak value detector is usually used. As we have already said, the I.F. amplifier in superheterodyne spectrometers usually has a bandwidth which considerably exceeds that necessary to transmit a line without distortion. However, from the point of view of reducing the noise, and correspondingly increasing the detection sensitivity, it is desirable that the effective bandwidth of the whole amplifier system be made as narrow as possible. In practice this is achieved by reducing the bandwidth of the L.F. amplifier following the second detector. If the ratio of the bandwidth of the I.F. amplifier and L.F. amplifier is designated as η, i.e. $\eta = \Delta f_{IF}/\Delta f_{LF}$, then with an ideal second detector the signal-to-noise ratio at the input and output is given by

$$\frac{(U_S)_{in}}{(U_R)_{in}} = \sqrt{\eta} \, \frac{(U_S)_{out}}{(U_R)_{out}}, \tag{2.52}$$

as according to equation (2.23), the effective noise voltages are proportional to $\sqrt{(\Delta f)}$. In a real peak detector, when the signal at the detector input is smaller than the noise level, there is a possibility that the signal will be suppressed by the noise,[19,20] and equation (2.52) is no longer applicable. For a superheterodyne spectrometer, the conditions of (2.34) and (2.44) imply that in the I.F. amplifier, the I.F. level lies far above the noise level (because $m \ll 1$). For this reason, equation (2.52) is always usable for superheterodyne spectrometers, and the overall bandwidth of the amplifier system is determined solely by the bandwidth of the L.F. amplifier.

The I.F. amplication necessary can be ascertained from the condition (2.34), and also from the fact that for efficient operation of the second detector, a voltage of 1 to 3 volts is necessary.[21,22] A calculation along these lines gives $V_{IF} = 10^3 - 3.10^3$. The block diagram of the amplifier of a double modulation spectrometer with direct microwave detection is shown in Fig. 2.10.

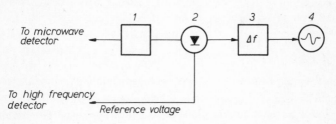

Fig. 2.10. Scheme of the amplifier section of a spectrometer with magnetic field double modulation.
1. High frequency amplifier
2. Phase-sensitive detector
3. Narrow band filter for reducing the frequency bandwidth Δf
4. Recorder

As may be seen from the figure, there is a phase-sensitive detector at the output of the high frequency amplifier. This is necessary as, to ensure a distortion-free line shape, the detector must be of correct phase. On the other hand, for large values of η, the E.S.R. signal and the input of the detector can be considerably smaller than the noise level. Here, $\eta = \Delta f_{HF}/\Delta f$, where Δf is the effective bandwidth of the overall amplifier system, which is determined by the filter at the output of the phase sensitive detector. If the phase-sensitive detector is replaced by a normal detector, then the E.S.R. signal is suppressed by the noise, and reducing the bandwidth with a filter placed after the detector will not give any improvement of the signal-to-noise ratio.

The amplifier bandwidth is determined by the requirement that the line shape must be undistorted when recorded at the smallest sweep time. If the sweep time of a spectral line is designated by τ, then the bandwidth of the high frequency amplifier must fulfil the following condition:

$$\Delta f_{HF} \gg \frac{1}{\tau} \tag{2.53}$$

If for example, the fastest tracing of the spectrum is made with a modulation of 50 Hz, i.e. if the spectral line is recorded in a time of the order of magnitude of $\tau \approx 10^{-2}$ s, then for an undistorted line shape, the bandwidth of the amplifier (and of the whole system) must be $\Delta f \approx 10^4 - 4.10^4$ Hz.

The recording device may be either a cathode ray oscilloscope or a pen recorder, depending on the rate at which the magnetic field is swept.

The double modulation technique is also used in superheterodyne spectrometers. In this case the circuit arrangement of Fig. 2.10 is fed to the second detector.

§2.4
ELECTRICAL INTERFERENCE AND MICROPHONIC EFFECTS

The working of a high frequency spectrometer is adversely affected by all forms of electrical interference and mechanical oscillations of its individual units. The main sources of electrical interference are the a.c. circuits and the circuitry for the magnetic field modulation. The large stray magnetic field from the modulation coils induces parasitic voltages in the neighbouring spectrometer components, and these find their way, through various paths, to the signal amplifier. As the stage most sensitive to these disturbances is the input stage of the amplifier, it is highly desirable to mount the microwave detector directly on the amplifier chassis. This allows the interconnecting lead to the amplifier to be kept very short, and so reduces the interference noise level. The klystron reflector circuit is also very sensitive to interference. Here, the interference produces a parasitic frequency modulation of the klystron, which leads to an amplitude modulation at the output of the microwave detector. As the reflector circuit is usually connected to a frequency stabilizing circuit, the klystron is mounted close to its corresponding electronic circuitry. All leads for the amplifier and the stabilizing circuits must be fed through filters. The magnetic modulation field produces strong eddy currents in the cavity walls and the neighbouring waveguide, by virtue of the interaction of the alternating currents with the static magnetic field, and this produces mechanical oscillations in the cavity and waveguide. These oscillations are particularly strong with low frequency modulation and produce a parasitic amplitude modulation of the signals reaching the microwave detector. Reducing the cavity wall thickness helps to reduce this effect, and is recommended in the literature.[3]

Interference and microphonics usually lead to a reduction in spectrometer sensitivity. If a pen-recorder is used, the stability of the zero line usually suffers. In addition to this, more time is required to balance the spectrometer, and measurement time is prolonged.

The sensitivity of a spectrometer to interference and microphonics depends to a large extent on the quality of its construction and its performance. Consequently, in the development of a spectrometer, careful attention should be paid to the following points.

§2.5

REASONS FOR DISTORTION OF THE SPECTRAL LINE SHAPE

Distortion of the spectral line shape may be caused by the following:

1. The bandwidth Δf of the amplifier system being too small for the time chosen to register the line. The following condition must be adhered to in order to prevent this type of distortion:

$$\Delta f \gg \frac{1}{\tau}$$

2. Too large a sweep rate of the static magnetic field (if high frequency modulation is used). Here, the following condition must be fulfilled:

$$\frac{dB}{dt} \ll \gamma(\Delta B_{1/2})^2$$

3. Too large a modulation amplitude in spectrometers using double modulation. Here the condition is

$$B_M \ll \Delta B_{1/2}$$

4. Saturation of the energy levels of the sample by too high a microwave power P_0. For a Lorentzian line shape, the following condition must be satisfied:

$$\gamma^2 B_1^2 T_1 T_2 \ll 1 \tag{2.54}$$

where T_1 and T_2 are the longitudinal and transverse relaxation times. If we calculate that the microwave power entering the cavity for the arrangements of Figs. 2.2 and, 2.3, with optimum coupling coefficients, is

$$P_{\text{cav}} = \tfrac{1}{2}P_0$$

we obtain from (2.3), by using (2.4a).

$$B_{1\max}^2 = \frac{\mu_0 Q_0 P_0}{V_{\text{eff}}\omega_0} \tag{2.55}$$

and condition (2.54) can be expressed in the following form:

$$\gamma^2 T_1 T_2 \frac{\mu_0 Q_0 P_0}{V_{\text{eff}} \omega_0} \ll 1 \tag{2.56}$$

5. Inhomogeneity of the magnetic field over the sample volume.
6. In systems using a waveguide bridge, distortion may be produced by a mixing of the absorption and dispersion signals, as we have already mentioned.

§2.6

SPECTROMETER SENSITIVITY

For calculation of the possible limiting sensitivity, equation (2.24) can in principle be used. This equation was deduced under the condition that χ'' was independent of P_0, i.e. under the assumption that saturation does not take place. Clearly, in order to calculate the actual limiting sensitivity, distortion of the line shape due to saturation may be ignored, and we can choose P_0 such that $\chi''_{\text{min,opt}}$ assumes its smallest value. For a sample with Lorentzian line shape, χ'' changes as a function of magnetic induction B in the following way:[12]

$$\chi''_B = \frac{\chi''}{1 + \gamma^2 B_1^2 T_1 T_2} \tag{2.57}$$

Here χ''_B is the suseptibility with existing saturation, and χ'' the susceptibility without saturation.

Using (2.57) and (2.55), we obtain from (2.24) the minimum detectable susceptibility as a function of P_0:

$$\chi''_{\text{min,opt}} = \left(1 + \gamma^2 T_1 T_2 \frac{\mu_0 Q_0 P_0}{\omega V_{\text{eff}}}\right) \frac{4 V_{\text{eff}}}{Q_0} \sqrt{\frac{2kT\Delta f}{P_0}} \tag{2.58}$$

This value reaches a minimum for

$$P_0 = (P_0)_{\text{opt}} = \frac{\omega V_{\text{eff}}}{\mu_0 Q_0 \gamma^2 T_1 T_2} \tag{2.59}$$

By using this equation, we obtain from (2.58) an expression for the limiting value of χ'':

$$\chi''_{\text{min,lim}} = 8\gamma \sqrt{\frac{2kT\Delta f \mu_0 V_{\text{eff}} T_1 T_2}{Q_0 \omega}} \tag{2.60}$$

At the same time we can establish that at $P_0 = P_{opt}$, the width of the spectral line is doubled because of saturation; i.e. the limiting sensitivity is achieved at the cost of distortion of the line shape.

The number of unpaired electrons depends on the magnitude of χ'', through the following equation:[12]

$$N = \frac{2kT_0\chi''}{\omega T_2 \beta^2} \tag{2.61}$$

Here T_0 is the sample temperature. Consequently the minimum number of detectable paramagnetic centres is

$$N_{min,\,lim} = \frac{16kT_0\gamma}{\omega\beta^2} \sqrt{\frac{2kT\Delta f\mu_0 V_{eff}T_1}{\omega Q_0 T_2}} \tag{2.62}$$

On the basis of this equation, we may make the following statements:

1. The cavity must be chosen so that the ratio V_{eff}/Q_0 is very small. Among the most frequently used cavities in E.S.R. spectrometers, the cyclindrical H_{011} cavity has the smallest value of V_{eff}/Q_0 (see Table 2.1). For example, a cylindrical H_{011} cavity made of copper with $\lambda = 3\cdot2$ cm and with dimensions $D = 4\cdot5$ cm and $L = 3\cdot2$ cm, has a $V_{eff} = 5\cdot4$ cm^3 and a theoretical $Q_0 = 3.10^4$. However, in choosing the type of cavity, one has to consider that an increase of Q_0 also increases the requirements on the stability of the alignment of the microwave generator and cavity with respect to each other. For this reason it is sometimes even desirable to reduce the value of V_{eff}/Q_0, and so make Q_0 substantially smaller. For example, a rectangular H_{011} cavity made of copper, for the same wavelength $\lambda = 3\cdot2$ cm and with dimensions $A = 2\cdot3$ cm, $B = 0\cdot5$ cm and $L = 2\cdot2$ cm, has a $V_{eff} = 1\cdot2$ cm^3 and $Q_0 = 2600$. Comparing these two cavities, the rectangular cavity has a ratio of V_{eff}/Q_0 which is only 2·5 times larger than that of the cylindrical cavity.

In contrast to this, the quality factor Q_0 is reduced by a factor 11·5. The sensitivity can therefore be decreased by a factor of only $\sqrt{2\cdot5}$, and the requirements on frequency stability reduced by an order of magnitude.

2. The bandwidth Δf is to be kept as small as possible. Even when stable samples are being investigated, a recording time of one hour can be exceeded only in exceptional cases. If we put $\tau_{max} = 3600$ s, then $\Delta f = 0\cdot1$ Hz.

3. $N_{min,lim}$ decreases with increasing ω. Since V_{eff}/Q_0 also decreases with increasing ω, we find that

$$N_{min,\,lim} = k_1\omega^{-11/4} \tag{2.63}$$

Table 2.1 Some important parameters of often-used cavities

Rectangular H_{01n}-mode	Cylindrical H_{011}-mode	Cylindrical H_{11n}-mode
$\lambda = \dfrac{2}{\sqrt{\left(\dfrac{1}{A^2} + \dfrac{n^2}{L^2}\right)}}$	$\lambda = \dfrac{2}{\sqrt{\left(\left(\dfrac{2\cdot45}{D}\right)^2 + \left(\dfrac{1}{L}\right)^2\right)}}$	$\lambda = \dfrac{2}{\sqrt{\left(\left(\dfrac{1\cdot17}{D}\right)^2 + \left(\dfrac{n}{L}\right)^2\right)}}$
$V_{\text{eff}} = V_{\text{cav}}\left[0\cdot25 + 0\cdot25\left(\dfrac{L}{nA}\right)^2\right]$	$V_{\text{eff}} = V_{\text{cav}}\left[0\cdot081 + 0\cdot136\left(\dfrac{D}{L}\right)^2\right]$	$V_{\text{eff}} = V_{\text{cav}}\left[0\cdot24 + 0\cdot33\left(\dfrac{L}{nD}\right)^2\right]$
$Q_0 = \dfrac{\lambda}{\delta}\cdot\dfrac{V_{\text{cav}}}{4}\cdot\dfrac{\left(\dfrac{1}{A^2}+\dfrac{n^2}{L^2}\right)^{3/2}}{\dfrac{L}{A^2}(A+2B) + \dfrac{n^2}{L^2}\cdot A(L+2B)}$	$Q_0 = 0\cdot61\dfrac{\lambda}{\delta}\cdot\dfrac{\left[1 + 0\cdot167\left(\dfrac{D}{L}\right)^2\right]^{3/2}}{1 + 0\cdot167\left(\dfrac{D}{L}\right)^3}$	$Q_0 = 2\cdot06\dfrac{\lambda}{\delta}\cdot\dfrac{\left[1 + 0\cdot73\left(\dfrac{nD}{L}\right)^2\right]^{3/2}}{1 + 0\cdot514\,n^2\left(\dfrac{D}{L}\right)^3 + 0\cdot216\left(\dfrac{nD}{L}\right)^2}$

H_{012} H_{012} H_{112}

λ the free-space wavelength corresponding to the resonant frequency
δ equivalent thickness of the conducting skin layer
V_{cav} geometrical volume of the cavity
n number of half-wavelengths along the length of the cavity

	k_1		k_1
silver	1·00	aluminium	1·4
copper	1·03	zinc	2·0
gold	1·20	brass	2·2

However, we must remember that equation (2.63) was deduced under the assumption that the geometrical dimensions of the sample are very small. In chemical investigations, the concentration of paramagnetic centres is often very small, and the sample must be made as large as possible. As ω increases, the cavity dimensions decrease, and so does the permissible sample size. In very special cases, high frequency spectrometers can even have a lower working sensitivity than low frequency spectrometers.[3]

Nowadays, the measure of spectrometer sensitivity is often given as the quantity of crystalline DPPH which gives a signal-to-noise ratio of unity. This measure does not always represent the real sensitivity of the spectrometer. The reason for this is that the concentration of paramagnetic centres in solid DPPH is unusually high, and so the condition of sample smallness, under which assumption equation (2.62) was calculated, is always satisfied. If however the concentration of paramagnetic centres is low, then this condition cannot usually be fulfilled. Hence the effective volume V_{eff} is enlarged, since in equation (2.4a) the following expression must be used in place of B_{1M}^2:

$$(B_1^2)_{av} = \frac{\int\limits_{sam} B_1^2 \, dV}{V_{sam}} \tag{2.64}$$

Apart from this, the dielectric losses in the sample usually increase, causing a decrease in Q. This results in a decrease in the overall sensitivity of the spectrometer, compared to the measure given by DPPH. Apart from this disadvantage, DPPH is still considered a very useful standard, since it permits a determination of the noise factor of the spectrometer.

If we use the following practical values in equation (2.26),

$$V_{eff}/Q_0 = 5 \cdot 4/3 \, . \, 10^4 \text{ cm}^3 \qquad \Delta f = 0 \cdot 1 \text{ Hz}$$

$$\gamma = 17 \cdot 7 \, . \, 10^6 \frac{\text{rad}}{\text{s} \, . \, 10^{-4} \text{ Wb m}^{-2}} \qquad T_0 = 300^\circ \text{K} \quad T_1/T_2 \approx 1$$

$$\omega = 2\pi \, . \, 9 \cdot 4 \, . \, 10^9 \frac{\text{rad}}{\text{s}} \qquad k = 1 \cdot 38 \, . \, 10^{-23} \text{ J K}^{-1}$$

$$\beta = 0 \cdot 93 \, . \, 10^{-23} \text{ Am}^2$$

then we obtain the value $N_{min, \, lim} \approx 3.10^9$, for the minimum number of unpaired electrons of a DPPH sample in a 3 cm wavelength spectrometer. This gives only a rough idea of the sensitivity, since the DPPH does not have a Lorentzian line shape.

A superheterodyne spectrometer, the sensitivity of which comes close to the calculated value, has been described in the literature.[23] This high sensitivity was obtained by using as a microwave source a double rhumbatron klystron, which has a higher power and stability than a reflex klystron. In addition to this, a cavity analogous to the measuring cavity was connected to arm D of the waveguide bridge in this spectrometer, so reducing the sensitivity of the waveguide bridge to frequency fluctuations of the microwave generator. It is our experience, however, that the use of two cavities makes the balancing of the spectrometer considerably more difficult, and also makes it very temperature-sensitive and microphonic.

For a calculation of the real limiting sensitivity, we have to introduce the noise figure of the spectrometer into equation (2.62). For a spectrometer with direct detection, we obtain, from equations (2.28) and (2.62),

$$N_{\min} = \frac{16kT_0\gamma}{\omega\beta^2} \sqrt{\frac{kT\Delta f\mu_0 V_{\text{eff}}T_1 t}{\omega Q_0 T_2 G}} \qquad (2.65)$$

For example, at $f_M = 10^6$ Hz and $G = 0\cdot25$, the coefficient $\sqrt{(t/2G)} \approx 10$ (for a diode of the type DK-S4), and the smallest detectable number of particles for a practical spectrometer is

$N_{\min} = 3.10^9 \cdot 10 = 3.10^{10}$

*An example of a spectrometer is given by the E.S.R. spectrometer ER9 of VEB Carl Zeiss, Jena. This instrument works with a magnetic field modulation frequency of 100 kHz. Phase-sensitive microwave detection and a wide-band bridge balance also allow sensitive detection of the dispersion signal. There is a choice of the first or second derivative of the signal. For performing investigations of anisotropy, the magnet can be rotated about the vertical axis.

References

1. Montgomery, C. G.: *Technique of Microwave Measurements* (Rad. Lab. Ser. Vol. 11), New York, London, 1947.
2. Southworth, G. C.: *Principles and Applications of Waveguides,* Soviet Radio, 1955.
3. Feher, G.: *Bell. Syst. Techn. J.* **36** (1957), 449.
4. Bresler, S. je., Saminski, je. M., Kasbekov, E. N.: *J. tech. Phys., Moscow,* **27** (1957), 2535.
5. Beringer, R., Castle, J. G.: *Phys. Rev.,* **78** (1950), 581.
6. See reference 1.
7. Torrey, H. C., Whitmer, C. A.: *Crystal Rectifiers* (Rad. Lab. Ser. Vol. 15), New York, London, 1948.
8. Van der Ziel, A.: *Noise,* New York, 1954.

9. Manenkov, A. A., Prochorov, A. M.: *Radiotechnika i Elektronika,* 1 (1956), 169.
10. Troizki, W. S., Chrulew, W. W.: *Radiotechnika i Elektronika,* 1 (1956), 831.
11. Hirshon, J. M., Fraenkel, G. K.: *Rev. Sci. Instr.,* 26 (1955), 34.
12. Andrew, E. R.: *Nuclear Magnetic Resonance,* Cambridge, 1955.
13. Buckmaster, H. A., Scovil, H. E. D.: *Canad. J. Phys.,* 34 (1956), 711.
14. Semenov, A. G., Bubnov, N. N.: *Pribory i Technika Eksperimenta,* 1 (1959), 92.
15. Tinkham, M.: *Proc. Roy. Soc.,* A 236 (1956), 535.
16. Llewellin, P. M.: *J. Sci. Instr.,* 34 (1957), 236.
17. Bowers, K. D., Kamper, R. A., Knight, R. B. D.: *J. Sci. Instr.,* 34 (1957), 49.
18. Bennet, R. G., Hoell, P. C., Schwenker, R. P.: *Rev. Sci. Instr.,* 29 (1958), 659.
19. Gutkin, L. S.: *Preobrazovanie sverchvysokich castot i detektirovanie* (Ultra High Frequency Mixing and Rectification). GEI 1953.
20. Sefirow, W. I.: *(Radiopriemnye ustrojstva* (Radio-receivers). Voenizdat, 1951).
21. Bunimowitsch, W. I.: *Fljuktuacionnye processy v radiopriemnych ustrojstvach* (Fluctuation Processes in Radio-receivers). Soviet Radio, 1951.
22. Sivers, A. P.: *Radiolokacionnye priemniki* (Radio-receivers). Soviet Radio, 1959.
23. Harihar Misra: *Rev. Sci. Instr.,* 29 (1958), 590.
24* Teaney, D. T., Klein, M. P., Portis, A. M.: *Rev. Sci. Instr.,* 32 (1961), 721.
25* Spry, W. J.: *J. appl. Phys.,* 28 (1957), 660.
26* Henning, J. C. M.: *Rev. Sci. Instr.,* 32 (1961), 35.
27* Laffon, J. L., Servoz-Gavin, P., Uchida, T.: *Phys. Radium,* 23 (1962), 951.
28* Holton, W. C., Blum, H.: *Phys. Rev.,* 125 (1962), 89.
29* Mehlkopf, A. F., Smidt, J.: *Colloque Ampère,* (1962) 758.
30* Redhardt, A.: *Z. ang. Phys.,* 13 (1961), 108.
31* Heuer, K.: Forschungsbericht 3-821/1 "Elektronenresonanz-Spektrometer" (Electron resonance spectrometer) des VEB Carl Zeiss, Jena.

Chapter 3

Theory of E.S.R. Spectra

This chapter aims at something rather less than a complete presentation of the theory of E.S.R. spectra, since to expound the subject fully would require considerably more space than is available to us in this monograph. Besides this, there are many questions in the theory of E.S.R. spectra which are not yet answered. The chapter is written for chemists who would like to familiarize themselves with the theory of the essential characteristics of E.S.R. spectra; but at the same time it can serve as an introduction, after a study of which the reader can follow the original theoretical papers on the subject. The necessary fundamentals of group theory, required for an understanding of some parts of the chapter, are included in the text.

§3.1

THE FREE PARAMAGNETIC ATOM

To a first approximation, neglecting the nuclear magnetic moments, the magnetic properties of atoms are determined by the orbital motion and spin of the electrons. The relationship between the orbital magnetic moment μ_{orb} and the mechanical moment p_ϕ is given by the well-known equation

$$\frac{\mu_{orb}}{p_\phi} = \frac{e}{2mc} \tag{3.1}$$

Here,

$$p_\phi = \sqrt{[l(l+1)]}\hbar \tag{3.2}$$

$$\mu_{orb} = \sqrt{[l(l+1)]}\beta \tag{3.3}$$

where l is the orbital quantum number, and $\beta = e\hbar/2mc$ is the Bohr magneton.

The relationship between the magnetic and mechanical moments, the so-called gyromagnetic ratio, and the g-factor, are usually measured in units of $e/2mc$. For the orbital magnetization we get

$$g_{orb} = 1 \tag{3.4}$$

In the case of pure spin magnetization, because of the gyromagnetic anomaly, we have

$$\mu_{spin} = 2\sqrt{[S(S+1)]}\beta \tag{3.5}$$

$$p_S = \sqrt{[S(S+1)]}\hbar \tag{3.6}$$

and

$$g = \frac{e}{mc} \tag{3.7}$$

In the units which we have chosen, this is

$$g_{spin} = 2 \tag{3.8}\dagger$$

If the free atom contains more electrons than it would by Russell-Saunders coupling, then the orbital and spin quantum members are added vectorially and form the total quantum numbers L and S and the total angular momentum quantum number J:

$$L = \sum_i l_i, \qquad S = \sum_i S_i, \qquad J = L + S$$

From the above equations, it can be easily shown that

$$P_S = \sqrt{[S(S+1)]}\hbar \qquad \mu_S = 2\sqrt{[S(S+1)]}\beta$$

$$P_L = \sqrt{[L(L+1)]}\hbar \qquad \mu_L = \sqrt{[L(L+1)]}\beta$$

$$P_J = \sqrt{[J(J+1)]}\hbar$$

$$\mu_J = \left[1 + \frac{J(J+1) + S(S+1) - L(L+1)}{2J(J+1)}\right]\sqrt{[J(J+1)]}\beta \tag{3.9}$$

The gyromagnetic ratio for the many-electron atom, in the case of Russell-Saunders coupling, is

$$g = 1 + \frac{J(J+1) + S(S+1) - L(L+1)}{2J(J+1)} \tag{3.10}$$

For $S = 0$, $g = 1$; for $L = 0$, $g = 2$; and for the in-between values, the following is valid:

$$1 < g < 2 \tag{3.11}$$

In a constant magnetic field B, a level with a particular value of J is split into $2J + 1$ components (Zeeman splitting):

$$E_{m_J} = m_J g \beta B \tag{3.12}$$

† A more accurate value of g_{spin}, taking into account the relativistic correction, is 2·0023.

The magnetic quantum number m assumes the values $J, J -,1, J - 2, \ldots,$ $- J$.

Under the influence of an alternating magnetic field B, transitions between the Zeeman levels may occur, where the following selection rules hold:

$$\vec{B}_1 \perp \vec{B}$$

$$\Delta m_J = 1 \tag{3.13}$$

In this way, under the influence of a microwave field, transitions between neighbouring levels will occur. Thus from this we arrive at the resonance condition:

$$h\nu = g\beta B \tag{3.14}$$

Here ν is the frequency of the alternating magnetic field, and B the induction of the constant magnetic field; g is determined from equation (3.10).

All the above refers to the case of the free atom, for which the positions of the E.S.R. lines correspond to a value of the g-factor of between 1 and 2, depending on the contribution of the orbital moment to the total magnetic moment of the system. However, generally speaking, the paramagnetic particles investigated by E.S.R. are not free atoms. The unpaired electrons are located in the relatively strong electric field of the crystal lattice or solvent (in the case of solutions of paramagnetic ions) or of neighbouring atoms and the valence electrons of chemical bonds. All of these fields only seldom exhibit spherical symmetry. The existence of an electric field can lead to a complete or partial lifting of the orbital motion, and influences the Zeeman splitting through the spin-orbit coupling. As we shall now see, this effect can show itself in the E.S.R. spectra of ligand or solid substances in such a way that the g-factor is shifted to values which considerably exceed the limits given in equation (3.11), so that an isotropy of the g-factor and a so-called fine structure of the E.S.R. spectra appear. In the following discussion, we shall designate all electric fields external to the unpaired electrons as 'crystal fields' and the whole surrounding region of the paramagnetic ion as the 'crystal lattice' or simply the 'lattice'. We shall also keep to this nomenclature when we are speaking about amorphous or liquid materials, or even about single molecules.

For a theoretical consideration of the influence of the neighbourhood of the paramagnetic particles on the E.S.R. spectrum, we need some knowledge of the theory of groups and their representation. The reason for this is that the behaviour of the paramagnetic particle in the crystal lattice depends significantly on such general features of the crystal lattice as its symmetry.

The use of group theory will thus frequently permit the interpretation of an E.S.R. spectrum without the necessity of an accurate calculation.

§3.2

FUNDAMENTALS OF THE THEORY OF GROUPS AND THEIR REPRESENTATION: GROUP THEORY†

Without going into abstract group theory, we will consider its basic concepts in their application to a concrete example of the symmetry group C_{3v}. Our example is the spatial configuration of the ammonia molecule, shown here schematically.

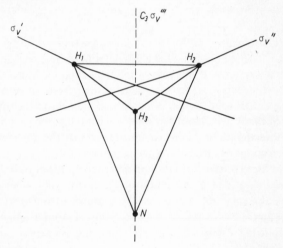

The three hydrogen atoms are at the base of the three-sided pyramid with equal sides, and the nitrogen atom is at the apex of the pyramid. In this way the NH_3 molecule exhibits a rather large degree of symmetry. This gives a whole range of symmetry operations which transform the molecule itself, i.e. which either do not change the positions of the individual atoms or which transform them into completely equivalent positions. We will now enumerate these symmetry operations. First we have the operation C_3, the clockwise rotation through $360 \div 3 = 120°$ about the third-order symmetry axis. The atom N remains in its place ($N \rightarrow N$), the atom H_1 goes into atom H_2, etc.:

$$H_1 \rightarrow H_2 \qquad H_2 \rightarrow H_3 \qquad H_3 \rightarrow H_1$$

† The reader can find a more detailed description of group theory and its application to quantum mechanics in references 1, 2, 3, 24* and 25*.

Then we have the operation C_3^2, the clockwise rotation about the same axis through $240°$ (or anti-clockwise through $120°$). For this,

$$N \rightarrow N \qquad H_1 \rightarrow H_3 \qquad H_2 \rightarrow H_1 \qquad H_3 \rightarrow H_2$$

The operation σ_v is the mirror reflection in the symmetry plane σ'_v, which goes through the points H_1, N and the middle of the line H_2–H_3:

$$N \rightarrow N \qquad H_1 \rightarrow H_1 \qquad H_2 \rightarrow H_3 \qquad H_3 \rightarrow H_2$$

The operation σ''_v gives

$$N \rightarrow N \qquad H_1 \rightarrow H_3 \qquad H_2 \rightarrow H_2 \qquad H_3 \rightarrow H_1$$

Finally, the operation σ'''_v gives

$$N \rightarrow N \qquad H_1 \rightarrow H_2 \qquad H_2 \rightarrow H_1 \qquad H_3 \rightarrow H_3$$

To these symmetry operations we can add the identity E, which does not alter the position of any of the spatial points:

$$N \rightarrow N \qquad H_1 \rightarrow H_1 \qquad H_2 \rightarrow H_2 \qquad H_3 \rightarrow H_3$$

The six symmetry operations enumerated form a group: E, C_3, C_3^2, σ'_v σ''_v, σ'''_v. The ammonia molecule belongs to this symmetry group, which is designated according to convention by the symbol C_{3v}.

We now give a rigorous definition of the idea of a group. Let G be a set of elements a, b, c, ... (the elements may be of any type: numbers, transformations, matrices, symmetry operations, spatial displacements, etc.). In addition to this, let a symbolical multiplication rule be defined, which assigns to each two elements a third one. The set G is a group if the following four conditions are fulfilled:

1. The product of any two elements a and b is an element c which belongs to the same set.
2. The associative law is valid:

   $$a(bc) = (ab)c$$

3. The set G contains an element e, called the unit element, for which the following equation is valid:

   $$ae = a$$

   where a is an arbitrary element of the set.
4. For each element there exists an inverse element a^{-1}:

   $$a \cdot a^{-1} = e$$

The commutative law, $ab = ba$, does not have to be valid. Groups for which the commutative law is valid are called *Abelian* groups. We now want to formulate the multiplication rule for symmetry operations. The product $a.b$ of two symmetry operations a and b is the symmetry operation obtained by carrying out first operation b and then operation a. As an example, we calculate the product $C_3\sigma_v'$ for the NH_3 molecule considered above. The application of the operations σ_v' and C_3 in that order can be written in the following way:

$$N \rightarrow N \rightarrow N \qquad H_1 \rightarrow H_1 \rightarrow H_2 \qquad H_2 \rightarrow H_3 \rightarrow H_1$$

$$H_3 \rightarrow H_2 \rightarrow H_3$$

We see that $C_3.\sigma_v' = \sigma_v'''$. In this manner we can now build up a multiplication table for the group C_{3v} (Table 3.1).

Table 3.1 Multiplication table for the group C_{3v} (NH_3 molecule)

b \ a	E	C_3	C_3^2	σ_v'	σ_v''	σ_v'''
E	E	C_3	C_3^2	σ_v'	σ_v''	σ_v'''
C_3	C_3	C_3^2	E	σ_v''	σ_v'''	σ_v'
C_3^2	C_3^2	E	C_3	σ_v'''	σ_v'	σ_v''
σ_v'	σ_v'	σ_v'''	σ_v''	E	C_3^2	C_3
σ_v''	σ_v''	σ_v'	σ_v'''	C_3	E	C_3^2
σ_v'''	σ_v'''	σ_v''	σ_v'	C_3^2	C_3	E

It is now not difficult to verify that the six elements E, C_3, C_3^2, σ_v', σ_v'', σ_v''' really do form a group. We leave this to the reader.

It can also easily be shown that the unit element on the left hand side is equal to that of the right hand side, and that the inverse element on the right and left hand sides are also equal. There can only be one unit element in each group.

Any subset of the set G which satisfies the four above requirements is called a *subgroup* of the group. Thus the three elements E, C_3 and C_3^2 form a subgroup of the group C_{3v}. The number h of group elements is called the *order* of the group. The order of the group C_{3v} which we have considered above is $h = 6$.

Let c be an arbitrary element of the group. Then the transformation cac^{-1} is called a *similarity transformation* of the element a. Elements convertible into one another by similarity transformations form a class. We

Table 3.2 Symmetry operations

Symbolic description of the operation	Explanation
E	Identity operation
C_n	Rotation through $2\pi/n$ about a symmetry axis
σ_v	Mirror reflection in a symmetry plane which lies in the main symmetry axis (axis of highest order)
σ_h	Mirror reflection in a symmetry plane perpendicular to the main axis
σ_d	Mirror reflection in a plane bisecting the angles between the second-order symmetry axes which are perpendicular to the main symmetry axis; the main symmetry axis lies in the plane σ_d
S_n	Rotation through $2\pi/n$ about a mirror rotation axis, followed by mirror reflection in a plane perpendicular to this axis
i	Inversion, mirror reflection at a centre of symmetry

see that the group C_3 consists of three classes: E; C_3, C_3^2; σ_v', σ_v'', σ_v'''. For reasons which will later be clear, it is expedient when writing down a group to combine the elements belonging to one class. The symmetry group C_{3v} can then be written in the following way:

$$E, 2C_3, 3\sigma_v$$

In Abelian groups each element forms its own class. Tables 3.2 and 3.3 summarize the classification of symmetry operations and symmetry groups.

A detailed classification of symmetry groups can be found, for example, in the monographs of G. Eyring, J. Walter and J. Kimbal.[1]

The groups T, T_h, T_d, O, O_h belong to the cubic system, the groups C_{3h}, C_{6h}, D_{3h}, C_{6v}, D_{6h} to the hexagonal, the groups C_{3v}, D_{3d} to the rhombohedric (trigonal), the groups C_{4h}, C_{4v}, D_{4h} to the tetragonal, and the groups C_{2v}, D_{2h} to the rhombic system.

Representation theory

If to each element of the group G can be uniquely assigned a particular element of the group G', in such a way that the product of any two elements of the group G corresponds to the product of the corresponding elements of group G', then one may say that group G corresponds *homomorphically* to group G'. In the case of a reversible one-to-one correlation, groups G and G' are called *isomorphs*.

Table 3.3 Some important symmetry groups

Basic symmetry operation	Description of the symmetry group	Examples
C_n, σ_v	C_{nv}	C_{2v} H_2O C_{3v} NH_3 $C_{\infty v}$ CO, HCl
C_n, σ_h	C_{nh}	C_{2h} $\left\{\begin{array}{l} \text{Trans-}C_2H_2Cl_2 \\[2em] \text{(benzene ring diagram with R, } R_1\text{)} \end{array}\right.$
C_{n^-}, σ_{d^-} and $2n$ axes of second order (D) perpendicular to the main axis	D_{nd}	D_{3d} left hand isomers of ethane
C_n, σ_v, σ_h	D_{nh}	D_{2h} naphthalene p dichlorobenzene D_{3h} trans isomers of ethane D_{6h} benzene
	T_d	CH_4
	O_h	cube, octahedron, SF_6

By a *representation* of group G, we mean any group of finite square matrices (or linear transformations), with non-zero determinants, to which group G can be made to correspond homomorphically. Isomorphism is not required here. For example, the number 1 is a representation of the symmetry group C_{3v} (NH_3 molecule), as it is, incidentally, of any group, if the symbolic group multiplication corresponds to the normal arithmetical multiplication:

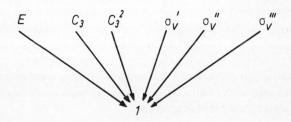

In the same way, the positive and negative units form a representation of the group C_{3v}, under the following correlation:

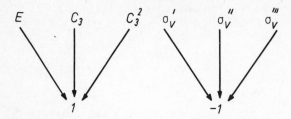

This can be easily verified by using the multiplication table of the group C_{3v} (Table 3.1).

These two representations can be written in more detail in the following way:

	E	C_3	C_3^2	σ_v'	σ_v''	σ_v'''
Γ_1	1	1	1	1	1	1
Γ_2	1	1	1	-1	-1	-1

$$(3.15)$$

The numbers 1 and -1 can be regarded here as square matrices of the first order. It is clear that Γ_1 and Γ_2 [see (3.15)] completely exhaust all possible representations of the group C_{3v} by first-order matrices, i.e. by numerals. We will now construct a second-order representation of the group C_3. For all symmetry operations of this group, the point of the pyramid (the nitrogen atom) remains in the same place. For this reason we can restrict ourselves to consideration of the base plane only, in which the three hydrogen atoms lie. An arbitrary symmetry operation corresponds to a transformation of coordinates in this plane:

$$x_2 = a_{11}x_1 + a_{12}y_1$$

$$y_2 = a_{21}x_1 + a_{22}y_1$$

The matrices of this transformation,

$$\begin{pmatrix} a_{11} & a_{12} \\ a_{21} & a_{22} \end{pmatrix}$$

form a natural representation of the group C_{3v}, the group multiplication being the usual matrix multiplication. The orthogonal coordinates are placed as shown in the following sketch:

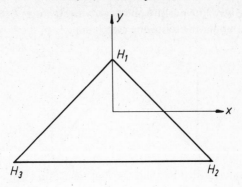

The operation E then corresponds to the matrix $\begin{pmatrix} 1 & 0 \\ 0 & 1 \end{pmatrix}$ and the operation σ'_v to the matrix $\begin{pmatrix} -1 & 0 \\ 0 & 1 \end{pmatrix}$

As is well known, the following transformation of the Cartesian coordinates corresponds to a rotation through an angle θ in the plane x, y:

$$x_2 = x_1 \cos \theta - y_1 \sin \theta$$
$$y_2 = x_1 \sin \theta + y_1 \cos \theta$$

The matrix of this transformation is

$$\begin{pmatrix} \cos \theta & -\sin \theta \\ \sin \theta & \cos \theta \end{pmatrix} \tag{3.16}$$

From (3.16) we can immediately find the matrices which correspond to the symmetry operations C_3 (rotation through 120°) and C_3^2 (rotation through 240°), and then by using the matrix multiplication rules we can find the remaining matrices of the representation. As a result of this, in addition to the representation Γ_1 and Γ_2 (3.15), we obtain the representation Γ_3:

$$
\begin{array}{cccccc}
E & C_3 & C_3^2 & \sigma'_v & \sigma''_v & \sigma'''_v \\
\begin{pmatrix} 1 & 0 \\ 0 & 1 \end{pmatrix} &
\begin{pmatrix} -\frac{1}{2} & -\frac{\sqrt{3}}{2} \\ \frac{\sqrt{3}}{2} & -\frac{1}{2} \end{pmatrix} &
\begin{pmatrix} -\frac{1}{2} & \frac{\sqrt{3}}{2} \\ -\frac{\sqrt{3}}{2} & -\frac{1}{2} \end{pmatrix} &
\begin{pmatrix} -1 & 0 \\ 0 & 1 \end{pmatrix} &
\begin{pmatrix} \frac{1}{2} & \frac{\sqrt{3}}{2} \\ \frac{\sqrt{3}}{2} & -\frac{1}{2} \end{pmatrix} &
\begin{pmatrix} \frac{1}{2} & -\frac{\sqrt{3}}{2} \\ -\frac{\sqrt{3}}{2} & -\frac{1}{2} \end{pmatrix}
\end{array}
$$

$$\tag{3.17}$$

It is easy to see that as many matrix representations of group C_{3v} can be written down as we wish. So if we assign numbers to the hydrogen atoms,

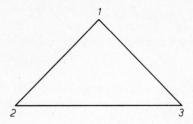

then a permutation can be assigned to each symmetry operation, and this again can be written in matrix form:

E	C_3	C_3^2	σ_v'	σ_v''	σ_v'''
100	010	001	100	001	010
010	001	100	001	010	100
001	100	010	010	100	001

If two coordinates (x_i, y_i) are used for each hydrogen atom, then a representation can be constructed from matrices of the sixth order, etc.

We shall see however, that the possible nonequivalent irreducible representations of the group C_{3v} are already exhausted by the representations we have so far obtained, Γ_1, Γ_2 and Γ_3 (see 3.15 and 3.17).

Let e, a, b, c, d, f, be a set of matrices which form a representation of group G (e.g. the representation Γ_3 of the group C_{3v}). Let β be an arbitrary matrix, and β^{-1} the inverse matrix.† Then we obtain, by similarity transformations such as

$$a' = \beta^{-1}a\beta \tag{3.18}$$

a new set of matrices

$$e', a', b', c', d', f'$$

$$\dagger \; \beta^{-1}\beta = \begin{pmatrix} 1 & 0 & . & . & . \\ 0 & 1 & . & . & . \\ . & . & . & . & . \\ . & . & . & 1 & 0 \\ . & . & . & 0 & 1 \end{pmatrix} \quad \text{is the unit matrix.}$$

These can be easily shown to form another representation of G. If for example $ab = e$, then $a'b' = e'$.

In fact, let us make $a'b' = e'$, and show that this implies $ab = e$. We get

$$\beta^{-1}a\beta\beta^{-1}b\beta = \beta^{-1}e\beta$$

Using the associative law of matrix multiplication, we obtain

$$\beta^{-1}ab\beta = \beta^{-1}e\beta$$

Multiplying both sides of the equation from the left by β and from the right by β^{-1}, we obtain

$$\beta\beta^{-1}ab\beta\beta^{-1} = \beta\beta^{-1}e\beta\beta^{-1}$$

i.e.

$$ab = e$$

which was to be proved.

Representations which may be obtained from each other by similarity transformations, are called *equivalent*. The sets of linear transformations of the space characterized by such representations are not linearly independent of each other.

Again, let e, a, b, c, d, f be a matrix representation of the group G. We choose a similarity transformation which transforms all matrices into diagonal form:

$$a' = \beta^{-1}a\beta = \begin{pmatrix} a_1' & 0 & 0 & . & . \\ 0 & a_2' & 0 & . & . \\ 0 & 0 & a_3' & . & . \\ . & . & . & . & . \\ . & . & . & . & . \\ . & . & 0 & 0 & a_n' \end{pmatrix} \tag{3.19}$$

Here a_i' are square matrices; the other matrices and matrix elements are equal to zero.

We can easily see that the matrix sets e_1', a_1', b_1', ..., e_2', a_2', b_2', ... are representations of the group G. Our representation Γ (or another representation Γ' equivalent to it, that is, obtained from Γ by a similarity transformation) is also a linear combination of the representations Γ_1, Γ_2, Γ_3, ..., Γ_n:

$$\Gamma = \sum_i \Gamma_i$$

If a representation Γ_i cannot be submitted to any corresponding operation, then it is said to be irreducible. Any other representation is reducible, i.e. a similarity transformation can be found which transforms it into diagonal form, so that it can be represented as a linear combination of irreducible representations.

We now consider again the representations Γ_1, Γ_2 and Γ_3 of the group C_{3v}, which we obtained earlier [see (3.15) and (3.17)]. It can easily be shown that they are non-equivalent irreducible representations. We designate the matrix in the i-th representation, corresponding to the symmetry operation R, by $\Gamma_i(R)$, and the matrix element mn (m being the column number and n the row number) of this matrix, by $\Gamma_i(R)_{mn}$.

The following can easily be shown to be valid:

$$\sum_R \Gamma_1(R)_{11}\Gamma_1(R)_{11} = 6 = h$$

$$\sum_R \Gamma_2(R)_{11}\Gamma_2(R)_{11} = 6 = h$$

$$\sum_R \Gamma_3(R)_{11}\Gamma_3(R)_{11} = \sum_R \Gamma_3(R)_{12}\Gamma_3(R)_{12} = \sum_R \Gamma_3(R)_{21}\Gamma_3(R)_{21}$$

$$= \sum_R \Gamma_3(R)_{22}\Gamma_3(R)_{22} = 3 = \frac{h}{l}$$

where h is the order of the group and l the dimension of the representation. By a generalization of the above equation, we get:

$$\sum_R \Gamma_i(R)_{mn}\Gamma_i(R)_{mn} = \frac{h}{l_i} \tag{3.20}$$

Analogously, we can also put

$$\sum_R \Gamma_i(R)_{mn}\Gamma_j(R)_{mn} = 0 \quad (i \neq j) \tag{3.21}$$

$$\sum_R \Gamma_i(R)_{mn}\Gamma_i(R)_{m'n'} = 0 \quad (m \neq m', n \neq n'). \tag{3.22}$$

Equations (3.20) to (3.22) can generally be written in the following form, which is valid for an arbitrary non-equivalent representation of an arbitrary group.†*

$$\sum_R \Gamma_i(R)_{mn}\sqrt{\left(\frac{l_i}{h}\right)}\Gamma_j(R)_{m'n'}\sqrt{\left(\frac{l_j}{h}\right)} = \delta_{ij}\delta_{mm'}\delta_{nn'} \tag{3.23}$$

† A rigorous analysis of the fundamental theorems of representation theory can be found, for example, in references 1, 2 and 3.

Here, δ is the Kronecker symbol:

$$\delta_{ij} = 1 \quad \text{for } i = j \qquad \delta_{ij} = 0 \quad \text{for } i \neq j$$

We see from (3.23) that $\Gamma_i(R_1)_{mn}$, $\Gamma_i(R_2)_{mn}$, ..., $\Gamma_i(R_h)_{mn}$, can be considered as components of an h-dimensional vector, which is orthogonal to any vector of another set, and to the vector derived analogously from any other representation Γ_j. This gives c non-equivalent irreducible representations with the dimension numbers l_i. Thus there are in all $l_1^2 + l_2^2 + \ldots + l_c^2$ such orthogonal vectors, since a matrix of grade l_i has l_i^2 matrix elements. On the other hand there are h h-dimensional orthogonal vectors. Thus we can put

$$\sum_i l_i^2 = h \tag{3.24}$$

In the case of the group C_{3v} considered above, $h = 6$ and consequently the non-equivalent irreducible representations obtained, Γ_1 $(l = 1)$, Γ_2 $(l = 2)$, and Γ_3 $(l = 3)$, are all possible irreducible representations of this symmetry group.

In all cases of the application of group theory to the problems relevant to us, it is quite sufficient to use not the matrices of the representations themselves, but their characters. The *character* (or *trace*) of a matrix is the sum of its diagonal elements:

$$\chi_i(R) = \sum_m \Gamma_i(R)_{mm} \tag{3.25}$$

The table of characters of the irreducible representations of the group C_{3v} is shown below:

	E	C_3	C_3^2	σ_v'	σ_v'	σ_v'''	
Γ_1	1	1	1	1	1	1	(3.26)
Γ_2	1	1	1	−1	−1	−1	
Γ_3	2	−1	−1	0	0	0	

The character of a matrix remains unchanged by similarity transformation. Assume that P is some matrix and Q is a matrix which results from P by a similarity transformation, $Q = X^{-1}PX$. Then

$$\chi(Q) = \sum_i Q_{ii} = \sum_i \sum_j \sum_k X_{ij}^{-1} P_{jk} X_{ki} = \sum_i \sum_j \sum_k X_{ki} X_{ij}^{-1} P_{jk}$$

$$= \sum_j \sum_k \delta_{jk} P_{jk} = \sum_j P_{jj} = \chi(P),$$

showing that the character is unchanged.

E.S.R. in Chemistry

From this, we can see that elements belonging to the same class have the same characters. The table of characters of the group C_{3v} can also be shown in the following way:

	E	$2C_3$	$3\sigma_v$
Γ_1	1	1	1
Γ_2	1	1	-1
Γ_3	2	-1	0

$$(3.27)$$

We now want to formulate some general statements, some of which have already been proved:

1. The number of irreducible representations is equal to the number of classes of a group.
2. The sum of the squares of the dimensions of irreducible representations of a group is equal to its order, or, since $l_j = \chi_j(E)$

$$\sum_j [\chi_j(E)]^2 = h \tag{3.28}$$

3. The characters of any two irreducible representations are orthogonal:

$$\sum_R \chi_i(R)\chi_j(R) = 0 \quad (i \neq j) \tag{3.29}$$

4. The character of an irreducible representation is normalized:

$$\sum_R [\chi_i(R)]^2 = h \tag{3.30}$$

Any matrix representation of a symmetry group is either one of the irreducible representations of the group or can be expressed as a linear combination of such irreducible representations.

Let $\chi(R)$ be the character of the matrix which in some reducible representation of the group G corresponds to the operation R. It follows from (3.19) that the following holds:

$$\chi(R) = \sum_{j=1}^{k} a_j \chi_j(R)$$

Here, $\chi_j(R)$ is the character of the corresponding matrix from the j-th irreducible representation, and the coefficient a_j determines how often this irreducible representation occurs in the decomposition of the representation. We multiply both sides of the equation by $\chi_i(R)$, and sum over all values of R. Then, from equations (3.29) and (3.30), we get

$$\sum_R \chi(R)\chi_i(R) = \sum_R \sum_{j=1}^{k} a_j \chi_j(R) \chi_i(R) = \sum_R a_i \chi_i^2(R) = a_i h \tag{3.31}$$

and

$$a_i = \frac{1}{h} \sum \chi(R)\,\chi_i(R) \tag{3.32}$$

Equation (3.32) enables us to perform the decomposition of a reducible representation into its irreducible components without having to use the extensive similarity transformations.

The irreducible representations of symmetry groups are usually classified in the following way. One-dimensional representation (so-called 'non-degenerate' representations) are designated by the symbols A and B, where A signifies a representation symmetric with respect to rotation about the symmetry axis, and B an antisymmetric one. Subscripts g and u signify symmetry and antisymmetry respectively, in relation to reflection in an inversion centre (if one exists). A two-dimensional ('doubly degenerate') representation is represented by the symbol E, and a triply degenerate one by the symbol T. Irreducible representations with a higher degree of degeneracy do not exist.

If the symbols shown above are not sufficient to designate the irreducible representations, then consecutive numbers are added to the index (e.g. A_1, A_2, B_{1g}, B_{2u} etc.). With these symbols we can now give a final representation for the character-table of the irreducible representations of the group C_{3v} (3.27):

	E	$2C_3$	$3\sigma_v$
A_1	1	1	1
A_2	1	1	-1
E	2	-1	0

Character-tables of irreducible representations of the most important symmetry groups are collected in Appendix 1 to this book, (p. 313)

§3.3

GROUP THEORY AND QUANTUM MECHANICS

The state of a quantum system is completely described by the Schrödinger equation. We write it here in the operator form:

$$\hat{H}\psi = E\psi. \tag{3.33}$$

Here $\hat{H}$ is the Hamiltonian operator of the system, ψ an eigenfunction, and E the corresponding eigenvalue.

An arbitrary transformation R of the symmetry group of the Hamiltonian operator transforms a system of points (coordinates) of the space q_1, q_2, q_3, ..., q_n into another system of points q'_1, q'_2, ..., q'_n, and the function ψ into another function ψ'. The Schrödinger equation is invariant so far as the symmetry operation is concerned (R transforms all nuclei and electrons of the system into equivalent positions and does not influence their interaction). For this reason the new function $\psi' = R\psi$ must belong to the same eigenvalue as ψ. From this it is evident that the eigenfunctions of each energy level are transformed linearly, and that the matrices of these transformations form irreducible representations of the symmetry group (reducible representations can always be broken down into irreducible ones). We may say that a specific energy level and a specific eigenvalue belong to a specific irreducible representation, and that the dimension of this representation is numerically equal to the value of $\chi(E)$ and equal to the degree of degeneracy of the level. if there is no degeneracy, then only one eigenfunction corresponds to each level, and this is $R\psi = \pm\psi$ ($|\psi|^2$ remains invariant). The corresponding matrices are simply represented by the numbers ± 1. If the level is doubly degenerate, then two eigenfunctions ψ_1 and ψ_2 exist which are transformed linearly by a symmetry operation:

$$R\psi_1 = a_{11}\psi_1 + a_{12}\psi_2$$

$$R\psi_2 = a_{21}\psi_1 + a_{22}\psi_2$$

The matrices of these transformations,

$$\begin{pmatrix} a_{11} & a_{12} \\ a_{21} & a_{22} \end{pmatrix}$$

form a representation of the symmetry group. We say that the set of functions ψ_1 and ψ_2 form the *basis* for the representation of the group.

Each eigenfunction of the group is also connected with one of the irreducible representations of the symmetry group of this system. The converse statement is in general untrue. No two eigenfunctions can belong to the same irreducible representation, since this case is forbidden by the Pauli principle.

The direct product

Let R be a symmetry operation of the group and let ϕ_1, ϕ_2, ..., ϕ_m and ψ_1, ψ_2, ..., ψ_n be two systems of functions which form the bases for two representations (of dimensions m and n).

From the foregoing it follows that

$$R\phi_i = \sum_{j=1}^{m} a_{ji}\phi_j$$

$$R\psi_k = \sum_{l=1}^{n} a_{lk}\psi_l$$

and clearly,

$$R\phi_i\psi_k = \sum_{j=1}^{m} \sum_{l=1}^{n} a_{ji}a_{lk}\phi_j\psi_l = \sum_{j} \sum_{l} c_{jl,ik}\phi_j\psi_l \qquad (3.34)$$

The function system $\phi_i\,\psi_k$, which consists of all possible products of the functions ϕ and ψ, also forms the basis for a representation of dimensions $m \cdot n$. The matrices of this representation have the character

$$\chi_{\phi\psi}(R) = \sum_{j} \sum_{l} c_{jl,jl} = \sum_{j=1}^{m} \sum_{l=1}^{n} a_{jj}b_{ll} = \chi_\phi(R)\,\chi_\psi(R) \qquad (3.35)$$

The function system $\phi_i\,\psi_k$ is called the direct product of the systems ϕ_i and ψ_k, and the corresponding matrices of the $m \cdot n$-dimensional representation are called the direct products of the given representation. The calculation of direct products is necessary for many problems in quantum mechanics. Thus it is necessary for the deduction of the selection rules to find out if an integral of the type $\int \psi_1 \bar{r}\, \psi_2 \, \mathrm{d}\tau$, which determines the transition probability between the states ψ_1 and ψ_2, is equal to zero or not.

ψ_1, ψ_2 and the radius vector $\bar{r}$ belong to a particular irreducible representation of the system. The direct product of this irreducible representation corresponds to the integrand. If this direct product belongs to another representation of the symmetry group, other than the total symmetric one,† then a symmetry operation can always be found which reverses the sign of $\psi_1 \bar{r}\, \psi_2$. This automatically leads to the integral of this expression over the entire space being identically zero. Only in the case when the direct product $\psi_1 \bar{r} \psi_2$ belongs to the total symmetrical representation, or to a reducible representation which contains the total symmetrical representation, is the integral $\int \psi_1 \bar{r} \psi_2 \, \mathrm{d}\tau$ different from zero and the corresponding transition is allowed.

† The symmetrical representation is an irreducible representation of the type A_1, which is symmetrical with respect to all symmetry operations of the group.

§3.4

THE SPLITTING OF LEVELS OF THE FREE PARAMAGNETIC ATOM IN CRYSTAL FIELDS OF DIFFERENT SYMMETRY

In a generalized crystal field, the atom is submitted to two types of disturbance:

(a) the exchange interaction with neighbouring atoms,

(b) the Stark effect splitting of levels in an electrical crystal field.

At this stage, we will consider the influence of electric fields, using the method of quantum mechanical perturbation theory. For the zero-th order approximation we will choose the free atom with Russell-Saunders coupling, i.e. the coupling most frequently occurring, in which the spin-orbit coupling is weak compared to the orbit-orbit and spin-spin coupling. For this type of coupling, the quantum states of the atom are built up from the quantum states of the individual electrons in the following way:

$$\Sigma \, l_j = L$$
$$\Sigma \, s_j = S$$
$$L + S = J$$

This means that the separation between the levels of a multiplet (with a particular value of L) will be smaller than the separation between neighbouring multiplets.

If we compare the magnitude of the Stark effect splitting with the separation between the levels of a free atom, then three cases can be distinguished.

1. *Strong crystal field.* The separation between the Stark levels is greater than the distance between the multiplets. For a first approximation, the interaction of the l_i-state with the electric field must be calculated. Here, it will be

$$l_i \rightarrow \lambda_i,$$

where λ_i is the mechanical orbital moment of the single electrons in the electric field. As a second approximation, the interaction of λ_i has to be calculated:

$$\Sigma \, \lambda_i = \Lambda$$

and as a third approximation, the interaction with the spin:

$$\Lambda + S = M$$

In this way the system is characterized in a strong electric field by the following set of quantum numbers:

$$n_i \quad l_i \quad \lambda_i \quad \Lambda \quad M \tag{3.36}$$

2. *Medium crystal field.* The Stark effect splitting is smaller than the separation of neighbouring multiplets. In this case L remains a good quantum number and the levels split according to the different orientations of L with respect to the crystal axes: $L \to \Lambda$. Accordingly the spin-orbit interaction is calculated: $\Lambda + S = M$. In this case we use the following set of quantum numbers:

$$n_i \quad l_i \quad L \quad \Lambda \quad M \tag{3.37}$$

3. *Weak crystal field.* The Stark effect splitting is smaller than the separation between the levels with a multiplet. The terms split in the crystal field according to the different orientations of J with respect to the crystal axes: $J \to M$. The system of quantum numbers is

$$n_i \quad l_i \quad L \quad J \quad M \tag{3.38}$$

Before we go on to accurate calculations, we would like to consider a more general problem: into how many levels, and which kinds of level, do the atomic terms split in crystal fields of different symmetries? This problem will be solved by the methods of group theory.

Continuous groups: the rotational group and its representations

The free atom exhibits completely spherical symmetry and belongs to the so-called rotational group K_n. The symmetry operations of this continuous group are the rotations by an arbitrary angle about an axis of arbitrary direction through the centre of the sphere. The individual elements of the group are characterized by two parameters, θ and ψ, which may take a continuous range of values. Here θ is the spatial angle between the rotational axis and a defined direction in the space (e.g. the z-axis),† and ψ the rotational angle about this axis. The group K_n is thus of infinitely high order. By using the definition of classes of a group given on p. 52, we can show that all rotations through a given angle of absolute value $|\psi|$ about an

† Here the angle θ represents a spatial direction and, as a result, naturally corresponds to two one-dimensional parameters, e.g. to the spherical coordinates of the point of penetration of the rotational axis through the unit sphere. The individual elements of the group K_n are thus characterized by three one-dimensional parameters.

arbitrary axis (for all values of θ) belong to the same class. Obviously each irreducible representation of a continuous group contains an infinite continuous range of matrices. There are infinitely many irreducible representations of the rotational group. However, the number of basis functions of each representation (the dimension or the degree of degeneracy of the representation) is finite, as we will now show. For the matrix elements and characters of this representation, generalized orthogonality relations are valid, analogous to equations (3.29) and (3.30) for the representation of discontinuous groups:

$$\int \chi^{(\alpha)}(G)\,\chi^{(\beta)}(G)\,\mathrm{d}\tau_G = \delta_{\alpha\beta} \int \mathrm{d}\tau_G \qquad (3.39)$$

In this case, summation is replaced by the 'invariant integration of the group'. We can express $\mathrm{d}\tau_G$ in the terms of the group parameters and their differentials; e.g. for the rotational group we have $\mathrm{d}\tau_G = \mathrm{d}\theta\,\mathrm{d}\psi$.

We will now construct the irreducible representations of the rotational group (or, to be more explicit, its characters). For this we shall digress slightly. We are looking for the wave functions of a system with a spherically symmetrical potential (free atom), which are transformed into themselves by symmetry operations of the group. It can be easily shown that these functions are eigenfunctions of the total angular momentum operator. The angular momentum operator is by its nature an operator of infinitely small rotation, and its eigenvalues characterize the behaviour of the wave function under rotation. Since, for a specific representation, the characters of the matrices which belong to the same class are equal, we can assume an arbitrary angle θ. The most convenient choice of angle is that of $\theta = 0$ (z-axis). In this case the operator $\hat{L}_z = (-h/2\pi)\mathrm{i}(\partial/\partial\phi)$, and its eigenvalues (in units of $h/2\pi$) are

$$L_z = L, L - 1, \ldots, -L$$

The moment of the system is defined by the quantum number j (which can be an orbital moment, a spin moment or a total moment). There are $2j + 1$ different eigenfunctions with $m = -j, -j + 1, \ldots, j-1, j$, which differ in the value of the z-component, but belong to one single $(2j + 1)$-fold degenerate level. On rotation through an angle ϕ, the wave functions with a given j and m are multiplied by $e^{im\phi}$, which does not change the squares of their absolute values. The transformation matrices of these $2j + 1$ wave functions (which belong to a given value of j) clearly form an irreducible representation of the rotational group. From this standpoint, the numeral j numbers the irreducible representations and $2j + 1$ is equal to their dimension. We can see that these matrices are diagonal; in fact, we will consider an example:

$$j = 1 \qquad m = -1 \qquad 0 \qquad +1$$
$$\psi_1 \quad \psi_2 \quad \psi_3$$

Under rotation by an angle ϕ, m does not change, and ψ_1, ψ_2 and ψ_3 are simply multiplied by $e^{im\phi}$, i.e. they are transformed in accordance with the following equations:

$$\psi_2' = e^{-i\phi}\psi \quad + 0\psi_2 + 0\psi_3$$
$$\psi_2' = 0\psi_1 \quad + 1\psi_2 + 0\psi_3$$
$$\psi_3' = 0\psi_1 \quad + 0\psi_2 + e^{i\phi}\psi_3$$

The matrix of these linear transformations, i.e. the matrix which corresponds to a rotation through an angle ϕ in the irreducible representation with $j = 1$, is as follows:

$$\begin{pmatrix} e^{-i\phi} & 0 & 0 \\ 0 & 1 & 0 \\ 0 & 0 & e^{+i\phi} \end{pmatrix}$$

Its character is

$$\chi^1(\phi) = e^{-i\phi} + 1 + e^{+i\phi} = \frac{\sin \frac{3}{2}\phi}{\sin \frac{1}{2}}$$

In the general case,

$$\chi^j(\phi) = \sum_{m=-j}^{j} e^{im\phi} = \frac{\sin (j + \frac{1}{2})\phi}{\sin \frac{1}{2}\phi} \qquad (3.40)\dagger$$

For the S-states of an atom, it is evident that

$$\chi^{(0)}(\phi) \equiv 1$$

and for the identity operation

$$\chi^{(j)}(0) = 2j + 1$$

We consider now an atom in a crystal field of non-spherical symmetry. For the time being, we will exclude consideration of the spin; this means we are limited to integral values of j. As an example, we will consider the behaviour of states with orbital quantum numbers $L = 0, 1, 2$, in a crystal field.

---

† In the derivation of (3.40), it should be noticed that $\sum_{m=-j}^{j} e^{im\phi}$ is nothing more than a geometrical series with $a_1 = e^{-ij\phi}$, $q = e^{i\phi}$ and $a_n = e^{ij\phi}$.

For a free atom, the states with $L = 0, 1, 2$ belong to the irreducible representation $\Gamma^{(L)}$ of the group K_n with one-, three- and five-fold degeneracy respectively. These representations can become reducible in a field of lower symmetry. They can then be resolved into the irreducible representations of a new symmetry group, the degenerate states being partially or completely lifted.

$$\Gamma^{(h)} = \Sigma\, a_i \Gamma_i. \tag{3.41}$$

Here Γ_i are the irreducible representations of the symmetry group of the crystal field.

We begin with a field of cubic symmetry. Since we are only interested in operations of pure rotation, we shall restrict ourselves to consideration of the corresponding symmetry classes. For this viewpoint, the different groups of the cubic system (O, O_h, T_d etc.) are equivalent. We give below a table of characters of the irreducible representations of the cubic system:

	E	$3C_3$	$6C_4$	$6C_2'$	$8C_3$	
A_1	1	1	1	1	1	
A_2	1	1	-1	-1	1	
E	2	2	0	0	-1	(3.42)
T_1	3	-1	1	-1	0	
T_2	3	-1	-1	1	0	

The rotation angles ϕ for the operations E, C_2, C_4, C_2' and C_3 are 0, π, $\pi/2$, π $2\pi/3$ respectively. From (3.40) we find the characters of the irreducible representations of the rotational group for the values of ϕ, for $L = j = 0, 1, 2$:

		E	$3C_2$	$6C_4$	$6C_2'$	$8C_3$	
	0	1	1	1	1	1	
L	1	3	-1	1	-1	0	(3.43)
	2	5	1	-1	1	-1	

We see that in a field of cubic symmetry, the state $L = 0$ (S-state) belongs to the representation A_1, and the state $L = 1$ (P-state) to the representation T_1. The D-state belongs to a reducible representation, which can be resolved by means of (3.41) and (3.31) into its irreducible components. This is:

$$a_{A_1} = \tfrac{1}{24}(5 + 3 - 6 + 6 - 8) = 0$$

$$a_{A_2} = \tfrac{1}{24}(5 + 3 + 6 - 6 - 8) = 0$$

$$a_E = \tfrac{1}{24}(10 + 6 + 8) = 1$$

$$a_{T_1} = \tfrac{1}{24}(15 - 3 - 6 - 6) = 0$$

$$a_{T_2} = \tfrac{1}{24}(15 - 3 + 6 + 6) = 1$$

$$\Gamma^{(L=2)} = E + T_2 \tag{3.44}$$

In a field of cubic symmetry, the level with $L = 1$ thus retains its three-fold degeneracy, and the five-fold degenerate level with $L = 2$ is split into a two-fold and a three-fold degenerate level, which belong to the representations E and T_2.

It is not difficult to extend these calculations to the cases of $L = 3$, 4, ...

Below are shown the results for fields of lower symmetry:

Hexagonal symmetry

	E	C_2	$2C_3$	$2C_6$	$3C_2'$	$3C_2''$	
A_1	1	1	1	1	1	1	
A_2	1	1	1	1	−1	−1	
B_1	1	−1	1	−1	1	−1	
B_2	1	−1	1	−1	−1	1	
E_1	2	−2	−1	1	0	0	
E_2	2	2	−1	−1	0	0	

$$\tag{3.45}$$

L		E	C_2	$2C_3$	$2C_6$	$3C_2'$	$3C_2''$	
	0	1	1	1	1	1	1	A_1
	1	3	−1	0	2	−1	−1	$A_2 + E_1$
	2	5	1	−1	−1	1	1	$A_1 + E_1 + E_2$

Tetragonal symmetry

	E	C_2	$2C_4$	$2C_2'$	$2C_2''$	
A_1	1	1	1	1	1	
A_2	1	1	1	−1	−1	
B_1	1	1	−1	1	−1	
B_2	1	1	−1	−1	1	
E	2	−2	0	0	0	

$$\tag{3.46}$$

L		E	C_2	$2C_4$	$2C_2'$	$2C_2''$	
	0	1	1	1	1	1	A_1
	1	3	−1	1	−1	−1	$A_2 + E$
	2	5	1	−1	1	1	$A_1 + B_1 + B_2 + E$

Rhombic symmetry

	E	C_2	C_2'	C_2''	
A_1	1	1	1	1	
A_2	1	1	−1	−1	
B_1	1	−1	1	−1	
B_2	1	−1	−1	1	(3.47)

L		E	C_2	C_2'	C_2''	
	0	1	1	1	1	A_1
	1	3	−1	−1	−1	$A_2 + B_1 + B_2$
	2	5	1	1	1	$2A_1 + A_2 + B_1 + B_2$

For groups with lower than rhombic symmetry, the orbital degeneracy is also, of course, completely lifted.

The case of non-integral values of j

If the Stark effect splitting is small compared to the separation of the multiplets (the 'weak field' case; see p. 65), then, as we have already seen, a total angular momentum j is formed. If the number of electrons is odd, then j will not assume integral values. In this case, from equation (3.40) we easily find that

$$\chi(2\pi \pm \varphi) = -\chi(\varphi) \tag{3.48}$$

This means that the characters change their sign under rotation through 360°. As a result of this, we obtain characters and representations both of which are double-valued. As an example,

$$\chi(0) = 2j + 1 \qquad \chi(2\pi) = -(2j + 1)$$

The character of the matrix is only single-valued when it corresponds to rotations through 180°:

$$\chi(\pi) = \chi(3\pi) = 0$$

It is clear that the double-valued characters of the representations satisfy the following equation:

$$\chi(\varphi) = \chi(4\pi - \varphi) \tag{3.49}$$

but not

$$\chi(\varphi) = \chi(2\pi \pm \varphi) \tag{3.50}$$

which is valid for the standard single-valued representations.

The double-valued representations of the rotational group, which become reducible in fields of lower symmetry, can evidently only be separated in irreducible representations with double value. On the other hand, all the representations of the cubic, tetragonal and other discontinuous symmetry groups are single-valued. A treatment which allows us to by-pass these difficulties was suggested in 1929 by von Bethe in his classical paper on the splitting of atomic terms in crystals.[4] Bethe introduced a new symmetry element R, which corresponds to a rotation of 2π. All elements of the group are multiplied by R; as a result, new classes are formed (for all elements other than rotations through π), and the number of representations is increased accordingly. The new representations are double-valued. In these, the characters of the matrices, which correspond to the symmetry classes, and which differ by the factor R, have opposite signs.

Below are given the corresponding character tables for the main symmetry groups, and also the reductions of the reducible representations of the rotational group for $j = \frac{1}{2}, \frac{3}{2}, \frac{5}{2}$ into irreducible representations of groups of lower symmetry. The tables only include characters of the new double-valued representations, designated by $\Gamma_1, \Gamma_2, \ldots$. The characters of the single-valued representations do not change (the characters of the new symmetry classes, which are formed by multiplication with R, exactly reproduce the characters of the original classes).

Cubic symmetry

	E	R	$6C_2$	$6C_4'$	$6C_4''$	$12C_2'$	$8C_3'$	$8C_3''$	j	Reduction
Γ_1	2	-2	0	$\sqrt{2}$	$-\sqrt{2}$	0	1	-1	$1/2$	Γ_1
Γ_2	2	-2	0	$-\sqrt{2}$	$\sqrt{2}$	0	1	-1	$3/2$	Γ_3
Γ_3	4	-4	0	0	0	0	-1	1	$5/2$	$\Gamma_2 + \Gamma_3$

$$(3.51)$$

Hexagonal symmetry

	E	R	$2C_2$	$2C_3'$	$2C_3''$	$2C_6'$	$2C_6''$	$6C_2'$	$6C_2''$	j	Reduction
Γ_1	2	-2	0	1	-1	$\sqrt{3}$	$-\sqrt{3}$	0	0	$1/2$	Γ_1
Γ_2	2	-2	0	1	-1	$-\sqrt{3}$	$\sqrt{3}$	0	0	$3/2$	$\Gamma_1 + \Gamma_3$
Γ_3	2	-2	0	-2	2	0	0	0	0	$5/2$	$\Gamma_1 + \Gamma_2 + \Gamma_3$

$$(3.52)$$

Tetragonal symmetry

	E	R	$2C_2$	$2C_4'$	$2C_4''$	$4C_2'$	$4C_2''$	j	Reduction
Γ_1	2	-2	0	$\sqrt{2}$	$-\sqrt{2}$	0	0	$1/2$	Γ_1
Γ_2	2	-2	0	$-\sqrt{2}$	$\sqrt{2}$	0	0	$3/2$	$\Gamma_1 + \Gamma_2$
								$5/2$	$\Gamma_1 + 2\Gamma_2$

$$(3.53)$$

Rhombic symmetry

	E	R	C_2	C_2'	C_2''	j	Reduction
Γ_1	2	-2	0	0	0	$1/2$	Γ_1
						$3/2$	$2\Gamma_1$
						$5/2$	$3\Gamma_1$

$$(3.54)$$

It follows from the above that the dimensions (degeneracy) of the double-valued representations are always a multiple of two. On the other hand, states with non-integral j always belong to double-valued representations of the rotational group, and in fields of lower symmetry, double-valued representations are converted only into double-values. Thus an electric field of arbitrary symmetry can never completely lift the spatial degeneracy of states with non-integral j. This is equivalent to Kramer's well-known theorem, which states that in systems with an odd number of unpaired electrons, the spatial degeneracy can be completely lifted only by an external magnetic field. In electric fields of arbitrary symmetry, there always remains at least one two-fold degeneracy (the so-called Kramer's doublet).[5]

§3.5

CALCULATION OF THE g-FACTOR OF A PARAMAGNETIC ION IN A CRYSTAL

We intend to perform this calculation on the copper ion Cu^{2+}, which has already been used as a classical example.[6,7] The ion Cu^{2+} has the electronic configuration $3d^9$ (for the outer shell), and consequently has one unpaired d-electron. The ground state of the ion can be represented by the term ^2D ($L = 2, S = \frac{1}{2}$). This term is split by spin-orbit interaction into the states $^2D_{5/2}$ and $^2D_{3/2}$ (with $j = \frac{5}{2}$ and $j = \frac{3}{2}$). However, since we do not want to consider the case of a weak crystal field, we must use as the zero-th approximation the ten-fold degenerate $[(2L + 1)(2S + 1) = 5 \times 2 = 10]$ ^2D-state of the free ion. The orbital degeneracy is lifted in the electric field of the crystal lattice. To a first approximation we assume that the crystal field exhibits cubic symmetry (as an example, the ions and dipoles of a solvent are located at the corners of an octahedron which encloses the Cu^{2+} ion).[†]

We have seen above [see (3.44)], that in a field of cubic symmetry a five-fold degenerate level ($L = 2$) is split into two levels of symmetries E and T_2; we now want to clarify their sequence. Instead of the usual sets of five d-functions with $m = 2, 1, 0, -1, -2$, we use their linearly independent combinations, which transform them by symmetry operations to simple functions of Cartesian coordinates. In the case of p-electrons, as is well known, this operation leads to the replacement of P_{+1}, P_0 and P_{-1} by

$$P_z = P_0 \qquad P_x = \frac{P_{+1} + P_{-1}}{\sqrt{2}} \qquad P_y = \frac{P_{+1} - P_{-1}}{\sqrt{2}}$$

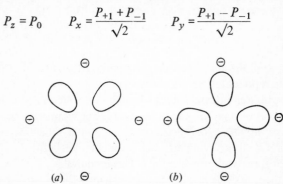

Fig. 3.1. Charge distribution around the Cu^{2+} ion in the x, y-plane.
   (*a*) state d_{xy}
   (*b*) state $d_{x^2-y^2}$; position of negative charges in the lattice [7]

In the case of d-electrons, we choose, as the most convenient set of basis functions, $d_{xy}, d_{xz}, d_{yz}, d_{x^2-y^2}, d_{2z^2-x^2-y^2}$. (The last two functions are linearly independent combinations of three functions which naturally suggest themselves: $d_{x^2-y^2}, d_{y^2-x^2}, d_{z^2-x^2}$.) It is clear that in a field of cubic symmetry, for which the directions x, y, z are completely equivalent, the states d_{xy}, d_{yz}, d_{xz} belong to the three-fold degenerate representation T_2, and the states $d_{x^2-y^2}, d_{2z^2-x^2-y^2}$ to the two-fold degenerate representation E. The sequence of these two levels can be determined in the following simple way.[7] The charge distribution around the Cu^{2+} ion in the x,y-plane is shown in Fig. 3.1. Since the distribution of the positive charges

[†] In aqueous solution we have $Cu^{2+}.6H_2O$, for example.

of the Cu^{2+}-ions are of interest to us, it is obvious that the system in the state $d_{x^2-y^2}$ has a lower energy than in the state d_{xy}. From this it follows that in a field of cubic symmetry the two-fold degenerate term E lies lowest.

This sequence of levels is valid for a cubic crystal field, which is produced by the negative charges situated at the corners of an octahedron (six-fold coordination). If the charges producing the field are at the corners of a tetrahedron (four-fold coordination) or a hexahedron (eight-fold coordination), then the sign of the cubic crystal field is reversed, and, hence, so are the relative positions of the terms.

According to the Jahn-Teller theorem, the degenerate ground-state of a symmetrical molecule (or complex) is unstable, the symmetry becoming so distorted that the ground state is no longer degenerate. It can easily be shown that this is readily achieved by lowering the symmetry to a tetragonal one (the deformation consists of an elongation along the z-axis).

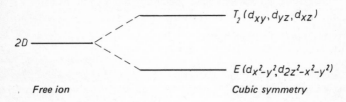

A lowering of symmetry is also naturally obtained by a compression along the z-axis. The field of axial symmetry thus added to the cubic crystal field then has the opposite sign, and because of this the position of the terms $d_{x^2-y^2}$ and $d_{2z^2-x^2-y^2}$, for example, are reversed (see below).

In actual fact the individual symmetry classes are transformed by a gradual lowering of the symmetry in the following way:

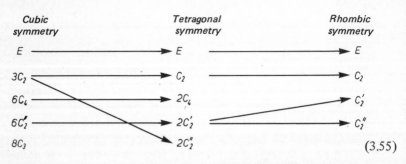

$$(3.55)$$

From this, and by using (3.31), (3.42), (3.46) and (3.47) we obtain the following diagram for the transitions of the irreducible representations:

Tetragonal symmetry	Rhombic symmetry	Cubic symmetry	Tetragonal symmetry
A	A_1	A_1	A_1
A_2	A_2	A_2	B_2
B_1	A_1	E	$A_1 + B_2$
B_2	A_2	T_1	$A_2 + E$
E	$B_1 + B_2$	T_2	$B_1 + E$

$$(3.56)$$

On the lowering of symmetry from the cubic to the tetragonal configuration, the two-fold degenerate ground-state E is thus split into two non-degenerate levels A_1 and B_2. As can easily be seen, the term $d_{x^2-y^2}$ belongs to the representation B_2, and the term $d_{2z^2-x^2-y^2}$ to the representation A_1. [Under the symmetry operations C_4 and C_2, we have $x \rightarrow y$ and the value of $x^2 - y^2$ changes its sign, which corresponds to the representation B_2, by (3.46).] It will also be clear that the term $d_{x^2-y^2}$ lies lower than $d_{2z^2-x^2-y^2}$, since the distortion leads to a removal of the negative charges on the z-axis. A diagram of the terms is shown below:

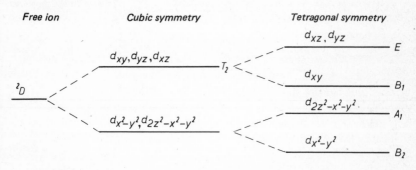

The ground state of the Cu^{2+} ion is now an orbital singlet. As we have already shown, the spin degeneracy (two-fold for one unpaired electron) can only be lifted in this case by the application of a magnetic field. If the crystal field is sufficiently strong (which it is in the case we are considering), the excited orbital levels lie so high above the ground state (at least as compared to the Zeeman splitting) that in the zero-th order approximation they may be neglected. Thus we may speak of the concept of magnetic spin resonance, in which the magnetic orbital moments are 'frozen in' by the action of the crystal field. This effect is called the *quenching* of the orbital moment. For this reason the g-factors of the E.S.R. signals of many paramagnetic atoms in the condensed phase, and of practically all organic free radicals, differ relatively very little from the pure free spin value, although the corresponding unpaired electrons can be in d- or p-states with orbital moments different from zero.

The excited orbital states can however change the wave functions of the ground state in the first order approximation of the theory of perturbation due to spin-orbit interaction. This leads to a change in the Zeeman splitting and to a deviation of the g-factor from the free spin value by a specific amount. Depending on the sign of the spin-orbit coupling constant λ, this deviation can be positive as well as negative.

We would now like to investigate how the spin-orbit interaction, which contributes the following Hamiltonian operator,

$$\hat{H}_{LS} = \lambda \hat{\vec{L}} \hat{\vec{S}}, \qquad (3.57)$$

will influence the degeneracy of the level E (d_{xz}, d_{yz}) in the above diagram. According to (3.53) a spin $S = \frac{1}{2}$ belongs to a double-valued representation Γ_1. We form the direct product $E \times \Gamma_1$, and obtain by the usual methods $E \times \Gamma_1 + \Gamma_2$. Thus the spin-orbit coupling acts in the same way as a field of axial symmetry. As a result of the joint action of the electric fields and the L-S interaction, the ten-fold degenerate term of the free Cu^{2+} ion is split into five spin doublets:

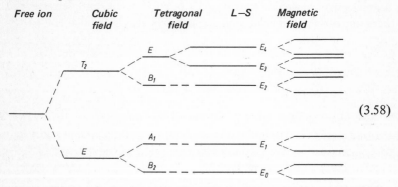

$$(3.58)$$

We are only interested in the behaviour of the lowest level E_0 in the magnetic field. The other levels lie so high that at normal temperatures they are not populated. We designate the trial wavefunctions of the ground state of the Cu^{2+} ion by $\psi_0(+\frac{1}{2})$ and $\psi_0(-\frac{1}{2})$, which correspond to the values $m_S = \pm\frac{1}{2}$. The electric field cannot change these functions. For this reason we will now consider the spin-orbit interaction as a perturbation (3.57). The first-order perturbation theory gives:

$$\psi'_n = \psi^0_n + \sum_m{}' \frac{\langle H_{nm} \rangle}{E_n - E_m} \psi_m \quad (m \neq n). \tag{3.59}$$

with

$$\langle H_{nm} \rangle = \int \psi^*_m \hat{H}_{LS} \psi_n \, d\tau.$$

Here, ψ^0_n is the wave function of the n-th state in the zero-th order approximation (unperturbed wave function), and ψ'_n is the perturbed wave function of the n-th state. The summation is over all unperturbed states.

By applying (3.59) to $\psi_0(+\frac{1}{2})$ and $\psi_0(-\frac{1}{2})$, we obtain the new wave functions of the ground state of the Cu^{2+} ion, perturbed by the spin-orbit interaction:

$$\psi_a = \psi_0(\tfrac{1}{2}) - \sum_n{}' \frac{\int \psi^*_n (\lambda \hat{L}\hat{S}) \, \psi_0(\tfrac{1}{2}) \, d\tau}{E_n - E_0} \psi_n \tag{3.60}$$

$$\psi_b = \psi_0(-\tfrac{1}{2}) - \sum_n{}' \frac{\int \psi^*_n (\lambda \hat{L}\hat{S}) \, \psi_0(-\tfrac{1}{2}) \, d\tau}{E_n - E_0} \psi_n \tag{3.61}$$

The correction for the spin-orbit interaction clearly has the order of magnitude $\lambda/(E_n - E_0)$; in our particular case this is ($\lambda \approx 10^{-3}$ cm^{-1}, $E_n - E_0 \approx 10^4$ cm^{-1}) $\approx 0 \cdot 1$. Thus the spin-orbit interaction does not lift the degeneracy of the ground state $d_{x^2-y^2}$ of the Cu^{2+} ion, but it changes the wave functions of this state, which correspond in zero-th order approximation to $S_z = \pm\frac{1}{2}$.

We now consider the action of a magnetic field, the operator $\hat{H}''$ of which is written in the following form:

$$\hat{H}'' = \beta\bar{B}(\hat{L} + 2\hat{S}) \tag{3.62}$$

As we have already stated above, this perturbation completely lifts the spatial degeneracy. Within the framework of the first-order approximation of the perturbation theory, the energy eigenvalues of the level are the roots of the secular equation:

$$\begin{vmatrix} \int \psi^*_a \hat{H}'' \psi_a \, d\tau - E & \int \psi^*_a \hat{H}'' \psi_b \, d\tau \\ \int \psi^*_b \hat{H}'' \psi_a \, d\tau & \int \psi^*_b \hat{H}'' \psi_b \, d\tau - E \end{vmatrix} = 0 \tag{3.63}$$

The magnetic field is directed along the z-axis, which should coincide with the four-fold symmetry axis of the ions in the lattice of tetragonal symmetry. The perturbation operator has the following form:

$$\hat{H}''_z = \beta B(\hat{L}_z + 2\hat{S}_z) \tag{3.64}$$

with

$$\hat{L}_z = i\left(y\frac{\partial}{\partial x} - x\frac{\partial}{\partial y}\right) \tag{3.65}$$

and

$$\hat{S}_z = \tfrac{1}{2}\begin{pmatrix} 1 & 0 \\ 0 & -1 \end{pmatrix} \tag{3.66}†$$

We now calculate the matrix elements in (3.63). In the first place it is clear that the functions ψ_a and ψ_b are eigenfunctions of the operator H''_z. Thus elements not on the diagonal of matrix (3.63) must be equal to zero. This can of course also be found by direct calculation. The diagonal elements of the matrix are

$$\int \psi_a^* \hat{H}'' \psi_a \, d\tau = \beta B \underbrace{\int \psi_a^* \hat{L}_z \psi_a \, d\tau}_{\text{I}} + 2\beta B \underbrace{\int \psi_a^* \hat{S}_z \psi_a \, d\tau}_{\text{II}} \tag{3.67}$$

Using equation (3.60), the first integral in (3.67), after a simple rearrangement, becomes

$$(\text{I}) = \beta B \underbrace{\int \psi_0^*(\tfrac{1}{2}) \hat{L}_z \psi_0(\tfrac{1}{2}) \, d\tau}_{\text{III}}$$

$$-2\beta B \sum_n{}' \underbrace{\frac{\int \psi_0^*(\tfrac{1}{2}) \hat{L}_z \psi_n \, d\tau \int \psi_n^*(\lambda\hat{L}\hat{S}) \psi_a(\tfrac{1}{2}) \, d\tau}{E_n - E_0}}_{\text{IV}}$$

$$+ \text{ higher order terms in } \lambda \tag{3.68}$$

The operator $\hat{L}_z$ does not act on the spin-function, and therefore in III we can separate the spin variables and the spatial variables. Thus III is equal to $\beta B \int \psi_0^* \hat{L}_z \psi_0 \, d\tau$. Here, ψ_0 is the spatial part of the function $\psi_0(\tfrac{1}{2})$. According to (3.58), ψ_0 belongs to the representation B_2 of the tetragonal symmetry group. On the other hand the operator $\hat{L}_z = i[y(\partial/\partial x) - x(\partial/\partial y)]$ belongs to the representation A_2 ($L_z \to L_z$ for symmetry operations E, C_2 and C_4, and $L_z \to -L_z$ for the operations C_2 and C_2). The direct product $\psi_0^* L_z \psi_0$ belongs to the representation A_2, and the integral $\int \psi_0^* L_z \psi_0 \, d\tau$ becomes identically equal to zero (see p. 63).

We now consider the integral $\int \psi_0^*(\tfrac{1}{2})\hat{L}_z \psi_n \, d\tau$. By an argument similar to the above, we find that this integral is equal to zero for all $n \neq 2$. In the

† See Appendix 2, p. 317.

case where $n = 2$, ψ_2 belongs to the representation B_1, the direct product $\psi_0^* \hat{L}_z \psi_2$ belongs to the representation $B_2 \times A_2 \times B_1 = A_1$, and the corresponding integral is different from zero. The sum in (3.68) reduces to a term with $n = 2$. The angular parts of functions ψ_0 and ψ_2 (the integration is performed in spherical coordinates) are proportional to $x^2 - y^2$ and xy. With this we obtain

$$\int \psi_0^* \hat{L}_z \psi_2 \, d\tau = i \int \psi_0^* \left[y \frac{\partial(xy)}{\partial x} - x \frac{\partial(xy)}{\partial y} \right] d\tau$$

$$= i \int \psi_0^* (y^2 - x^2) \, d\tau = -i \int \psi^{*2} \, d\tau = -i$$

where it has been taken in account that the functions $\psi_0, \psi_1, \psi_2, \ldots$ are ortho-normalized. By analogy, we also get

$$\int \psi_2^* (\lambda \hat{L} \hat{S}) \, \psi_0(\tfrac{1}{2}) \, d\tau = \lambda \int \psi_2^* (\hat{L}_z \hat{S}_z + \hat{L}_x \hat{S}_x + \hat{L}_{yy}) \, \hat{S} \psi_0(\tfrac{1}{2}) \, d\tau$$

The operators $\hat{L}_x = i[z(\partial/\partial y) - y(\partial/\partial z)]$ and $\hat{L}_y = i[x(\partial/\partial z) - z(\partial/\partial x)]$ belong to the representation E [see (3.46)]. The integrals $\int \psi_0^* \hat{L}_x \psi_0 \, d\tau$ and $\int \psi_2^* \hat{L}_y \psi_0 d\tau$ are therefore identically equal to zero.

On the other hand†

$$\lambda \int \psi_2^* \hat{L}_z \hat{S}_z \psi_0(\tfrac{1}{2}) \, d\tau = \lambda \int \psi_2^*(\tfrac{1}{2}) \, \hat{S}_z \psi_0(\tfrac{1}{2}) \, d\tau \, . \int \psi_2^* \hat{L}_z \psi_0 \, d\tau$$

$$= \frac{\lambda i}{2} \int \psi_2^* \left[y \frac{\partial(x^2 - y^2)}{\partial x} - x \frac{\partial(x^2 - y^2)}{\partial y} \right] d\tau$$

$$= \frac{\lambda i}{2} \int \psi_2^* 4xy \, d\tau = \frac{4\lambda i}{2} \int \psi_2^2 \, d\tau = 2\lambda i$$

So for the sum (IV) in (3.68) we get $4\lambda \beta B/(E_2 - E_0)$, and hence the whole term (I) in (3.67) becomes equal to $-4\lambda \beta B/(E_2 - E_0)$.

The second integral in (3.67) is calculated in the same way. With an accuracy of up to second-order terms in $\lambda/(E_n - E_0)$, this is

$$\text{II} = 2\beta B \int \psi_a^* \hat{S}_z \psi_a \, d\tau = 2\beta B \int \psi_0(\tfrac{1}{2}) \, \hat{S}_z \psi_0(\tfrac{1}{2}) \, d\tau = \beta B$$

The first diagonal element of the matrix in (3.63) is finally found to be

$$\int \psi_a^* \hat{H}'' \psi_a \, d\tau \approx \beta B \left(1 - \frac{4\lambda}{E_2 - E_0} \right) = E_a. \tag{3.69}$$

† See equation (3) in Appendix 2, p. 317.

Since, as we have already seen, the matrix elements not on the diagonal are equal to zero, this value is one of the roots of equation (3.63). By analogy we can calculate the other diagonal element in (3.63):

$$\int \psi_b^* \hat{H}'' \psi_b \, d\tau = -\beta B \left(1 - \frac{4\lambda}{E_2 - E_0} \right) = E_b \tag{3.70}$$

On the basis of these calculations, we can say that under the influence of an external magnetic field B_z directed along the electric axis of the system, the ground state of the Cu^{2+} ion splits into two Zeeman levels, with

$$\Delta E = E_a - E_b = 2\beta B \left(1 - \frac{4\lambda}{E_2 - E_0} \right) \tag{3.71}$$

If we compare (3.71) with the fundamental equation of magnetic resonance,

$$\Delta E = g\beta B$$

we get

$$g_z = 2 \left(1 - \frac{4\lambda}{E_2 - E_0} \right) \tag{3.72}$$

There are also no further difficulties in calculating the matrix elements of the secular equation for a magnetic field directed along the x- and y-axes (i.e. perpendicular to the main axis of the electric field). All calculations are performed in the same way, substituting L_x (or L_y) and S_x (or S_y) for L_z and S_z respectively. In our particular case, because of the tetragonal symmetry the directions x and y are equivalent. Therefore we obtain for both orientations the same secular equation:

$$\begin{vmatrix} -E & \beta B \left(1 - \dfrac{\lambda}{E_3 - E_0} \right) \\ \beta B \left(1 - \dfrac{\lambda}{E_3 - E_0} \right) & -E \end{vmatrix} = 0 \tag{3.73}$$

From this it follows that

$$g_x = g_y = 2 \left(1 - \frac{\lambda}{E_3 - E_0} \right) \tag{3.74}$$

As a result of the action of the electric crystal field, of the spin-orbit coupling and of the magnetic field, the g-factor of the paramagnetic particle becomes anisotropic. If two or three of the g-factors are equal, as in the previous case, then we usually use the equations

$$g_z = g_\parallel \qquad g_x = g_y = g_\perp \tag{3.75}$$

The indices ‖ and ⊥ refer respectively to the parallel and perpendicular orientations of the main axis of the electric field with respect to the constant magnetic field.

For Cu^{2+}, $\lambda = -828$ cm^{-1} (for atoms whose outer electron shell is more than half filled, $\lambda < 0$, and in the opposite case $\lambda > 0$). The optical absorption spectra of aqueous solutions of Cu^{2+} give $E_2 - E_0 \doteq E_3 - E_0 \doteq 12\ 300$ cm^{-1}. From this we obtain $g_{\parallel} \doteq 2 \cdot 4$ and $g_{\perp} \doteq 2 \cdot 08$, which agrees well with the experimental values.†

§3.6
THE ANISOTROPY OF THE g-FACTOR

The fine structure of the E.S.R. spectra

The secular equation (3.68) is valid for arbitrary orientations of the external magnetic field with respect to the electric crystal axis (the term 'crystal' must be understood here in the general sense; see p. 48). We have seen above that in the parallel orientation only the diagonal elements of the matrix in (3.63) are different from zero, and in the perpendicular orientation only the elements not on the diagonal are different from zero. In the calculation for arbitrary orientation of the crystal in the magnetic field it is useful to introduce the so-called effective spin-Hamiltonian[8] instead of the Hamiltonian operator $\beta \bar{B}(\hat{L} + 2\hat{S})$. We also saw that the orbital moment becomes quenched and that the action of the operator of the orbital moment $\hat{L}$ leads to the introduction of an anisotropic g-factor with the components g_x, g_y and g_z instead of the usual value of $g = 2$. The arbitrarily orientated field $\bar{B}$ has the components B_x, B_y and B_z. We can then write, instead of the Hamiltonian operator,

$$\hat{\mathcal{H}} = \beta\{g_z B_z \hat{S}_z + g_x B_x \hat{S}_x + g_y B_y \hat{S}_y\} \tag{3.76}$$

where the introduction of g_x, g_y and g_z instead of $g = 2$ reflects the action of the operator $\hat{L}$. For the case of axial symmetry $g_x = g_y = g_{\perp}$ and $g_z = g_{\parallel}$, and if θ is the angle between $\bar{B}$ and the z-axis, this becomes

$$\hat{\mathcal{H}} = \beta B\{g_{\parallel}\hat{S}_z\cos\theta + g_{\perp}\hat{S}_x \sin\theta\} \tag{3.77}$$

† The energy levels, which by spin-orbit interaction influence the ground state of the ion, can correspond to very different energies in other crystal fields. The values $g_{\parallel}$ and $g_{\perp}$ always remain larger than $g_{el} = 2 \cdot 0023$, but they can assume very different values, such that $g_{\parallel}$ can be smaller than $g_{\perp}$ (see the compilation of experimental data in reference 23).

In (3.76) and (3.77), $\mathcal{H}$ is described as the spin-Hamiltonian operator. The secular equation can now be written in the following way:

$$
\begin{vmatrix}
\int \psi_a^* \hat{\mathcal{H}} \, \psi_a \, d\tau - E & \int \psi_a^* \hat{\mathcal{H}} \, \psi_b \, d\tau \\[2ex]
\int \psi_b^* \hat{\mathcal{H}} \, \psi_a \, d\tau & \int \psi_b^* \hat{\mathcal{H}} \, \psi_b \, d\tau - E
\end{vmatrix} = 0 \qquad (3.78)
$$

Here ψ_a and ψ_b mean simply the functions $\psi(+\tfrac{1}{2})$ and $\psi(-\tfrac{1}{2})$ (see Appendix B to Chapter 3).

By using (3.77), and equation (3) of Appendix B, the matrix elements in (3.78) can be easily calculated. We obtain

$$
\begin{vmatrix}
\tfrac{1}{2}\beta B g_\parallel \cos \theta - E & \tfrac{1}{2}\beta B g_\perp \sin \theta \, (1 - i) \\[2ex]
\tfrac{1}{2}\beta B g_\perp \sin \theta \, (1 + i) & \tfrac{1}{2}\beta B g_\parallel \cos \theta - E
\end{vmatrix} = 0 \qquad (3.79)
$$

From this it follows that

$$
\Delta E = \beta B \{ g_\parallel^2 \cos^2 \theta + g_\perp^2 \sin^2 \theta \}^{+1/2}
$$

and

$$
g(\theta) = \{ g_\parallel^2 \cos^2 \theta + g_\perp^2 \sin^2 \theta \}^{+1/2} \qquad (3.80)
$$

The anisotropy of the g-factors leads to a change in the transition probabilities. In fact, transitions between Zeeman levels take place under the action of the magnetic component of the microwave field, which is perpendicular to $\bar{B}$. If the B-field is at its strongest in the perpendicular orientation ($g_\perp > g_\parallel$), then the microwave field has a weaker effect at this orientation than in the parallel case, and it follows from this that for the transition probabilities, $P_\perp < P_\parallel$. Bleaney[9] deduced a formula for the transition probability of a crystal with axial symmetry at arbitrary orientation:

$$
P \sim \tfrac{1}{2} g_\perp^2 \left\{ \left(\frac{g_\parallel}{g} \right)^2 + 1 \right\} \qquad (3.81)
$$

with

$$
g_\perp \lessgtr g \lessgtr g_\parallel
$$

Until now we have limited ourselves to consideration of the case $S = \tfrac{1}{2}$ ($m_s = \pm \tfrac{1}{2}$), and in our calculations we have ignored all second-order terms in λ. If we take into account all terms in λ^2, then we obtain, e.g. for parallel orientation, the following expression for the energy of the Zeeman level:

$$E = Dm_s^2 + g_\| \beta B m_S \qquad (3.82)$$

The coefficient D is proportional to λ^2. Let $m_s = n \pm \frac{1}{2}$, where n goes through the $2S$ values from $S - \frac{1}{2}$ to $S + \frac{1}{2}$. Then the separation between the consecutive Zeeman levels will be

$$\Delta E = g_\| \beta B + 2nD \qquad (3.83)$$

From (3.82) and (3.83) it can be seen that at $S = \frac{1}{2}$ ($n = 0$) the consideration of further terms (second approximation) leads only to a shift of both Zeeman levels and not to a change in their separation. For $S \geqslant 1$ the separations ΔE of the $2S$ possible transitions with $\Delta m_s = 1$ are in the first approximation all equal to $g\beta B$, so that only one line is observed. However, from (3.83) we see in the second approximation that the splittings for lines with different m_s (different n) have different values, and that for $B = 0$ a splitting $2nD$ appears. In the case of a non-integral spin (odd number of unpaired electrons), and on the basis of Kramer's theorem, for $B = 0$ a double degeneracy remains for $m_s = \pm \frac{1}{2}$, and the E.S.R. line is in principle observable. For an even number of unpaired electrons, the degeneracy of the ground state can be completely lifted. In this case, ΔE can become larger than $h\nu$, so that observation of the E.S.R. spectrum is impossible.

The following statement is valid for a fixed frequency source of approximately 9 GHz. By increasing the observation frequency, materials with quite large values of zero-field splitting can be studied. Corresponding investigations have been carried out at frequencies of up to approximately 100 GHz.

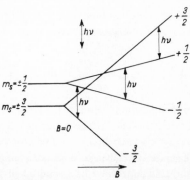

Fig. 3.2. The formation of E.S.R. lines of Cr^{3+} in chrome alum.

From (3.83) it is easily shown that resonance lines can be observed at the following values of the external magnetic field B:

$$B_{res} = \frac{h\nu}{g_\parallel \beta} - n\frac{2D}{g_\parallel \beta} \tag{3.84}$$

In the case of $S \geqslant 1$, a fine-structure of the E.S.R. lines can be formed by the action of the electric crystal field and the spin-orbit coupling, producing a splitting into $2S$ components with a separation of $2D/g_\parallel\beta$. All that we have said above is naturally also valid for any other orientations of the electric and magnetic field. As an example, we give the fine structure of the E.S.R. spectrum of the Cr^{3+} ion in chrome alum. For the Cr^{3+} ion (configuration ^4F, $3d^3$), $S = \frac{3}{2}$ ($n = 1, 0, -1$), $D \approx -0.07$ cm^{-1}. In a field with lower than cubic symmetry, the lowest term is split into two Kramer's doublets, with $\Delta E \approx 0.15$ cm^{-1}. The fine structure so formed is shown in Fig. 3.2.

If we take D into consideration, the spin-Hamiltonian operator can be written in the following form:

$$\hat{\mathcal{H}} = D\hat{S}_z^2 + g_\parallel\beta B_z \hat{S}_z + g_\perp\beta(B_x\hat{S}_x + B_y\hat{S}_y) \tag{3.85}$$

§3.7

ANISOTROPY AND SHIFT OF THE g-FACTOR FOR ORGANIC FREE RADICALS

In the case of organic free radicals, the above considerations are completely valid. The orbital degeneracy (of the p-electrons) is nearly always completely abolished, since the orientation of the orbital moments is strongly coupled to that of the wave functions of the electrons, which are determined by the covalent bonds and the total geometry of the radical molecule. In the case of planar aromatic free radicals of the semi-quinones (see Chapter 8), for example, the unpaired electrons are $2p_z\pi$-electrons. The orbital levels corresponding to the p_x and p_y orientations lie considerably higher than the ground state. These orbital levels correspond to an excitation of the type $\pi \to \sigma^*$ (an excitation of an unpaired π-electron into a localized σ-orbital), and to an excitation of the type $\sigma \to \pi$ (an excitation of a bound σ-electron into a π-orbital).

Since the spin-orbit coupling constant λ is small for the light atoms from which free radicals are built (e.g. for C, $\lambda = 28$ cm^{-1}),[10] and since on the other hand the excited orbital levels lie very high ($10^4 - 10^5$ cm^{-1}), the deviation of the g-factor from the free spin value, and the anisotropy of the g-factor $(g_\perp - g_\parallel)$, for hydrocarbon radicals are very small and seldom exceed a few parts per thousand. The presence of nitrogen atoms lowers the energy of the excited orbital states and can increase these values a little. A localization of an unpaired electron on an S-atom $(\lambda \approx 382 \text{ cm}^{-1})$ leads to a shift in the g-factor by a few per cent from the free spin value, and to a large anisotropy. A qualitative theory which explains the observed shifts and anisotropies of the g-factors for aromatic free radicals, was suggested by McConnell and Robertson.[11]

§3.8

THE HYPERFINE STRUCTURE OF E.S.R. SPECTRA

If the paramagnetic system which is to be investigated contains, in addition to the unpaired electrons, atomic nuclei which have a magnetic moment (H^1, D^2, N^{14}, C^{13} etc.), then a so-called hyperfine structure (H.F.S.) of the E.S.R. spectrum is formed, due to the interaction of the electron moments with the nuclear moments. In the theoretical consideration of the H.F.S. one has to keep in mind that the induction of the external magnetic field B is usually completely sufficient to lift the S-I coupling. I and S then precess independently of each other about the direction of B (Paschen-Back effect). In this section we will consider this case, which although simple is most important. We will not go into the complications which are present in measurements in low fields, and under other conditions whereby deviations from the usual Paschen-Back effect are possible. *The contributions of the splitting which are produced by the remaining S-I coupling, are of the order of magnitude $A^2/g\beta H$. For a very large hyperfine splitting of 10 mWb m^{-2} and an observation frequency of 9 GHz, they are approximately 3 per cent of the total splitting.* The unpaired electron produces a magnetic field which interacts with the nuclear magnetic moment. This interaction can be represented by adding the following term to the spin-Hamiltonian operator:

$$\sum_i A_i \hat{\vec{I}}_i \hat{\vec{S}}$$

Here A_i is the H.F.S. constant of the i-th magnetic nucleus, and $\hat{\vec{I}}$ the nuclear spin operator.

If the nuclear spin is equal to I, then this interaction leads to a splitting of each Zeeman level into $2I + 1$ sub-levels, with energies $E_0 + A_i m_I$, where

$m_I = I, I-1, \ldots, -I$. For a transition between the electronic Zeeman levels, the following selection rules hold:

$$\Delta m_S = 1$$

$$\Delta m_I = 0 \qquad (3.86)$$

This is the same as saying that for electronic transitions the orientations of the nuclear magnetic moments with respect to the external field do not change. When H.F.S. is present we can therefore write the resonance condition in the following way:

$$h\nu = g\beta B_0 + \sum_i 2A_i m_i \qquad (3.87)$$

Here B_0 is the resonance induction without H.F.S.

This equation may be usefully solved for the induction at which the H.F.S. components appear:

$$B = B_0 + \frac{2}{g\beta} \sum_i A_i m_i = B_0 + \sum_i \Delta B_i m_i \qquad (3.88)$$

Figure 3.3 shows schematically the formation of H.F.S. for a magnetic nucleus with $I = 1$. In Chapter 5 we will consider in detail the H.F.S. of E.S.R. spectra when there is interaction of the unpaired electron with many magnetic nuclei with different values of I. In this chapter we will consider the basic concepts concerning the nature of this interaction.

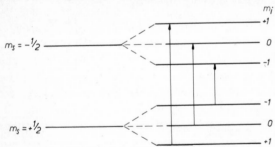

Fig. 3.3. Diagram of the formation of the H.F.S. for $I = 1$.

The isotropic H.F.S. interaction

There are two basic types of H.F.S. interaction: the anisotropic H.F.S. interaction, which is produced by the dipole-dipole interaction of the magnetic moments of the electron and nucleus, and the isotropic or contact H.F.S. interaction, which is produced when there is a real probability (other than zero) of the unpaired electron being at the site of the

nucleus. As we shall now see, in a large number of cases the anisotropic
H.F.S. interaction does not contribute to the formation of a resolved
H.F.S. Thus the H.F.S. is frequently determined entirely by the contact
interaction. The density of the electron cloud at the nucleus, which is
equal to $(\psi \cdot \psi^*)_{\lambda=0}$, is naturally different from zero only for S-states.
The formation of H.F.S. is therefore generally dependent on these factors,
that either the unpaired electron is actually an S-electron, or it is described
by a mixed wave function which contains an S-component. The H.F.S.
constant of a pure S-electron can be calculated from the following
equation:

$$A_S = \frac{8}{3} \frac{R\alpha^2 g(I) z^3}{n_0^3} \tag{3.89}$$

Here R is the Rydberg constant, α the fine structure constant, $g(I) = \mu_I/I$
the nuclear g-factor (μ_I being the nuclear magnetic moment), n_0 the
effective principal quantum number, and Z the effective nuclear charge.

The anisotropic H.F.S. interaction

We will now consider the dipole-dipole interaction of the magnetic
moments of the nucleus and electron. For this, we must calculate the
mean induction $\langle \Delta B \rangle_m$ produced by the magnetic nucleus at the site of
the electron. We will consider first the case where the electron is located in
an atomic orbital of the magnetic nucleus.

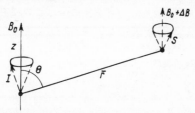

Let μ_I be the nuclear magnetic moment and $\bar{r}$ the radius vector connecting
the electron and nucleus. Then the magnetic potential produced by the
nucleus at the site of the electron is

$$U = \frac{\mu_1 r}{r^3}$$

From this it follows that

$$\Delta B = -\text{grad } U = -\text{grad } \frac{\mu_I \bar{r}}{r^3} = -\frac{1}{r^3}\text{grad }(\bar{\mu}_I \bar{r}) - (\bar{\mu}_I \bar{r})\text{grad }\frac{1}{r^3}$$

$$= \frac{\bar{\mu}_I}{r^3} + 3\bar{\mu}_I \bar{r} \frac{\bar{r}}{r^5} = \frac{3(\bar{\mu}_I \bar{r})\bar{r} - \bar{\mu}_I r^2}{r^5} = \frac{3\mu_I r \cos\theta \, \bar{r} - \bar{\mu}_I r^2}{r^5}$$

If we split $\bar{\mu}_I$ into the three components μ_I^x, μ_I^y and $\mu_I^z = \mu_I^B$, we see that the fields produced by μ_I^x and μ_I^y are averaged out as a result of the precession of the magnetic moments about the B direction. The component of the nuclear magnetic moment in the direction of the magnetic field is

$$\mu_I^{(B)} = \mu_I \frac{m_I}{I}. \tag{3.90}$$

Here I is the nuclear spin, and $m_I = I, I - 1, \ldots, -I$ is the nuclear magnetic quantum number.

Thus we obtain

$$\Delta B = \mu_I^{(B)} \frac{3\cos^2\theta - 1}{r^3} \quad \text{and} \quad \langle \Delta B \rangle_m = \mu_I^{(B)} \left\langle \frac{3\cos^2\theta - 1}{r^3} \right\rangle_m \tag{3.91}$$

with

$$\left\langle \frac{1}{r^3} \right\rangle_m = \int \psi_r^* \left(\frac{1}{r^3} \right) \psi_r \, d\tau$$

and

$$\langle 3\cos^2\theta - 1 \rangle_m = \int \psi_\theta^* (3\cos^2\theta - 1) \psi_\theta \, d\tau$$

For an S-electron ($l = 0$), the wave function of which is generally symmetric, $\langle \cos^2\theta \rangle_m = \frac{1}{3}$ and $\langle \Delta B \rangle_m = 0$. The E.S.R. spectra of unpaired S-electrons therefore do not show any anisotropic H.F.S. For $l \neq 0$ we obtain as an approximation for hydrogen-type wave functions of the electron,

$$\left\langle \frac{1}{r^3} \right\rangle_m = \frac{z^3}{a_0^3 n^3 l(l+1)(l+\frac{1}{2})} \tag{3.92}$$

Here Z is the effective nuclear charge (after Slater)[1], $a_0 = 0.528 \cdot 10^{-8}$ cm is the Bohr radius, and n is the principal quantum number.

If into (3.91) we put the expressions (3.92) and (3.90) and the numerical values of the constants, we get

$$\langle \Delta B \rangle_m \approx 34 \frac{\mu_I m_I z^3 \langle 3\cos^2\theta - 1 \rangle_m}{I n^3 l(l+1)(l+\frac{1}{2})} \cdot 10^{-4} \text{ Wb m}^{-2} \tag{3.93}$$

where μ_I is measured in nuclear magnetons.

As an example, we will consider the H.F.S. which an unpaired electron would give, if completely localized in a non-hybridized $2P$-orbital of an N^{14}-atom of a nitrogen-containing radical.

In this case, $n = 2$, $l = 1$, $I = 1$, $\mu_I = 0.40$, $m_I = +1, 0, -1$, and $Z \approx 3.5$.

For the H.F.S. components corresponding to $m_I = \pm 1$ we get

$$\langle \Delta B \rangle_m \approx \pm 34 \, \frac{0 \cdot 40 \cdot 3 \cdot 5^2 \langle 3 \cos^2 \theta - 1 \rangle_m}{2^3 \cdot 2 \cdot 1 \cdot 5}$$

$$\approx \pm 24 \langle 3 \cos^2 \theta - 1 \rangle_m \cdot 10^{-4} \; \text{Wb m}^{-2}$$

The p-orbital of the unpaired electron in a molecular radical has a fixed orientation with respect to the system of valence bonds, and the angle θ, which is single-valued, is determined by the orientation of the molecule in the external magnetic field. For a polycrystalline sample the angle θ can thus assume arbitrary values between 0 and $\pi/2$, and the value $\langle \Delta B \rangle_m$, for example for H.F.S. components given by radicals with $m_I = +1$, will assume arbitrary values between $+4 \cdot 8$ mWb m^{-2} ($\theta = 0$) and $-2 \cdot 4$ mWb m^{-2} ($\theta = \pi/2$). In this particular example, the outermost H.F.S. components are therefore broadened so strongly that they envelop the other components, and the H.F.S. cannot be resolved.

For calculations on actual radicals the values deduced above must be multiplied by the electron density at the nucleus in question, i.e. by approximately C_a^2, where C_a is the normalized coefficient of the atomic function ϕ_a in the linear combination of atomic functions which form the molecular orbital of the unpaired electron. Although the width of the individual components is in this case always larger than their separation, the absolute values calculated can become considerably smaller (often $C_a^2 \ll 1$).

Even though the H.F.S. parameters are determined by the isotropic interaction, the anisotropic dipole-dipole interaction can prove to be a factor determining the widths of the individual H.F.S. components, particularly in the case of viscous liquids.† In normal liquids the fast chaotic change of orientation of the individual molecules causes an averaging-out of the anisotropic H.F.S., and in solids the exchange interaction is often the dominating factor (see §3.9).

The H.F.S. of aromatic free radicals

The aromatic free radicals (semiquinones, negative ions of carbohydrates and others, see Chapter 8) give E.S.R. spectra with well-resolved proton H.F.S. McConnell suggested the following empirical formula which gives the magnitude of the splitting ΔB_i due to the i-th proton of the aromatic

---

† From (3.93) it follows that the broadening due to the anisotropic hyperfine structure is at its largest for the outermost components with the largest absolute values of m_I.

radical, in terms of the density of the unpaired $2p_z$-electrons of the C-atom (q_i) bound to this proton:

$$\Delta B_i = Q\rho_i \tag{3.94}$$

Here Q is a constant which is virtually the same for the majority of aromatic radicals:

$$Q = 2 \cdot 25 \text{ mWb m}^{-2} \tag{3.95}$$

This poses the question of the physical nature of H.F.S. and the justification of equation (3.94), since the resolvable H.F.S. cannot be caused by the anistotropic dipole-dipole interaction, which in non-viscous liquids is zero because of averaging-out. On the other hand, the unpaired electron is a $2p_z$-electron, and the $2p_z$-function has a node in the plane of the aromatic ring in which the hydrogen atoms lie. An isotropic H.F.S. due to indirect contact interaction is also therefore excluded. Weissman and his co-workers[12] suggest that the H.F.S. in this case is caused by the stress vibrations of the C—H bond, through which the protons are concentrated in the plane of the aromatic ring; however, this would give rise to a splitting which is an order of magnitude below the observed value.[13]

The theory of the H.F.S. of aromatic free radicals has been studied by many workers who have used the method of localized pairs as well as the molecular orbital process (M.O.) with regard to configurational interaction. However, since the quantitative calculations involve a large number of approximations and hardly appear very reliable, and since the qualitative physical models are completely equivalent, we shall consider this problem only within the framework of the method of localized pairs.[14]

We will restrict ourselves to consideration of the part-molecule $>$C—H.

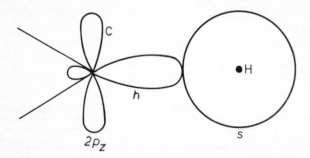

In the diagram, h is the sp^2-orbit of the C-atom of the aromatic ring which is directed towards the hydrogen atom, s is the 1s-orbital of the hydrogen atom and p the $2p_z$-orbital of the C-atom localized on the unpaired electron. By the exchange interaction of the h- and s-electrons, the σ-bond C—H is formed. We write the wave function of zero-th order corresponding to this state $\phi_1^{(0)}$ (bonding by h- and s- electrons; p-electron unpaired) as one usually does in the method of localized pairs in quantum chemistry:

$$\phi_1^{(0)} = \bar{p}\left\{\frac{1}{\sqrt{2}}\frac{1}{(1+S_0^2)^{1/2}}p(1)\,h(2)\,s(3)[\alpha(1)\alpha(2)\beta(3)\right.$$
$$\left. - \alpha(1)\beta(2)\alpha(3)]\right\} \qquad (3.96)$$

Here S_0 is the non-orthogonality integral, and $\bar{p}$ the anti-symmetry operator: $\bar{p} = (1/\sqrt{3!})\,\Sigma\,(-1)^p$ when it is summed over all $3!$ permutations of the three electrons.

This state obviously gives no H.F.S., since the unpaired electron is a $2p_z$-electron. We write the wave function of the excited doublet term which can combine with $\phi_1^{(0)}$:

$$\phi_2^{(0)} = \bar{p}\left\{\frac{1}{\sqrt{6}}\frac{1}{(1+S_0^2)^{1/2}}\,phs(\alpha\alpha\beta + \alpha\beta\alpha - 2\beta\alpha\alpha)\right\} \qquad (3.97)$$

In the excited state $\phi_2^{(0)}$ is the bond influenced by the first and second electron, and the unpaired electron is in the $1s$-state. The actual state of the system can be described by the following wave function:

$$\phi = \phi_1^{(0)} + \lambda\phi_2^{(0)} \qquad (\lambda \ll 1) \qquad (3.98)$$

Solving the Schrödinger equation for this system gives

$$\hat{H}\phi = \epsilon\phi$$

with

$$\epsilon = \frac{\int \phi^*\hat{H}\phi\,d\tau}{\int \phi^*\phi\,d\tau}$$

If we neglect the normalization, we obtain

$$\epsilon = H_{11} + 2\lambda H_{12} + \lambda^2 H_{22} \equiv 2\lambda H_{12} + \lambda^2(\Delta E_{12})$$

where

$$H_{11} = \int \phi_1^{*(0)}\hat{H}\phi_1^{(0)}\,d\tau$$
$$H_{12} = \int \phi_1^{*(0)}\hat{H}\phi_2^{(0)}\,d\tau$$
$$H_{22} = \int \phi_2^{*(0)}\hat{H}\phi_2^{(0)}\,d\tau$$

The energy is numbered from the energy of the state $\phi_1^{(0)}$ ($H_{11} \equiv 0$, $H_{22} - H_{11} \equiv \Delta E_{12}$).

By using the variation principle, we obtain

$$\frac{d\epsilon}{d\lambda} = 2(H_{12} + \lambda \Delta E_{12}) = 0 \qquad \left(\lambda = -\frac{H_{12}}{\Delta E_{12}} \right) \qquad (3.99)$$

The molecular integrals H_{11}, H_{12} and H_{22} in (3.99) can be expressed by atomic integrals of the functions p, h and s, and calculated approximately. In this way it is possible in principle to calculate the value λ. If the unpaired electron were a pure 1s-electron, then the constant Q in (3.94) would be equal to Q_H, the H.F.S. constant for atomic hydrogen ($Q_H \approx$ 0·05 Wb m^{-2}). Clearly, in our case it is

$$Q = \lambda^2 Q_H$$

This calculation gives a value which is in approximate agreement with the experimental one.

The H.F.S. of E.S.R. spectra of aromatic free radicals is thus of a contact nature and originates from the interaction of the unpaired $2p_z$-electron with the σ-electrons of the CH-bond.

Negative spin densities

Equation (3.94) is equivalent to the statement that in aromatic free radicals the separation between the outermost H.F.S. components (i.e. the total splitting of the spectrum) is constant and equal to Q.† This is actually observed in a large number of cases, but there are some remarkable exceptions, and these are the alternating aromatic radicals with an odd number of bonded C-atoms (e.g. perynaphthene, triphenylmethyl etc.). In such unusual radicals the total splitting is always larger than that given by equation (3.99).

The spin density ρ_i at the i-th C-atom is usually taken as the square of the coefficient a_i, assuming we write the molecular function of the unpaired electron $\psi = \sum_i a_i \phi_i$ as a linear combination of atomic functions, as is necessary for the simple M.O. method in the Hückel form. This will clearly give only positive values for ρ_i. In this simple form the M.O. method does not take into account the configurational interaction, i.e. the perturbation of the ground state by excited states, corresponding to π–π transitions, in

† This of course only applies to aromatic hydrocarbons without alkyl groups. In other cases the splitting can assume considerably larger values (see Chapter 7).

which the unpaired electron may occupy other molecular orbits (either higher or lower). In the case of the allyl radical (three electrons and three centres) there are, for example, nine possible configurations which correspond to the spin $\frac{1}{2}$:

$$\psi_0 \quad \psi_1 \quad \psi_2 \quad \psi_3 \quad \psi_4 \quad \psi_5 \quad \psi_6 \quad \psi_7 \quad \psi_8$$

If configurational interaction is taken into account, ρ_i is no longer taken as the square of a_i in ψ_0, but as a complicated combination of products of $a_i^{(j)}$ for different molecular orbits (in the different configurations the unpaired electron assumes different molecular orbits). The coefficients a_i can have different signs for different orbits and ρ_i can become negative. Since all configurations belong to the same total spin and all wave functions are normalized, then clearly $\sum_i \rho_i = 2S$ (for $S = \frac{1}{2}$, $\sum_i \rho_i = 1$).

However, the splitting due to the i-th hydrogen atom depends on the absolute value of ρ_i and therefore the total splitting can become larger.

We will take as an example the allyl radical:

The simple calculation without considering configurational interaction gives $\rho_1 = \rho_3 = 0.5$, $\rho_2 = 0$, and the unpaired electron can interact with only three equivalent protons (two at atom C_1 and one at atom C_3). We should then obtain an E.S.R. signal consisting of four equidistant components with intensity ratios $1:3:3:1$ and a separation between the components $\Delta B \approx 2.25 \times 0.5 = 1.125$ mWb m^{-2}. A more rigorous calculation of the $\pi-\pi$ configurational interaction[15] gives $\rho_1 = \rho_3 = 0.622$, $\rho_2 = -0.231$. Thus on the central C-atom there is a small additional splitting due to the proton. The spectrum consists of four main components with a mutual separation $\Delta B_1 = 2.25 \times 0.622 \approx 1.4$ mWb m^{-2}, each of which is split into two equal components with $\Delta B_2 = 2.25 \times 0.231 \approx 0.5$ mWb m^{-2}. This spectrum is in excellent agreement with the experimental results.

The calculation according to the method of localized pairs, and considering only the most important canonical structure,

$$
\begin{array}{c}
\overset{\uparrow}{C}-C=C \\[2pt]
C=C-\overset{\uparrow}{C}
\end{array}
$$

gives

$$\rho_1 = \rho_3 = \tfrac{1}{2} \qquad \rho_2 = 0$$

However, we have already seen that if we consider the perturbing action of the unpaired electron on the orbits of the remaining π-electrons, i.e. the first approximation of the perturbation theory, we get

$$\rho_1 = \rho_3 = \tfrac{2}{3} \qquad \rho_2 = -\tfrac{1}{3}$$

So, generally speaking, the unpaired electron has a perturbing action on the π-bonds which in effect leads to a de-pairing of the bonds. Since here a strong exchange interaction is present, the total spin, and also the number of unpaired electrons (obtained from the intensity of the E.S.R. lines), remain unchanged. The effective additional de-pairing shows itself only as an increase in the absolute value of the H.F.S. constant. This effect can most easily be observed experimentally in those cases where, ignoring the π–π configurational interaction on the proton in question, the skin density and thus the H.F.S. constant would be equal to zero without such an interaction.

§3.9

WIDTH AND SHAPE OF THE E.S.R. LINES

Spin-lattice interaction†

From the uncertainty principle, we can state that

$$\Delta E \,.\, \Delta t \approx h \tag{3.100}$$

The line width (ΔE) is inversely proportional to the lifetime of the excited particles (Δt). We will consider the simplest example, in which the E.S.R. spectrum is produced by a paramagnetic particle with $S = \tfrac{1}{2}$, with a small spin-orbit interaction and without interaction with a magnetic nucleus. In this particular case, two Zeeman levels are formed in the external magnetic field, which we will designate as '+' and '−' (according to the values $m_s = \pm\tfrac{1}{2}$).

† Here, as before (see p. 48), we are talking about the lattice in general.

The separation between the levels is $\Delta E = g\beta H$, and the ratio of their populations at equilibrium is

$$\frac{N_+}{N_-} = e^{g\beta B/kT} \tag{3.101}$$

We will write P_- for the probability of the transition $(-) \to (+)$, transferring energy ΔE to the lattice in unit time, and P_+ as the probability of the transition $(+) \to (-)$, by which the spin takes energy from the lattice. At equilibrium, the following clearly holds:

$$P_- N_- = P_+ N_+$$
$$\frac{P_-}{P_+} = \frac{N_+}{N_-} = e^{g\beta B/kT} \approx 1 + \frac{g\beta B}{kT} \tag{3.102}$$

We now introduce the mean transition probability $P = (P_+ + P_-)/2$. Thus

$$P_- \approx P\left(1 + \frac{g\beta B}{2kT}\right)$$
$$P_+ \approx P\left(1 - \frac{g\beta B}{2kT}\right) \tag{3.103}$$

All that we have so far said refers to a paramagnetic particle in a constant magnetic field. If we now subject the sample to a microwave resonance field, then the induced transitions $N_+ \to N_-$ and $N_- \to N_+$ will *a priori* take place with equal probability. As $N_+ > N_-$, this causes N_+/N_- initially to become smaller than $\exp(g\beta H/kT)$. We can now introduce the spin temperature T_s of the system, which is defined by the following equation:

$$\frac{N_+}{N_-} = e^{g\beta B/kT_s} \tag{3.104}$$

Thus in our case $T_s > T$.

We now switch off the microwave field. After a specific time the system returns to an equilibrium state and T_s becomes equal to T. We can now write down the kinetic equation of this process. Let $n = N_+ - N_-$ be the excess population of the lower Zeeman level. At each transition n changes by 2:

$$\frac{dn}{dt} = 2N_- P_- - 2N_+ P_+$$

At equilibrium $dn/dt = 0$. Using (3.103), we obtain

$$\frac{dn}{dt} = 2N_-P\left(1 + \frac{g\beta B}{2kT}\right) - 2N_+P\left(1 - \frac{g\beta B}{2kT}\right)$$

$$= 2P\left[N_- - N_+ + (N_+ + N_-)\frac{g\beta B}{kT}\right] = 2P\left(\frac{g\beta BN}{kT} - n\right)$$

with $N = N_+ + N_-$.

Since at equilibrium we have $N_+ \approx N(\frac{1}{2} + g\beta H/2kT)$ and $N_- \approx N(\frac{1}{2} - g\beta H/kT)$ we obtain $g\beta BN/kT = (N_+ - N_-)_0 = n_0$ as the population difference of the levels (+) and (−) in the state of Boltzmann equilibrium. This gives

$$\frac{dn}{dt} = 2P(n_0 - n)$$

and

$$n_0 - n = (n_0 - n_a)\,e^{-2Pt} \tag{3.105}$$

Here, n_a is the difference in population between the levels (+) and (−) at the instant $t = 0$, i.e. at the moment of switching off the microwave field.

The time in which $(n - n_a)$ decreases by the factor e, in the above case, is called the *spin-lattice relaxation time,*† and is designated by the symbol T_1:

$$T_1 = \frac{1}{2P}$$

Here T_1 plays the role of Δt in equation (3.100), and can therefore determine the width of the E.S.R. line.

The considerations employed above naturally have a certain degree of formal character. The possibility of adjusting the equilibrium depends on the possibility of energy exchange between the spin system and the lattice. In the case of the spin system, the question reduces to the energy change of spin moments in a magnetic field, and in the case of the lattice, to the energy of oscillating electric charges. An interaction between the two systems can therefore occur only‡ through the spin-orbit coupling (only the orbital motion of the electron, it being a charged particle, can interact directly with the electrical lattice vibrations).

---

† This time is also called the *longitudinal relaxation time,* since the relaxation in question is that of the magnetization components in the direction of the external magnetic field.

‡ If we do not consider cases of strong exchange interaction (see below).

We can picture the lattice as a system of oscillators with a constant separation $\Delta E = g\beta H$ between the neighbouring energy levels. (Naturally, in the energy spectrum of the lattice, there is also a large number of other energy levels, but for the moment these are not important). For the transition $(+) \rightarrow (-)$, the lattice delivers energy, i.e. the energy of one of the oscillators decreases by one quantum $(g\beta B)$. This can occur with all oscillators of the lattice, with the exception of those already in the lowest level. The number of oscillators which are not in the lowest level, is proportional to the value

$$e^{-g\beta B/kT} \approx 1 - \frac{g\beta B}{kT}$$

and thus

$$P_+ \approx 1 - \frac{g\beta B}{kT}$$

For the $(-) \rightarrow (+)$ transition there are no other limitations. Thus, in agreement with (3.102), we obtain

$$\frac{P_-}{P_+} \approx \frac{1}{1 - \dfrac{g\beta B}{kT}} \approx 1 + \frac{g\beta B}{kT}$$

We may distinguish here two principal mechanisms.[16]

1. The frequencies $g\beta B/h$ agree numerically with the eigenfrequencies of the lattice oscillators. In this case the relaxation is caused by the resonance exchange of quanta between the spin system and the lattice vibrations. Kronig[16] has shown that the following relation holds:

$$T_1 \approx \frac{10^4 \Delta_L^4}{\lambda^2 B^4 T} \tag{3.106}$$

Here T_1 is measured in seconds, ΔL is the separation between the lowest orbital levels, λ the spin-orbit coupling constant is in cm^{-1}, and B is in 10^{-4} Wb m^{-2}.

2. The values $g\beta B$ agree numerically with the energy differences of the lattice vibrations, which have considerably higher frequencies. In this case we can assume that this relaxation is caused by a Raman scattering of the lattice phonons, and is analogous to the Raman scattering of light. Here, the following relation holds:

$$T_1 \approx \frac{10^4 \Delta_L^6}{\lambda^2 B^2 T^7} \tag{3.107}$$

We see that down to very low temperatures, $\Delta L > 10^3$ cm^{-1}, the actual process is Raman scattering, i.e. the T_1 of equation (3.107) is considerably smaller than that calculated from equation (3.106).

If T_1 is sufficiently small, then the spin-lattice interaction is the principal factor in the determination of the line width. However, in most cases of interest in chemistry, T_1 is large, and the line width caused by other factors exceeds the natural line width caused by the spin-lattice interaction. Materials with a large value of T_1 have an important practical value; at microwave frequencies which are not particularly high, saturation occurs, resulting in a broadening and distortion of the E.S.R. lines. The only method of preventing this saturation is to reduce the microwave power level.

Spin-spin interaction: Line shape

The lifetime of a spin in an excited state is limited not only by the spin-lattice interaction. Let us consider two spins, j and k. In a magnetic field they precess about the direction of the magnetic induction B at the Larmor frequency $g\beta B/h$. At the same time, the spin j produces an alternating magnetic field B_{loc} in the region of the spin k, with a frequency $g\beta B/h$. If the spin j goes into the higher Zeeman level by the absorption of a microwave quantum, then the alternating field B_{loc} can induce the corresponding transition of the spin k, as a result of which the spin j returns again to the ground state and passes on its excitation to the spin k. A spin-spin interaction of this type limits the lifetime of the spin in the excited state and disperses the power absorbed by the spin in question over the entire spin system. This can only result in a transfer of excitation energy, whenever, as a result of dipole-dipole interaction between the spins of the system, the phases of the precessing spins coincide. If $\Delta\nu_0$ is the frequency of the phase change, then $1/2\pi\Delta\nu_0$ is called the *phase memory time*. After this mean time, the energy transfer process can repeat itself. In this way the average lifetime of a spin in an excited state equals $1/2\pi\Delta\nu_0$, and this produces a line width $h\Delta\nu_0$. The time $1/2\pi\Delta\nu_0$, which determines the relaxation time of a spin with respect to the transfer of excitation energy to other spins of the system, is usually designated by T_2.†

One may approach the problem of spin-spin interaction from another

---

† This time is also called the *transverse relaxation time*, since the energy transfer occurs through the components m_x and m_y of the magnetic spin moments perpendicular to B.

point of view. Each spin is a magnetic dipole with a moment μ_0. Therefore it produces in the region of another spin a local field $B_{loc} \approx \mu_0/r^3$, which varies by a value of the same magnitude. As a result of this the effective value of the magnetic field varies for different spins, and the E.S.R. lines are broadened (in energy) to approximately $g\beta B_{loc}$. So, clearly

$$h\Delta\nu_0 = g\beta B_{loc}$$

We now pass to the quantitative consideration of the problem, and begin with the Lorentzian model.[17] This model is used for the analysis of spectral line widths of gases, but can also serve as a starting point for a general consideration of the problem.

In this model the absorbing particle is considered as a harmonic oscillator which undergoes collisions, of very short impact time, with other particles. At the moment of impact, the oscillators undergo a sudden phase change in their oscillations (actually this sudden phase change is called impact). The system does not exhibit any 'phase memory' whatsoever: the phases after the collisions all have equal probability. This model also describes paramagnetic centres which do not interact with each other, which are far away from each other and which only come together for a time which is small compared with the time between collisions. The system is located in a periodic field $E\cos 2\pi\nu t$ (in our case in a microwave field). The equation of the harmonic oscillators in this case is:

$$m\ddot{x} + ax = -eE \cos 2\pi\nu t \tag{3.108}$$

The general solution of (3.108) can be described as the real part (Re) of the following expression:

$$x = \mathrm{Re}\left[\frac{eE \exp(2\pi\nu it)}{4\pi^2 m(\nu^2 - \nu_0^2)} + A \exp(2\pi\nu_0 it) + B \exp(-2\pi\nu_0 it) \right] \tag{3.109}$$

where $\nu_0 = (1/2\pi)\sqrt{(a/m)}$ is the eigenfrequency of the oscillator, and A and B are integration constants. For random distribution of the phase oscillation, it can be shown that, after impact, on the average $x = \dot{x} = 0$. The last impact of the oscillators takes place at a time $t = t_0$. Then for this oscillator, on the average,

$$x(t, t_0) = \mathrm{Re}\left\{ \frac{eE}{4\pi^2 m(\nu^2 - \nu_0^2)} \left[\exp(2\pi\nu it) - \exp(2\pi\nu it_0) \right] \times \right.$$
$$\left. \times \cos 2\pi\nu_0(t - t_0) - i\frac{\nu}{\nu_0} \exp(2\pi\nu it_0) \sin 2\pi\nu_0(t - t_0) \right\} \tag{3.110}$$

We form the mean value of (3.110) over all t_0. If τ is the average time between impacts, then for the time t, the probability that the last collision took place at the time t_0 is equal to $(1/\tau) \exp [-(t - t_0)/\tau]$. From this we can obtain, as a mean value,

$$\overline{x(t)} = \frac{1}{\tau} \int\limits_{-\infty}^{t} x(t, t_0) \exp [-(t - t_0)/\tau] \, dt_0 \qquad (3.111)$$

If here we substitute the value from (3.110), and neglect the integration terms $\sim 1/(\nu + \nu_0)$ (which are small compared with terms $\sim 1/(\nu - \nu_0)$, as the amplitude of x rapidly decreases far from resonance), we obtain

$$\overline{x(t)} = \mathrm{Re} \left\{ \frac{eE \exp [2\pi\nu it] [2\pi i(\nu - \nu_0)]}{4\pi^2 m(\nu^2 - \nu_0^2)[(1/\tau) + 2\pi i(\nu - \nu_0)]} \right\} \qquad (3.112)$$

The line intensity at the frequency ν is proportional to the rate of energy absorption at this frequency, and equals

$$I(\nu) = \left\langle -eE \cos 2\pi\nu t \frac{dx(t)}{dt} \right\rangle_m = \frac{e^2 E^2}{4m} \cdot \frac{1/\tau}{(1/\tau)^2 + 4\pi^2(\nu - \nu_0)^2} \qquad (3.113)$$

The line shape described by equation (3.113) is of Lorentzian form. In the case of E.S.R. lines it is more useful to describe $I(\nu)$ in the form $I(B)$ and to normalize the line to unit area: $\int_{-\infty}^{\infty} I(B) \, dB = 1$. We then obtain

$$I(B) = \frac{1}{\pi \Delta B_L} \frac{1}{1 + \left(\dfrac{B - B_0}{\Delta B_L}\right)^2} \qquad (3.114)$$

where ΔB_L is the line-width parameter of the Lorentzian line. For lines which are not normalized we get

$$I(B) = I_0 \frac{1}{1 + \left(\dfrac{B - B_0}{\Delta B_L}\right)^2} \qquad (3.114')$$

Here I_0 is the intensity at maximum absorption ($B = B_0$).

The Gaussian model

In the calculation of the line shape $I(\nu)$ in the previous model, we made the basic assumption that the impact duration T was small compared to the reciprocal of the deviation of the frequency from the resonance value, i.e. $T \ll |\nu - \nu_0|^{-1}$. A statistical model has been suggested by Van

Vleck;[18] described as the Gaussian model, it represents the other limiting case, i.e. $T \gg |v - v_0|^{-1}$. The fundamental assumption in this model is that the paramagnetic centres are located in differing effective magnetic fields, which change slowly compared to the line width. From the above criterion, it is clear that at a sufficiently large distance from its centre, each line must have a shape which corresponds to this statistical model. In the following section this will be developed further.

The assumption of a Gaussian distribution of the local magnetic fields is obviously the most correct one. We can then write the normalized line shape $I(v)$ in the following form:

$$I(v) = \frac{1}{\sqrt{(2\pi)} \langle \Delta v^2 \rangle_m^{1/2}} \exp \left\{ -\frac{(v - v_0)^2}{2\langle \Delta v^2 \rangle_m} \right\} \qquad (3.115)$$

or

$$I(B) = \frac{1}{\sqrt{(2\pi)} \langle \Delta B^2 \rangle_m^{1/2}} \exp \left\{ -\frac{(B - B_0)^2}{2\langle \Delta B^2 \rangle_m} \right\} \qquad (3.116)$$

Here, $\langle \Delta B^2 \rangle_m^{1/2}$ is the second moment of the line,

$$\langle \Delta B^2 \rangle_m^{1/2} = \left\{ \int\limits_{-\infty}^{+\infty} (B - B_0)^2 I(B) \, dB \right\}^{1/2} \qquad (3.117)$$

with the condition for normalization,

$$\int\limits_{-\infty}^{+\infty} I(B) \, dB = 1. \qquad (3.118)$$

For a line which is not normalized, we can write

$$I(B) = I_0 \, e^{-(B - B_0)^2 / 2\langle \Delta B^2 \rangle_m} \qquad (3.119)†$$

with

$$I_0 = I(B_0)$$

The theoretical calculation of the only parameter of the Gaussian line, the second moment, leads to the solution of the Schrödinger equation with a Hamiltonian operator which contains the spin dipole-dipole interaction:

$$\hat{H} = g\beta B \sum_j \hat{S}_{zj} + \sum_{k>j} \tilde{B}_{jk} \{ (\hat{\vec{S}}_j \hat{\vec{S}}_k) - 3r_{jk}^{-2} (\vec{r}_{jk} \hat{\vec{S}}_j)(\vec{r}_{jk} \hat{\vec{S}}_k) \} \qquad (3.120)$$

with $\tilde{B}_{jk} = g^2 \beta / r_{jk}^2$; r_{jk} being the separation of the spins j and k.

† The line-width parameter $\langle \Delta B^2 \rangle_m^{1/2}$ is obviously related to the parameter ΔB_G, used in Chapter 4, by the following relationship:

$$\Delta B_G = \sqrt{2} \langle \Delta B^2 \rangle_m^{1/2}$$

The same equation was solved by Van Vleck,[18] who obtained

$$\langle \Delta v^2 \rangle_m = \tfrac{1}{3}S(S+1)h^{-2} \sum \tilde{B}_{jk}^2 \tag{3.121}$$

The summation in (3.121) does not depend on j, since all the centres are assumed to be identical.

For a simple cubic lattice (3.121) becomes

$$\langle \Delta v^2 \rangle_m = 36 \cdot 8 g^4 \beta^4 \, d^{-6} h^{-2} \left[\tfrac{1}{3}S(S+1)\right] \left[(\lambda_1^4 + \lambda_2^4 + \lambda_3^4) - 0 \cdot 187\right] \tag{3.122}$$

where λ_1, λ_2 and λ_3 are the direction cosines of the field B with respect to the main axes of the cube, and d is the distance between the neighbouring magnetic centres in the cubic lattice.

For a polycrystalline powder, the direction cosines can be averaged over a sphere. Thus we get

$$\langle \Delta v^2 \rangle_m = \tfrac{3}{5} g^4 \beta^4 h^{-2} S(S+1) \sum_k r_{jk}^{-6} \tag{3.123}$$

The analysis of the Gaussian line shape, using the Van Vleck method of moments, is described in considerably greater detail in Chapter 4.

The frequency modulation model: delocalization and exchange narrowing

The previous model dealt with a case found relatively infrequently in practice, in which the local magnetic fields produced by the nuclei or electrons may be viewed as quasi-stationary. The interaction with the magnetic nuclei produces a splitting of the E.S.R. lines (H.F.S.), and the spin-spin interaction produces a broadening of the lines. Various processes cause a frequency change in the local fields, which is large enough to be effectively averaged, and this leads to a change in the line shape and to a narrowing of the lines. Such processes are the rapid movement of paramagnetic particles relative to each other, the delocalization of the unpaired electrons, and the exchange interaction. The effective narrowing is extremely significant. It has been shown[19] in the case of solid aromatic free radicals, that as a result of exchange interaction T_2 becomes equal to the spin-lattice relaxation time T_1. This effect may be explained by saying that for a strong exchange interaction, the coupling of the spin system with the lattice occurs by exchange interaction, and not through the spin-orbit coupling.

We will give a short summary of the quantitative theory put forward by Anderson and Weiss,[21] and by Anderson.[22] In this model the Hamiltonian operator of the system is written in the form

$$\hat{H} = \hat{H}_0 + \hat{H}_R + \hat{H}_m \qquad (3.124)$$

where $\hat{H}_0$ and $\hat{H}_R$ are respectively the unperturbed Hamiltonian operator $(g\beta \sum_j \hat{S}_j \, \bar{B})$ and the perturbation through the interaction with the magnetic electron and nuclear dipoles [see (3.120)]. $\hat{H}_m$ is the 'motional Hamiltonian operator', e.g. the Heisenberg exchange operator:

$$\hat{H}_m = \sum_{jk} \vec{J}(\tau_{jk}) \hat{S}_j \hat{S}_k$$

$\hat{H}_R$ is not exchangeable with $\hat{H}_0$, and can change the resonance frequency, as a result of which the line becomes broadened or split.

$\hat{H}_m$ is exchangeable with $\hat{H}_0$ and cannot influence the frequency directly. Alternatively, $\hat{H}_m$ and $\hat{H}_R$ are not exchangeable, which according to the equation

$$i\hbar\dot{\hat{H}}_R = [\hat{H}, \hat{H}_R] = [\hat{H}_0, \hat{H}_R] + [\hat{H}_m, \hat{H}_R] \qquad (3.125)$$

leads to a time-dependence of $\hat{H}_R$ and to a reduction of the broadening. The model suggested by Anderson and Weiss is called the *frequency modulation model*. We would like now to consider a simple example of its use.

Let there be an unpaired electron with two possible localization positions, which differ in the value of the local magnetic field. For example, these two positions could represent two protons with opposite orientation of the nuclear spin $(m_I = \pm\frac{1}{2})$ in an external magnetic field B_0. In either position the unpaired electron has a well-defined, but different, Larmor frequency, and thus it gives two discrete E.S.R. lines. As a model, we can assume an oscillator, with two eigenfrequencies ν_1 and ν_2. Sometimes the oscillator has the frequency ν_1, and at other times the frequency ν_2. The frequency change, which is equivalent to the 'collision' of the Lorentzian model, occurs at random. This implies that there is a certain value τ, the mean time between two consecutive collisions (the reciprocal value of the mean delocalization—or exchange—frequency) around which the actual times between consecutive collisions are statistically distributed (approximately according to a Gaussian distribution).

We will designate the mean 'collision frequency' by ν_e (exchange frequency). Anderson[22] calculated the shape and position of the line as a function of the ratio ν_e/ν_0, where ν_0 is the value of the splitting. The results of this calculation are shown in Fig. 3.4.

The frequency of the central line was chosen as the starting point for numbering the abscissa values, and put equal to zero. The natural width of each line, without exchange, was assumed to be negligibly small. From Fig. 3.4 it can be seen that for $\nu_e/\nu_0 < 1$ the exchange or the delocalization broadens the individual components and brings them naturally closer. For

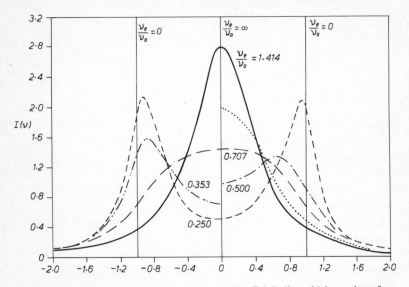

Fig. 3.4 Influence of the exchange interaction on an E.S.R. line which consists of two H.F.S. components.[22]

$\nu_e/\nu_0 > 1$ we obtain a line which has a resonance character (at least at its central point). Finally it should be noted that at $\nu_e/\nu_0 < 1$ the width of each individual line at half value is equal to ν_e, so that under these conditions the exchange leads to a broadening.

This model was extended to the case of an infinitely large number of frequencies, i.e. to the case of the spin-spin interaction, which leads to a Gaussian distribution of the local fields. The random 'collisions' lead to a random 'Gaussian' frequency modulation of this Gaussian 'signal'. As a result of this, the central part of the line becomes narrower (for which $|\nu - \nu_0| \ll \nu_e$) and takes on a Lorentzian shape. Anderson and Weiss[21] obtained the following expression for the normalized line shape:

$$I(\nu) = \frac{1}{2\pi^2 \langle \Delta\nu \rangle_G^2} \frac{1}{1 + \dfrac{(\nu - \nu_0)^2}{(\langle \Delta\nu \rangle_G^2 / \nu_e)^2}} \tag{3.126}$$

where $\langle \Delta\nu \rangle_G^2$ is the square of the second moment of the original Gaussian line in the absence of exchange [see (3.115)].

The value $\langle \Delta\nu \rangle_G^2 / \nu_e$ for a line which is made narrower by exchange or delocalization, plays the rôle of the line-width parameter. From (3.126) we can easily obtain an expression for the half-width of the resulting Lorentzian line:

$$\Delta\nu_{1/2} = \frac{2 \langle \Delta\nu \rangle_G^2}{\nu_e} \tag{3.127}$$

The shoulders of the line, for which $| \nu - \nu_0 | \gg \nu_e$, retain their Gaussian character. In Chapter 4 we will use this fact in the analysis of experimental E.S.R. lines.

§3.10
SUMMARY

From the material compiled in this chapter one can see that the theory of E.S.R. spectra is developed most completely for paramagnetic ions in crystalline fields of different symmetries. The theory of E.S.R. spectra of organic free radicals, which are of chemical interest, is still only in its initial stages of development. One extremely disappointing aspect is the state of the theory of the shift of the *g*-factor and its anisotropy for organic structures, in which the lifting of the orbital degeneracy is caused not by the electric fields of the crystalline lattice, but by exchange interaction. Through the absence of a suitable theory, the chemist loses an important additional source of information, the E.S.R. spectra of organic free radicals. The question of the ratio of spin density to charge density, which has a direct bearing on the mechanism and kinetics of radical reactions, is also not yet clear. The list of such unsolved problems could be continued. Electron spin resonance spectroscopy is also a profitable field for the theoretical physicist interested in using this technique to help in his investigations of important chemical problems.

References

1. Eyring, H., Walter, J., Kimball, G. E.: *Quantum Chemistry,* New York, 1944.
2. Van der Waerden, B. L.: *Die gruppentheoretische Methode in der Quanten-mechanik* (The Group Theory Method in Quantum Mechanics), Berlin 1932.
3. Bhagavantam, S., Venkatarayudu, T.: *Theory of Groups and its Application to Physical Problems,* Waltar 1951.
4. Bethe, H.: *Ann. d. Phys.,* 3 (1930), 133.
5. Kramers, H. A.: *Proc. Amsterdam Acad.,* 33 (1930), 959.
6. Polder, D.: *Physica,* 9 (1942), 709.
7. Pryce, M. H. L.: *Nuovo Cimento,* 6/3 (1957), 817.
8. Abragam, A., Pryce, M. H. L.: *Proc. roy. Soc.,* A 205 (1951), 135.
9. Bleaney, B.: *Proc. Phys. Soc.,* 75 (1960), 621.
10. McClure, D. S.: *J. Chem. Phys.,* 17 (1949), 905.
11. McConnell, H. M., Robertson, R. E.: *J. Phys. Chem.,* 61 (1957), 1018.
12. Weissman, S. J., Townsend, J., Paul, D., Pake, G.: *J. Chem. Phys.,* 21 (1953), 2227.
13. Venkataraman, B., Fraenkel, G. K.: *JACS,* 77 (1955), 2707.
14. McConnell, H. M., Chesnut, D. B.: *J. Chem. Phys.,* 28 (1958), 107.
15. Lefkovitz, H. C., Fain, J., Matsen, F. A.: *J. Chem. Phys.,* 23 (1955), 1690.
16. Kronig, R.: *Physica,* 6 (1939), 33.
17. Van-Vleck, J. H.: *Nuovo Cimento,* 6 (1957), 1081.
18. Van-Vleck, J. H.: *Phys. Rev.,* 74 (1948), 1168.
19. Lloyd, J. P., Pake, G. E.: *Phys. Rev.,* 92 (1953), 1576.
20. Bloembergen, H., Wang, S.: *Phys. Rev.,* 93 (1954), 72.
21. Anderson, P. W., Weiss, P. R.: *Rev. Mod. Phys.,* 25 (1953), 269.
22. Anderson, P. W.: *J. Phys. Soc. Japan,* 9 (1954), 316.
23. Altschuler, S. A., Kosyrev, B. M.: *Paramagnetische Elektronenresonanz* (Electron Paramagnetic Resonance), Leipzig 1963.
24* Wigner, E.: *Gruppentheorie und ihre Anwendung auf die Quantenmechanik der Atomspektren* (Group Theory and its Application to the Quantum Mechanics of Atomic Spectra), Braunschweig, 1931.
25* Heine, V.: *Group Theory in Quantum Mechanics,* London-Oxford-New York-Paris, 1960.

Chapter 4

Isolated, Symmetric Lines in E.S.R. Spectra

The simplest type of E.S.R. spectrum consists of a single isolated symmetric line. Although such simple spectra are seldom found in practice, we will nevertheless consider this case, as the analysis can be carried out by very simple procedures.

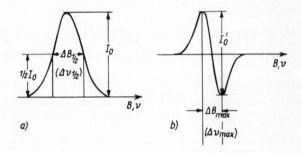

Fig. 4.1 Isolated symmetric line.
(*a*) Absorption line. (*b*) First derivative of the absorption line.

The samples which give this characteristic line come under the following general headings: various carbons and carbonized products of organic compounds, aromatic free radicals in the solid state, defects in solids with high crystal field symmetry in the absence of magnetic nuclei in the region of the defects, and various free radicals and paramagnetic centres in the liquid state at sufficiently high concentration (see Part II). In this chapter we will show, on the basis of an analysis of the line shape, how, from the interaction of the paramagnetic particle in the sample, we can determine such important characteristics as the spin-lattice, spin-spin and exchange interaction.

The isolated symmetric line is characterized by four parameters: the integrated intensity, the width, the shape and the g-factor. In this chapter we will limit ourselves to a discussion of the first three parameters, since the g-factor was considered in detail in Chapter 3.

As we have already pointed out, the limiting cases are lines described by the equations of Gauss and Lorentz. These equations can also be written as functions of frequency (at constant magnetic field B_0) and magnetic field (at constant frequency ν_0):

$$I_\nu^G = I_{\nu_0}^G \cdot e^{-(\nu - \nu_0)^2 / \Delta \nu_G^2} \left.\begin{array}{l}\\\\\end{array}\right\} \text{Gaussian shape} \tag{4.1a}$$

$$I_B^G = I_{B_0}^G \cdot e^{-(B - B_0)^2 / \Delta B_G^2} \tag{4.1b}$$

$$I_\nu^L = I_{\nu_0}^L \left(1 + \frac{(\nu - \nu_0)^2}{\Delta \nu_L^2}\right)^{-1} \left.\begin{array}{l}\\\\\end{array}\right\} \text{Lorentzian shape} \tag{4.2a}$$

$$I_B^L = I_{B_0}^L \left(1 + \frac{(B - B_0)^2}{\Delta B_L^2}\right)^{-1} \tag{4.2b}$$

As the equations (a) and (b) are completely identical in form, we will use only equations (4.1b) and (4.2b), since, in the practical case, B represents the variable.

In both limiting cases, the line is completely described by the value of the maximum intensity I_{B_0} and one of the parameters ΔB_G or ΔB_L. The width of the line at half height, $\Delta B_{1/2}$, can be measured directly from the spectrum (see Fig. 4.1a). The value $\Delta B_{1/2}$ depends uniquely on the parameters ΔB_G and ΔB_L in the following way:

For a Gaussian line

$$\Delta B_G = \frac{1}{2 \ln 2} \Delta B_{1/2} \approx 0{\cdot}6 \, \Delta B_{1/2} \tag{4.3}$$

For a Lorentzian line

$$\Delta B_L = 0{\cdot}5 \, \Delta B_{1/2} \tag{4.4}$$

If the line is recorded as a first derivative (see Fig. 4.1b), then equations (4.1b) and (4.2b) change to

$$\frac{dI_G}{dB} = -I_0^G \frac{2(B - B_0)}{\Delta B_G^2} e^{-(B - B_0)^2 / \Delta B_G^2} \tag{4.1$'$}$$

$$\frac{dI_L}{dB} = -I_0^L \frac{2(B - B_0)}{\Delta B_L^2} \left(1 + \frac{(B - B_0)^2}{\Delta B_L^2}\right)^{-2} \tag{4.2$'$}$$

However, as the values I_0^G and I_0^L cannot be measured directly from the curve of the first derivative, it is useful to introduce instead the amplitudes between the extreme values of this curve (I_0', see Fig. 4.1b). We carry out the corresponding calculations, and obtain for the Gaussian curve

$$\frac{\mathrm{d}I_G}{\mathrm{d}B} = -(I_0')_G \cdot \sqrt{\left(\frac{\mathrm{e}}{2}\right)} \cdot \frac{(B-B_0)}{\Delta B_G} \mathrm{e}^{-(B-B_0)^2/\Delta B_G^2} \qquad (4.1'')$$

and for the Lorentzian curve

$$\frac{\mathrm{d}I_L}{\mathrm{d}B} = -(I_0')_L \cdot \frac{8}{3\sqrt{3}} \cdot \frac{(B-B_0)}{\Delta B_L} \left(1 + \frac{(B-B_0)^2}{\Delta B_L^2}\right)^{-2} \qquad (4.2'')$$

Also by analogy, it is useful to introduce the separation between the maxima $\Delta B_{\max}$ (see Fig. 4.1b), as a measure of the line width. Similarly, by calculation we obtain

$$\Delta B_G = \frac{\sqrt{2}}{2} \Delta B_{\max} \qquad (4.5)$$

$$\Delta B_L = \frac{\sqrt{3}}{2} \Delta B_{\max} \qquad (4.6)$$

The original equations for I and $\mathrm{d}I/\mathrm{d}B$ can thus be written in terms of the parameters which are measured experimentally:

$$I_G = I_0 \, \mathrm{e}^{-(B-B_0)^2/0 \cdot 36 \Delta B_{1/2}^2} \qquad (4.7)$$

$$I_L = I_0 \left(1 + 4 \frac{(B-B_0)^2}{\Delta B_{1/2}^2}\right)^{-1} \qquad (4.8)$$

$$\frac{\mathrm{d}I_G}{\mathrm{d}B} = -I_0' \sqrt{\mathrm{e}} \frac{(B-B_0)}{\Delta B_{\max}} \mathrm{e}^{-2(B-B_0)^2/\Delta B_{\max}^2} \qquad (4.9)$$

$$\frac{\mathrm{d}I_L}{\mathrm{d}B} = -I_0' \frac{(B-B_0)}{\Delta B_{\max}} \left(1 + \frac{4}{3} \frac{(B-B_0)^2}{\Delta B_{\max}^2}\right)^{-2} \qquad (4.10)$$

To obtain the number of paramagnetic particles N in the sample, we have to calculate the integral from $-\infty$ to $+\infty$ over the absorption line (see Fig. 4.1a), or the double integral over the differentiated absorption line (Fig. 4.1b). From equation (4.1), in the case of a Gaussian line for the absorption curve it follows that

$$N_G = a \int_{-\infty}^{+\infty} I_G(B) \, \mathrm{d}B = a\sqrt{\pi} \, I_0^G \Delta B_G = 0 \cdot 6 \sqrt{\pi} a I_0^G \Delta B_{1/2} \qquad (4.11)$$

for the curve of the first derivative

$$N_G = \frac{1}{4} \sqrt{\left(\frac{\pi e}{2}\right)} a(I_0')_G \Delta B_{max}^2 \qquad (4.12)$$

Similarly for the Lorentzian line, we obtain

$$N_L = 0 \cdot 5 \pi a I_0^L \Delta B_{1/2} \qquad (4.13)$$

or

$$N_L = \frac{\pi}{\sqrt{3}} a(I_0')_L \Delta B_{max}^2 \qquad (4.14)$$

If we are only interested in the ratios of the integral intensities of E.S.R. lines, which may change as the result of some process or other whilst the line shape and width remain constant, then it is sufficient to measure only the value of I_0 or I_0'. If the line shape is preserved, then changes in line width and related changes in intensity are determined uniquely by the products $I_0 \Delta B_{1/2}$ or $I_0' \Delta B_{max}$ respectively. If the line shape is not preserved, then this may lead to errors of from 50 to 100 per cent.

In the general case, besides the quantities I_0 and $\Delta B_{1/2}$ (or I_0' and ΔB_{max}) directly measurable from the spectrum we require a calibration factor a in equations (4.11) to (4.14). This coefficient is uniquely determined by the experimental conditions and does not depend on the shape of the measured line. In principle, its value can be calculated from the electrical characteristics of the instrument [see equation (2.61)]. However, as we have already seen, the accuracy of such calculations is very poor, and is acceptable only for a rough calculation of the order of magnitude. Thus for the majority of cases, the measurement of the absolute concentration of paramagnetic particles N is determined by comparing the spectrum of the sample under investigation with that of a calibrated sample containing a known number of unpaired electrons. The spectra must be recorded under identical conditions, in order to guarantee a constant value of the parameter a.†

If the sample and the calibrated standard have the same line shape, then the number of unpaired electrons in the sample N_x is calculated from the equation

$$N_x = N_{st} \frac{(I_0 \Delta B_{1/2})_x}{(I_0 \Delta B_{1/2})_{st}} \qquad (4.15)$$

† As a standard for simultaneous comparative measurements, it is best to use a paramagnetic sample with a different g-factor, so that there is no overlap between the calibrated standard and the sample to be investigated.

or

$$N_x = N_{st} \frac{(I_0' \Delta B_{max}^2)_x}{(I_0' \Delta B_{max}^2)_{st}} \tag{4.16}$$

By comparison with equations (4.11) to (4.14), we obtain the value of a for the Gaussian line shape

$$a = \frac{N_{st}}{0 \cdot 6 \sqrt{\pi} (I_0 \Delta B_{1/2})_{st}} = \frac{4\sqrt{2} \cdot N_{st}}{\sqrt{\pi} \, e (I_0' \cdot \Delta B_{max}^2)_{st}} \tag{4.17}$$

and for a Lorentzian shape,

$$a = \frac{2 N_{st}}{\pi (I_0 \Delta B_{1/2})_{st}} = \frac{\sqrt{3} \cdot N_{st}}{\pi (I_0' \Delta B_{max}^2)_{st}} \tag{4.18}$$

Thus if we know the coefficient a from the data of the calibrated standard, we can calculate the number of unpaired electrons directly from the spectrum of the unknown sample, assuming that the line shape is pure Gaussian or pure Lorentzian.

In practice, real line shapes can only seldom be accurately described by the equations of Lorentz and Gauss, and generally represent a combination of both limiting cases. However, the E.S.R. signal of the stable free radical diphenyl-picryl-hydrazyl (D.P.P.H.), which is very often used as a calibration standard, can be described with high accuracy by the Lorentzian equation, and for this reason may be used for the determination of a.

It follows from equations (4.11) to (4.14) that for the determination of N from the values I_0 and $\Delta B_{1/2}$ (I_0' and ΔB_{max}), the calculated value cannot be in error by more than a factor of $1 \cdot 36$ (from measurement of the absorption line) or $2 \cdot 3$ (from measurement of the derivative) respectively. In this case the error will naturally always be in the same direction, and in many cases such an accuracy is adequate. By this method, the accuracy of measurement of the experimental parameters is independent of the noise level, which constitutes a big advantage. If for some reason another method of normalization is used, the line shape of which is unknown, then the reliability of this method decreases, since the sign of the error cannot be determined in advance. However, even in the worst case, the error is no more than 36 per cent.

In addition to the procedure described above, we can also use the method of graphical integration:

$$N_x = N_{st} \frac{\displaystyle\int_{-\infty}^{+\infty} I_x(B)\, dB}{\displaystyle\int_{-\infty}^{+\infty} I_{st}(B)\, dB} = N_{st} \frac{\displaystyle\int_{-\infty}^{+\infty}\int I_x'(B)\, dB^2}{\displaystyle\int_{-\infty}^{+\infty}\int I_{st}'(B)\, dB^2} \tag{4.19}$$

A major error in this method of data analysis is produced by the noise. This form of error is particularly large in cases where the values of I_0 and I_0' are comparable with the noise amplitude (I_R and I_R' in Fig. 4.2). As can be seen from the figure, with a graphical integration, that part of the area under the curve which lies below the noise level cannot be taken into account (and hence the wings of the line will be cut off).

The error in graphical integration is most simply calculated for the case of the absorption line.† Its maximum value, which results from completely ignoring that part of the curve which goes below the noise level, can be calculated from the following equations:

$$\left(\frac{\Delta N}{N}\right)_G = 1 - \frac{2}{\sqrt{\pi}} \int_0^{\sqrt{(\ln I_0/I_R)}} e^{-z^2}\, dz \tag{4.20}$$

$$\left(\frac{\Delta N}{N}\right)_L = 1 - \frac{2}{\pi} \arctan \sqrt{\left(\frac{I_0}{I_R} - 1\right)} \tag{4.21}$$

The numerical calculation gives:

for $\dfrac{I_0}{I_R} = 10,$ $\left(\dfrac{\Delta N}{N}\right)_G \approx 0\cdot13$ and $\left(\dfrac{\Delta N}{N}\right)_L \approx 0\cdot21$

for $\dfrac{I_0}{I_R} = 3,$ $\left(\dfrac{\Delta N}{N}\right)_G \approx 0\cdot29$ and $\left(\dfrac{\Delta N}{N}\right)_L \approx 0\cdot39$

The calculation of the error in the case of the plot of the derivative, that is the double graphical integration, is somewhat more complicated. In the derivation of these formulae, we have to take into account that the total error arises from two factors. For the first integration the area under the wings of the curve must be added to all coordinates of the absorption curve, which in this case is represented by the first integral. The error on the

---

† In this case, we are not calculating an error in the usual meaning of the word, but the value of the maximum reduction of N.

second integration is calculated according to the above procedure, where we assume the following equation:†

$$\frac{I'_R}{I'_0} \approx \frac{I_R}{I_0}$$

The equations for the calculation of the total error have the following form:

$$\left(\frac{\Delta N}{N}\right)_G = 1 - \frac{2}{\sqrt{\pi}}\left(1 - 0\cdot48\,\frac{I'_R}{I'_0}\right)\int\limits_0^{\sqrt{(\ln I'_0/I'_R)}} e^{-z^2}\,dz \qquad (4.22)$$

$$\left(\frac{\Delta N}{N}\right)_L = 1 - \frac{2}{\pi}\left(1 - 1\cdot31\,\frac{I'_R}{I'_0}\right)\arctan\sqrt{\left(\frac{I'_0}{I'_R} - 1\right)} \qquad (4.23)$$

For the special cases which we have considered, we get

for $\quad\dfrac{I'_0}{I'_R} = 10,\qquad \left(\dfrac{\Delta N}{N}\right)_G \approx 0\cdot21\quad$ and $\quad\left(\dfrac{\Delta N}{N}\right)_L \approx 0\cdot31$

for $\quad\dfrac{I'_0}{I'_R} = 3,\qquad \left(\dfrac{\Delta N}{N}\right)_G \approx 0\cdot40\quad$ and $\quad\left(\dfrac{\Delta N}{N}\right)_L \approx 0\cdot65$

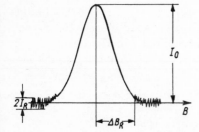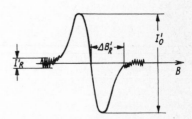

Fig. 4.2. The cutting-off of the wings of the line by noise.

The determination of the concentration of paramagnetic particles, by graphical integration as well as by calculation with analytical formulae, is thus quite inaccurate in cases where the line cannot be proved to be strictly at a limiting case (Lorentzian or Gaussian). Thus a knowledge of the line shape is an essential requirement for the determination of concentration,

† This equation is only a very rough approximation, but can be very helpful in all stages of the analysis. A more accurate calculation carried out by Molin,[1] shows that the computation method used by us in the case of a Lorentzian line gives values which come close to the actual ones, while in the case of a Gaussian line, the error calculated according to our equation is too large by a factor of 2 to 4.

and it will be clear that an analysis of the line shape will give important
information about exchange and other interactions. ·

The simplest and most useful procedure for the determination of the line
shape is direct comparison of the recorded line with theoretical lines having
the same parameters I_0 and $\Delta B_{1/2}$ (I'_0 and ΔB_{max}) , which can be
calculated from equations (4.7) to (4.10).

Fig. 4.3 shows that the limiting cases differ very little from each other in
their central region. The essential differences can be observed only in the
wings. In these parts of the line, an accurate comparison is again made
difficult by the reduced intensity. Small changes of the line shape, which, as
we have seen above, are essential for an accurate determination of the
concentration, are almost undetectable.

The first attempt to formulate a method of analysis of the lineshape was
made over twenty years ago by Van Vleck, and he used the so-called
method of moments.[2] The n-th order moment of a symmetric curve $I(B)$
which tends asymptotically to zero as $B \to \pm \infty$, is given by

$$M_n = \langle \Delta B^n \rangle^{1/n} = \left(\frac{\int_{-\infty}^{+\infty} I(B)(B - B_0)^n \, dB}{\int_{-\infty}^{+\infty} I(B) \, dB} \right)^{1/n} \tag{4.24}$$

For a Gaussian line, the ratio of the fourth order moment to the second
order moment is equal to 1·32. For a Lorentzian line, the corresponding
integrals diverge and the ratio $\alpha = M_4/M_2$ tends to infinity. It is therefore
usually concluded that a value of α of over 1·32 indicates a deviation from
the Gaussian law and an approach to the Lorentzian law. It was shown
above that this indicates the presence of exchange interaction. A distortion
of the Gaussian line as a result of strong dipole-dipole interaction or of
unresolved hyperfine structure leads to a value of α smaller than 1·32.

However, we must take into account that we are speaking here of very
small effects. For example, a transition from a Gaussian shape to the
extreme case of a rectangular shape only decreases the value of α to 1·16.
On the other hand, the most important limitation of the method of
moments for the determination of line shape is the accuracy with which α
can be determined from the experimental curve. We have already seen that
for the determination of concentration, graphical integration is inaccurate
with a relatively high signal-to-noise ratio (up to 10). The error, due to
neglecting the wings of the line hidden beneath the noise, increases with the
increasing order of the moment.

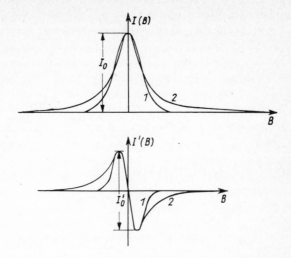

Fig. 4.3. Comparison of Gaussian and Lorentzian lines for equal I_0 and I'_0.
(1) Gaussian line   (2) Lorentzian line

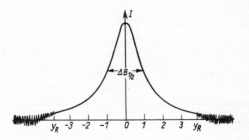

Fig. 4.4 Sketch of an isolated absorption line, in the coordinates $I(y)$.

Thus, in the case where I_0/I_R is not very large, it is impossible to obtain from α a quantitative prediction of the line shape. However, there is a quantitative procedure for the analysis of the line shape, based on the method of moments, which is practicable even when the wings of the line are neglected. This procedure is based on the fact that if we neglect the edges of the line outside a certain value ΔB_0, then the integrals of the form $\int_0^{\Delta B_0} I(B)\Delta B^n \, d\Delta B$ can be used for a Gaussian as well as for a Lorentzian line. Naturally, for this procedure, values of ΔB_0 are chosen which are smaller than ΔB_R. For this calculation it is preferable to measure the abscissa of the curve $I(B)$ using units of $\Delta B_{1/2}$, and in place of ΔB_0 we use the dimensionless parameter $y = 2\Delta B_0/\Delta B_{1/2}$ (Fig. 4.4). The processing of the experimental data involves graphical computation of the integrals in the expression for M_2 and M_4, taken not from $-\infty$ to $+\infty$, but between the limits $-y$ and $+y$, where y is chosen so that the corresponding point on the absorption line can be measured sufficiently accurately. The quotient of the effective 'moments' obtained in this way, for the selected value of y, is a function of the parameter y, and we can designate it by the symbol α_y. For a line of Lorentzian shape, this value, for large y, may be described by the following expression:

$$\alpha_y^L = 0.84 \sqrt[4]{y} \tag{4.25}$$

For a line of Gaussian shape, we get

$$\alpha_y^G = 1.32 \left(\int_0^{0.83y} e^{-z^2} \, dz \right)^{1/4} F(y) \tag{4.26}$$

Here $F(y)$ is a complicated function, which for $y \geqslant 2$ rapidly approaches unity.

Table 4.1

$y = \dfrac{2\Delta B_0}{\Delta B_{1/2}}$	α_y^L	α_y^G	$y = \dfrac{2\Delta B_0}{\Delta B_{1/2}}$	α_y^L	α_y^G
0	1·19	0	12	1·54	1·28
2	1·26	1·19	14	1·58	1·29
4	1·32	1·24	16	1·62	1·30
6	1·38	1·25	18	1·66	1·31
8	1·44	1·26	20	1·69	1·31
10	1·49	1·27	30	1·84	1·32

In Table 4.1 the values of α_y^G and α_y^L are given for values of y between 0 and 30. These values are shown graphically in Fig. 21. It can be seen from Fig. 4.5 that the value of α obtained from the experiment is insufficient by itself to permit decision on the line shape; in addition we must also know the value of y for which α was determined. For example, for $y = 2$ a value of $\alpha = 1.25$ is obtained; this means that the line in question is Lorentzian. If the same value of α is obtained for $y = 4$, then the line is Gaussian. Line-shape determination using this method is most easily carried out for large values of y. However, this is not always possible, since the method is naturally applicable only for $y < 2\Delta B_0/\Delta B_{1/2}$, and for signals of smaller intensity, the maximum value of y can be too small. In this case, we must make the measurement for several small values of y, as it can be seen from Fig. 4.5 that for $y \to 0$, the curves α_y^G and α_y^L diverge sufficiently for this purpose.

Another simple and accurate method for the analysis of line shape was recently put forward by Tichomirova and Voevodski.[3] This uses the construction of the linear anamorphoses of the experimental data which results from equations (4.7) to (4.10). In the case of the absorption line, the experimental points $I = f(B)$ are plotted in two coordinate systems:

$$\ln \frac{I_0}{I} = f[(B - B_0)^2]$$ (4.27)

and

$$\frac{I_0}{I} - 1 = f[(B - B_0)^2]$$ (4.28)

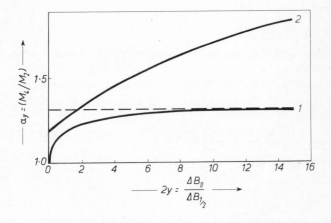

Fig. 4.5 Graph of the dependence between α_y and y for different line shapes.
(1) Gaussian line   (2) Lorentzian line.

From a simple transformation of equation (4.7) it can be seen that according to (4.27), the experimental points for a Gaussian line form a straight line. For a Lorentzian line, the transformation to a straight line follows by application of the coordinates (4.28). The possibility of straightening out either one or other of the coordinates thus permits the clear-cut determination of the line shape. From the slope of the straight lines, the parameter $B_{1/2}$ can be determined with considerably higher accuracy than is otherwise possible. The accurate equations of the linear anamorphoses which correspond to the two limiting cases have the following form:

$$\ln \frac{I_0}{I} = \frac{1}{0.36 \Delta B_{1/2}^2} (B - B_0)^2$$ (4.29)

$$\frac{I_0}{I} - 1 = \frac{4}{\Delta B_{1/2}^2} (B - B_0)^2 \tag{4.30}$$

We can easily see that this method may also be used if only one side of the line is usable for measurements. This occurs for example if a narrow line overlaps the central part of a wide line, so preventing a direct measurement of I_0. In this case, the following expressions must be used in place of (4.29) and (4.30):

$$\ln I = \ln I_0 - \frac{1}{0 \cdot 36 \Delta B_{1/2}^2} (B - B_0)^2 \tag{4.29'}$$

and

$$\frac{1}{I} = \frac{1}{I_0} + \frac{4}{I_0 \Delta B_{1/2}^2} (B - B_0)^2 \tag{4.30'}$$

In the case of the straightening in one of the two coordinate systems, we can, from the parameters of the straight lines, determine the values of the straight lines, determine the values of $\Delta B_{1/2}$ and I_0 very accurately. Once the line shape is known, it is possible from these values to calculate the concentration of parámagnetic centres.

If the curve is given in the form of the first derivative, then a completely analogous procedure is adopted. In this case, equations (4.9) and (4.10) must be written in the following way:

$$\ln \frac{I'}{(B - B_0)} = \ln \left(\sqrt{e} \, \frac{I_0'}{\Delta B_{max}} \right) - 2 \frac{(B - B_0)^2}{\Delta B_{max}^2} \tag{4.31}$$

$$\frac{B - B_0}{I'} = \frac{9}{16} \frac{\Delta B_{max}}{I_0'} + \frac{3}{4} \frac{(B - B_0)^2}{I_0' \Delta B_{max}} \tag{4.32}$$

If we plot the experimental data in the following coordinates,

$$\ln \frac{I'}{(B - B_0)} = f[(B - B_0)^2]$$

and

$$\frac{(B - B_0)}{I'} = f[(B - B_0)^2]$$

then the line shape and its parameters can be found with the help of the above procedure.

At first sight, it may appear that the method of linear anamorphosis above is only applicable in one or other of the limiting cases (4.7) or (4.8). Since the cases of most interest are those where a normal Gaussian distribution is transformed by exchange interaction, which leads to a mixing of the line shapes, then the anamorphosis method would appear to be very limited in application. However, a detailed consideration of the problem shows that this is not the case. Several years ago it was shown by Van Vleck,[4] that for an arbitrary finite exchange frequency ν_e the only part of a Gaussian curve which changes is that for which ν lies in the interval $\nu_0 - \nu_e < \nu < \nu_0 + \nu_e$, or, in the coordinates used by us, within the range $B_0 \pm B_e$ (Fig. 4.6). To simplify this, we may say that the exchange interaction cannot average out the local magnetic fields for those particles when the fields differ greatly from the mean field. Accordingly, the central part of the line, $|B - B_0| < B_e$, is described by a Lorentzian curve, and the wings, $|B - B_0| > B_e$, by a Gaussian curve. If we now use the anamorphosis method, we see that by the application of equations (4.30) or (4.32) a straight line will result only for $|B - B_0| < B_e$. In the coordinates of equations (4.29) or (4.31), the results are reversed, and the straightening occurs for the range $|B - B_0| > B_e$. The position of the transition range allows an approximate calculation of the exchange frequency.†

As an example of the application of this method, we will consider the E.S.R. line of sugar carbon (Fig. 4.7).[3] From the two curves obtained, we find the values of $\Delta B_{\max}^L$ and $\Delta B_{\max}^G$, and from the transition region we calculate the value of B_e.

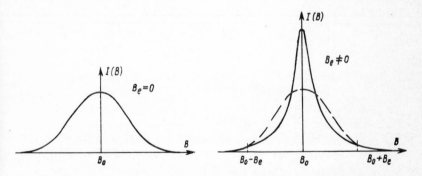

Fig. 4.6. Narrowing of a Gaussian line as a result of exchange interaction.

---

† From extrapolation of the linear sections we can ascertain I_0^L and I_0^G [or $(I_0')_L$ and $(I_0')_G$ respectively], and in this way, by integration between the corresponding limits, the concentration of paramagnetic particles can be determined with an accuracy considerably better than by other methods.

Only the value ΔB^G_{max} has any physical meaning, and this is determined by the actual Gaussian distribution of the paramagnetic particles, by the value B_e, and by the frequency of the exchange interaction of the particles. The value ΔB^L_{max} is determined from the ratio of the aforementioned parameters. Van Vleck[4] has shown theoretically that these three values satisfy the following simple relation:

$$\frac{(\Delta B^G)^2}{(\Delta B^L)B_e} \approx 1 \tag{4.33}$$

How well equation (4.33) is satisfied can serve as a criterion for the validity of the analysis performed on the line shape. In this way, for the example given in Fig. 4.7, we get

$$B^L = 0.093 \text{ mWb m}^{-2} \qquad B_e \approx 0.3 \text{ mWb m}^{-2}$$

$$\Delta B^G = 0.17 \text{ mWb m}^{-2}$$

from which it follows that

$$\frac{(\Delta B^G)^2}{\Delta B^L B_e} \approx 1.03$$

In connection with the above method, the following very important condition has to be taken into account. In the case of a paramagnetic sample with strong exchange interaction, the observable part of the line is described essentially by a Lorentzian equation. The directly measurable parameter ΔB^L is a derived value (one and the same value of ΔB^L can originate from different values of the actual parameters ΔB^G and B_e), and thus it cannot serve as a criterion for the character of the interaction within the sample.

Through the determination of the shape of the line and its parameters, it is possible, as we have shown above, to substitute an analytical method for the graphical integration, which considerably reduces the possible error in the concentration measurement. Nevertheless, there are still many more possible sources of error—inaccuracy in the measurement of signal amplitude, inhomogeneity of the microwave field, errors in the positioning of the sample and standard in the cavity, inhomogeneity of the high frequency modulation field, saturation of the signal, and instability of the magnetic field, to mention but a few. A detailed analysis of all these errors, carried out by Molin,[1] shows that even for a known line shape, the error of an absolute measurement of concentration can reach ± 40 per cent. Comparative measurements can be made with an accuracy of ± 15 to ± 20

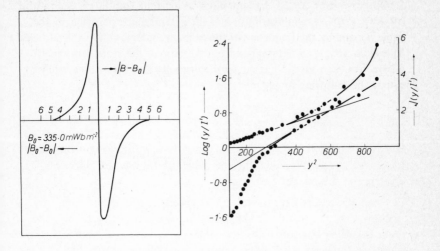

Fig. 4.7. Analysis of an isolated line with exchange interaction, by the method of linear anamorphosis.

per cent. It would appear to us that in the present state of the art of experimental techniques, statements which claim a higher accuracy do not make sense.

References

1. Molin, Ju. N.: *Diss. Inst. f. Chem. Kinet. u. Brennst. Sib. Abt. Akad. Wiss. USSR Nowosibirsk* (1961).
2. Van-Vleck, J. H.: *Phys. Rev.*, 74 (1948), 1168.
3. Tichomirowa, N. N., Voevodski, V. V.: *Optika i Spektroskopija*, 7 (1959), 829.
4. Van-Vleck, J. H.: *Nuovo Cimento*, 6 (1957), 1081.

Chapter 5

Asymmetric E.S.R. Lines

The symmetric E.S.R. lines considered in the last chapter are obtained only in cases where the crystalline field is negligibly small, or where it exhibits spherical symmetry, i.e. for $g_x = g_y = g_z$. In the general case the influence of the crystalline field can lead to the formation of a fine structure, as we saw in Chapter 3, and to dependence of the position of the line on the orientation of the electric crystal axis with respect to the static magnetic field. We will consider first the cases where the position of the E.S.R. line is dependent on orientation although it has no fine structure, i.e. the separation between neighbouring Zeeman levels is equal (for example, this case is automatically fulfilled for $S = \frac{1}{2}$). We will limit ourselves to the analysis of lines in crystalline fields of axial symmetry, i.e. in the case $g_x = g_y = g_\perp$, $g_z = g_\parallel$. It was shown in Chapter 3 that for an arbitrary orientation of the crystal in the magnetic field, the observed g-factor and transition probability $W(g)$ could be determined from the following formulae:

$$g = (g_\perp^2 \sin^2 \theta + g_\parallel^2 \cos^2 \theta)^{1/2} \tag{5.1}$$

and

$$W(g) \approx \frac{1}{2} g_\perp^2 \left[\left(\frac{g_\parallel}{g} \right)^2 + 1 \right] \tag{5.2}$$

Here θ is the angle between the electric crystalline axis and the direction of the static magnetic field.

In this chapter we will give the methods for the determination of the values $g_\parallel$ and $g_\perp$ for single crystals and polycrystalline samples, and also a method for the calculation of the width and shape of the true E.S.R. lines from the asymmetric lines obtained from measurement of the E.S.R. spectrum of a polycrystalline sample.

§5.1

SINGLE CRYSTALS WITH AXIAL SYMMETRY

In a single crystal the directions of the electric axes of all lattice units coincide with the paramagnetic centres, and as a result of this, the angles θ

for all centres of a particular type are equal. Thus at an arbitrary orientation of the crystal with respect to the magnetic field, there is one single symmetric line, the shape of which is described by the same laws as the symmetric lines considered in the last chapter.

We will consider the simplest possible case, that in which the crystalline symmetry coincides with the symmetry of a rotational ellipsoid. Here, there are two limiting values of the g-factor: $g_\parallel$ and $g_\perp$, where $g_\parallel$ corresponds to the parallel orientation of the crystal axis with respect to the magnetic field ($\theta = 0$), and $g_\perp$ to the perpendicular orientation ($\theta = \pi/2$).

It is clear from the above that for values of θ between 0 and $\pi/2$, the symmetric resonance line corresponding to equation (5.1) lies between the two limiting positions. The intensity of these lines, which is proportional to the transition probability $W(\theta)$ and the number n of paramagnetic particles in the sample, may be expressed by the equation

$$S(\theta) = \alpha . n . W(\theta) = \frac{\alpha n}{2} g_\perp^2 \left[1 + \frac{1}{1 + \left(\dfrac{g_\perp^2}{g_\parallel^2} - 1 \right) \sin^2 \theta} \right] \qquad (5.3)$$

By changing from θ to g with the help of equation (5.1), we find

$$S(g) = \frac{\alpha n}{2} g_\perp^2 \left(\frac{g_\parallel^2}{g^2} + 1 \right) \qquad (5.4)$$

Here, $S(\theta)$ and $S(g)$ are the integral values of the intensity of the individual lines at specific values of θ and g respectively. From Chapter 4, the following equation holds:

$$S(g) = I_{(g)}^{max} \Delta B_{1/2} \rho \qquad (5.5)$$

where $I_{(g)}^{max}$ is the intensity at the maximum of the absorption line, $\Delta B_{1/2}$ the half width and ρ a numerical form factor.

Equations (5.4) and (5.5) can be used for the determination of the total number of particles n. The calibration follows the procedure as in Chapter 4, except for a correction relative to the position of the line, which brings in another factor $\frac{1}{2} g_\perp^2 (g_\parallel^2/g^2 + 1)$. This correction, however, only has a meaning for very large values of the difference $(g_\perp - g_\parallel)$. In the case of Cr^{3+} ions in the MgO lattice,[1] with $g_\parallel = 1.980$ and $g_\perp = 1.986$, the difference $(g_\perp - g_\parallel)$ is very small, and the change in line intensity in the single crystal on going from the parallel to the perpendicular orientation is expressed by the factor $2(1 + g_\parallel^2/g_\perp^2)^{-1} = 1.0003$. In the case of the very wide asymmetric line of copper acetate, $(g_\parallel - g_\perp) = 0.34$,[2] and the corresponding value of the correction factor is 0.87.

The problem of measuring $g_\perp$ and $g_\parallel$ in a single crystal can be solved experimentally if the crystal can be oriented at will with respect to the magnetic field. In principle there are many ways of rotating the crystal. Experimentally, it is very simple to carry out such a rotation about an axis which lies in a plane perpendicular to the magnetic field. To place the crystal in an arbitrary orientation, we must be able to rotate it about two mutually perpendicular axes lying in this plane. To do this, we usually resort to the technique of rotating the crystal about the axis of the sample holder, and also to the rotation of the magnet.† If the crystal has a distinct crystallographic alignment, we can, in general, restrict ourselves to a rotation about one single axis. If this is done a sufficient number of times, then we obtain the values of $g_\perp$ and $g_\parallel$ corresponding to the limiting positions.

It follows from the arguments which we are presenting that the larger the *g*-factor of a line, the smaller the intensity of that line. But from this it cannot be concluded which of the two limiting values of *g* corresponds to $g_\perp$ and which to $g_\parallel$. If we consider the simplest case, this problem can be solved if the measurements are carried out in the following way. Firstly, the crystal must be oriented in the magnetic field so that we obtain one of the two limiting positions of the absorption line. Naturally this position may correspond to either parallel or perpendicular orientation of the electric crystal axis with respect to the magnetic field. We then rotate the crystal about one of the two chosen rotation axes (see above) through $\pi/2$, and after returning it to the initial position, rotate it about the same angle with respect to the other axis. If in both cases we obtain identical *g*-values, which are equal to the other limiting value, then the electric crystal axis in the initial state is oriented parallel to the magnetic field, and the position of the observed line corresponds to $g_\parallel$.

If on rotation about both axes, different positions of the line are obtained, or if they are equal but do not correspond to the other limiting position, then this means that at the initial state the line is observed at $g_\perp$. Analogous reasoning can also be used if after the establishment of the first limiting position, the second has to be found. For this, it suffices to rotate the crystal with respect to one of the rotation axes through $\pi/2$ and then, without reversal, to rotate the crystal into the original position about the second axis until the limiting position of the line is reached, which then corresponds to the second limiting value of *g*.

† In the following section, for simplicity, we will talk about the rotation of the crystal about two mutually perpendicular axes.

§5.2

ASYMMETRIC E.S.R. LINES IN POLYCRYSTALS: METHOD FOR THE DETERMINATION OF $g_\perp$ AND $g_\parallel$

The term polycrystal in this section covers the following cases:

(*a*) Polycrystalline powder, which consists of a large number of randomly distributed single crystals, each acting in its own right as a single crystal.

(*b*) Amorphous bodies, in which the anisotropy of the *g*-factor results from the anisotropy of the individual molecule, or from the complexes formed between the molecule in question and the molecules of the solvent.

In all these cases, we will assume an even distribution of the orientations of the microcrystals (molecules).

The E.S.R. spectrum of the polycrystal is formed by the overlapping of a large number of individual symmetric lines, the positions of which are determined by the orientation of the individual microcrystals (molecules) with respect to the magnetic field. The intensity of the envelope at each of its points is determined by the number of particles having that particular orientation, and by the transition probability as determined from equations (5.2) and (5.4).

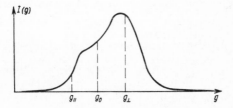

Fig. 5.1. Asymmetric line $I(g)$.

The number of particles for which the angle between the electric axis and the direction of the magnetic field lies between the values θ and $\theta + d\theta$, is

$$dn(\theta) = n \sin \theta \; d\theta \tag{5.6}$$

or, as a function of g,

$$dn(g) = \frac{n}{\sqrt{(g_\perp^2 - g_\parallel^2)}} \cdot \frac{g\,dg}{\sqrt{(g_\perp^2 - g^2)}} \qquad (5.7)$$

where n is the total number of particles.

The actual problem is to find the dependence of the absorption intensity I of the polycrystalline spectrum on the magnetic induction, i.e. the function $I(g)$ (Fig. 5.1).†

The intensity at any point, e.g. for g_0, is obtained by the overlapping of all lines from $g_\parallel$ to $g_\perp$. We will consider first the line whose centre coincides with g_0. To be more precise, this is actually the group of lines which lie between $g_0 + \frac{1}{2}dg$ and $g_0 - \frac{1}{2}dg$. The total number of lines comprising this group, is, from equation (5.7).

$$dn(g_0) = \frac{n}{\sqrt{(g_\perp^2 - g_\parallel^2)}} \cdot \frac{g_0\,dg}{\sqrt{(g_\perp^2 - g_0^2)}} \qquad (5.8)$$

The probability for the absorption of high frequency energy at $g = g_0$ is proportional to

$$P(g_0) = \frac{1}{2}\,g_\perp^2 \left(\frac{g_\parallel^2}{g_0^2} + 1 \right) \qquad (5.9)$$

The group of particles in question thus gives a symmetric E.S.R. line with its centre at g_0 and an integrated intensity

$$dS(g_0) = \alpha P(g_0)\,dn(g_0) = Kn\,\frac{g_\parallel^2 + g_0^2}{g_0} \cdot \frac{dg}{\sqrt{(g_\perp^2 - g_0^2)}} \qquad (5.10)$$

Here K is a constant which is dependent upon the spectrometer characteristics and the values of $g_\parallel$ and $g_\perp$.

Equation (5.10) can be considerably simplified if we take into account that in the majority of cases $(g_\perp - g_\parallel) \ll g_\perp, g_\parallel$. With $g_\parallel < g_0 < g_\perp$, (5.10) becomes

$$dS(g_0) = K'n\,\frac{dg}{\sqrt{(g_\perp - g_0)}} \qquad (5.11)$$

with $K' = K\sqrt{(2g_\perp)}$.

---

† In this calculation and the resulting arguments, we assume that $g_\perp > g_\parallel$, and correspondingly $B_\parallel > B_\perp$, although the calculations are also valid for the opposite condition. One should note that in the case of the anisotropic line of a polycrystal, in contrast to that of the single crystal, the sign of the inequality $g_\perp \gtrless g_\parallel$ follows directly from the appearance of the spectrum: the line intensity in the vicinity of $g_\perp$ is always larger than in the vicinity of $g_\parallel$.

The development of the analysis from here depends essentially on how large is the anistropy of the g-factor, i.e. on the value of $\delta = (B_\| - B_\perp)/\Delta B_{1/2}$. In the case of $\delta \gg 1$ (strong anistropy) the shape of the envelope in the entire interval $g_\| < g_0 < g_\perp$ will be independent of the shape of the individual line. Such a dependence is observed only on the edges of the asymmetric line in the region close to $g_\perp$ and $g_\|$ (see below). In the case of $\delta \ll 1$ (weak anisotropy), the shape of the individual line is the determining factor for the entire interval $g_\perp - g_\|$.

In the first case, the calculation can be performed by neglecting lines of arbitrary shape; in the second case a solution consistent for the whole envelope is possible only for a Lorentzian line, as is shown in reference 3.

We will now consider the condition $\delta \gg 1$ in more detail. In equation (5.11) we will substitute the value $g_\perp$ for all factors of the same order of magnitude, i.e. $g_\|$, g_0 and g. The differential intensity of the group of lines which is produced by the $dS(g_0)$ particles at a point B between $B_\|$ and $B_\perp$ is equal to

$$d\mathscr{I}(B, g_0) = \frac{q}{\Delta B_{1/2}} f\left(\frac{(B - B_0)^2}{\Delta B_{1/2}^2}\right) dS(g_0) \tag{5.12}$$

Here q is a shape-dependent numerical factor, and f the function describing the shape of the individual line.

For reasons of clarity we will consider a Gaussian line. This will make a detailed analysis of the edges of the asymmetric line somewhat easier for us. In this case we obtain from (5.12), with g as variable, for the contribution of a line with its centre at g_0 and with an ordinate on the curve at a point g:

$$d\mathscr{I}(g, g_0) = \frac{k''n}{\sqrt{(g_\perp - g_0)}}\, e^{-\gamma^2 (g - g_0)^2}\, dg \tag{5.13}$$

with

$$k'' = \frac{\alpha g_\perp^2}{0{\cdot}6\sqrt{\pi}\sqrt{(g_\perp - g_\|)}\,\Delta B_{1/2}}$$

$$\gamma = \frac{h\nu}{0{\cdot}6\,\Delta B_{1/2}\,\beta g_\perp^2}$$

At the point $g = g_0$, the contribution of the group of lines in question will be

$$d\mathscr{I}(g_0, g_0) = k''n \frac{dg}{\sqrt{(g_\perp - g_0)}} \tag{5.14}$$

In order to find the total intensity at the point g_0, we must add to the value of $d\mathscr{I}(g_0,g_0)$ the contributions of all the other lines, the centres of which lie between $g_\parallel$ and $g_\perp$. Here we can use an equation of the type (5.13). From Fig. 5.2 we see that in the calculation of $d\mathscr{I}(g_0,g_1)$, i.e. the contribution of the line with the centre at g_1 to $d\mathscr{I}(g_0)$, g_0 plays the role of the variable coordinate g in (5.13). In other words

$$d\mathscr{I}(g_0,g_1) = \frac{k''n}{\sqrt{(g_\perp - g_1)}}\, e^{-\gamma^2 (g_0 - g_1)^2}\, dg_1 \tag{5.15}$$

For the determination of the total intensity at the point g_0, (5.15) must be integrated with respect of dg_1 from $g_\parallel$ to $g_\perp$.†

From (5.15) it follows that for $g \to g_\perp$, both $d\mathscr{I}(g_0,g)$ and $(g_\perp - g)^{-1/2}$ tend to infinity. However, it can be easily shown that the integral which is of interest to us actually converges. Departures from the range $g \approx g_\perp$ have little effect on the results of our calculations.

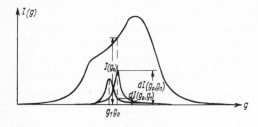

Fig. 5.2. Diagram of the overlapping of components with different g.

Since the function $\mathscr{I}(g_0)$, which describes the anisotropy of the line, changes considerably slower within the interval $g_\perp - g_\parallel$, as the edges of the individual lines fall off, we can with reasonable accuracy substitute g_0 for g in the factor before the exponential function. Thus the slight changes in the contributions of the lines which lie in the immediate vicinity of g_0 are ignored. As these changes are of opposite signs to the left and to the right of g_0, they are also partially self-compensating. For lines further away this error is considerably larger, but it is unimportant, as the rapid decrease of

† In the following calculations we will omit the index 1 in g_1.

the individual lines farther from their centre makes these contributions negligibly small.†

The expression (5.15) now takes the following form:

$$d.\mathscr{I}(g_0, g) = \frac{k''n}{\sqrt{(g_\perp - g_0)}} e^{-\gamma^2(g - g_0)^2} \, dg \tag{5.16}$$

An integration in closed form of this equation over the interval $g_\parallel \leqslant g \leqslant g_\perp$ is not possible. However, in the above situation we can fortunately overcome this difficulty.

We now carry out a substitution of variables:

$$\gamma(g_0 - g) = z$$

Then (5.16) becomes

$$d.\mathscr{I}(g_0, g) = \frac{k''n}{\gamma\sqrt{(g_\perp - g_0)}} e^{-z^2} \, dz \tag{5.17}$$

The function of interest to us, $\mathscr{I}(g_0)$, we obtain by integration of the expression (5.17) from $z(g_\parallel)$ to $z(g_\perp)$, i.e.

$$\mathscr{I}(g_0) = \frac{k''n}{\gamma\sqrt{(g_\perp - g_0)}} \int\limits_{+\gamma(g_0 - g_\parallel)}^{\gamma(g_\perp - g_0)} e^{-z^2} dz \tag{5.18}$$

If g_0 lies in the interval $g_\parallel - g_\perp$, and is not near those limits, and considering that $\delta \gg 1$ and there is a rapid convergence of the Gaussian error integral (as also of corresponding integrals for lines of arbitrary form), then we can replace the integration limits by $+ \infty$, with which we obtain

$$\mathscr{I}(g_0) \approx \lambda \frac{n}{\sqrt{(g_\perp - g_0)}} \tag{5.19}$$

with

$$\lambda = \sqrt{\pi} \frac{k''}{\gamma} = \frac{\alpha g_\perp^4 \beta}{\sqrt{(g_\perp - g_\parallel)} h\nu} \tag{5.20}$$

Equation (5.19) is the basic expression for the shape of the central part of the asymmetric line. As we would expect, the final expression contains neither the character of the line shape nor $\Delta B_{1/2}$, the width at half height.

---

† For this very reason we could assume that for $\delta \gg 1$, the deviations from the calculation in the region $g \approx g_\perp$ operate only on a very small part of the overall line.

Note that for $g_0 = g_\parallel$, the lower limit of the integral in equation (5.18) becomes zero. Thus we obtain

$$\mathscr{I}(g_\parallel) = \frac{\lambda n}{2\sqrt{(g_\perp - g_\parallel)}}$$

a value half as large as that which followed from equation (5.19). This result follows directly from the approximation which we used in the deduction of (5.19). At the point $g_0 = g_\parallel$ the line integral actually results from contributions of lines which lie on one side only of $g_\parallel$ (viz. in the direction of $g_\perp$). For the derivation of (5.19) it was assumed, however, that lines lying on both sides of g_0 contributed to the total intensity. Thus according to (5.19), the calculation gives a value of $I(g_\parallel)$, which is twice as large as the actual value.

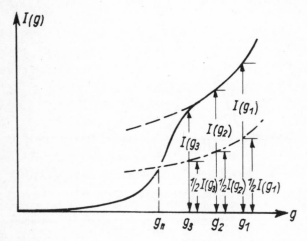

Fig. 5.3. Graph for the determination of $g_\parallel$ from the sloping edges of an asymmetric absorption line.

On the basis of the above argument, the following simple procedure can be given for the approximate determination of $g_\parallel$ from the asymmetrical absorption line (assuming δ is sufficiently large). To do this, it is necessary to extrapolate the central part of the curve over the limits of the experimental line (Fig. 5.3, dashed line). We also draw on the same graph a line whose ordinates are half those of the original line (dashed and dotted line). The point where this curve crosses the experimental line must lie in the vicinity of the value $g_\parallel$, as precisely at this point the actual ordinate is half the ordinate calculated from equation (5.19) (the actual contribution from the right and the fictitious one from the left are equal in size).

In the region near $g_\perp$, equation (5.19) is no longer valid, since

$$(g_\perp - g_0)^{-1/2} \to \infty$$

To derive the true line shape for a small range of values of g_0 in the vicinity of $g_\perp$, we can put $\exp[-\gamma^2(g - g_0)^2] \approx 1$, and integrate only the function $(g - g_0)^{-1/2}$, which in principle does not present any difficulties. But since the interval in question is very small, we can consider this edge of the line in the same way as the region in the vicinity of $g_\parallel$. The

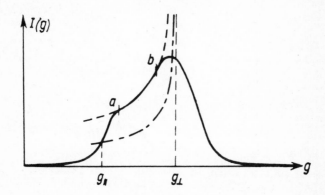

Fig. 5.4. Diagram of an asymmetric absorption line for the approximate calculation of $g_\perp$.

value of $g_\perp$ can be determined with sufficient accuracy by means of the same extrapolation of the central part of the curve (Fig. 5.4).

Another approximate method for the determination of $g_\parallel$ and $g_\perp$ is based on the analysis of the central part of the asymmetric line (in the region ab in Fig. 5.4). Over this interval, equation (5.19) must be valid, and therefore the following linear relation must be fulfilled:

$$\frac{1}{[\mathscr{I}(g_0)]^2} = \frac{1}{(\lambda n)^2}(g_\perp - g_0) \tag{5.21}$$

If we plot $[\mathscr{I}(g_0)]^{-2}$ as a function of g_0, we can determine $g_\perp$ and λn. If n, $g_\perp$ and α are known, $g_\parallel$ can be obtained from equation (5.20).

The second method which we will give is also suitable for the calculation of $g_\perp$ and $g_\parallel$ from the curve of the first derivative. It follows from (5.19) that the range $a'b'$ of the spectrum in the coordinates $\mathscr{I}' = f(g_0)$ (Fig. 5.5) is described by the following equation:

$$\mathscr{I}'(g_0) = \frac{\lambda n}{2} (g_\perp - g_0)^{-3/2} \qquad (5.22)$$

From this it follows that the graph of $[\mathscr{I}'(g_0)]^{-2/3} = f(g_0)$ in the range $a'b'$ must be a straight line, the parameters of which will again give $g_\perp$ and λn.

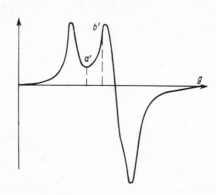

Fig. 5.5. Curve of the first derivative of an asymmetric absorption line.

In order to verify that it is possible to apply expressions (5.21) and (5.22) in the determination of $g_\perp$, our young scientific colleague in ICK, W. K. Yermolayev, recorded, at our request, the E.S.R. spectra of (I) polycrystalline $CuSO_4 . 5H_2O$ and (II) the peroxide radical $\sim CF_2 - CF(O\dot{O})-CF_2 \sim$ (irradiated Teflon), for which the values of $g_\perp$ are known from other measurements.[4,5]

Figure 5.6 shows the linear anamorphosis of the central part of the absorption curve of the sample (I) in coordinates $\mathscr{I}^{-2} = f(g_0)$. The extrapolation of the central part gives $g_\perp = 2.26 \pm 0.02$. According to reference 4, $g_\perp = 2.27$.

Figure 5.7 shows a series of anamorphoses of the curves $\mathscr{I}'(g)$ for the peroxide radical (II) in the coordinates $\mathscr{I}(g_0)^{-2/3} = f(g_0)$. The average value of $g_\perp$ obtained was 2.0193 ± 0.0002. From reference 5 we get $g_\perp = 2.023 \pm 0.005$.

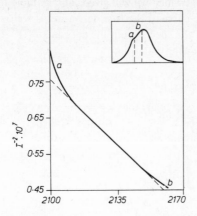

Fig. 5.6. Linear anamorphosis of the central part of the asymmetric absorption line of polycrystalline $CuSo_4 \cdot 5H_2O_4$

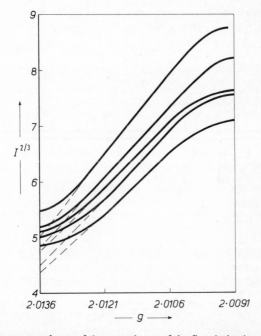

Fig. 5.7. Linear anamorphoses of the central part of the first derivative of the peroxide radical $\sim CF_2 - CF - CF_2 \sim$
$$\underset{\displaystyle O-O}{\mid}$$

It follows from these examples, that with the aid of the graphical method given, $g_\perp$ can actually be determined with reasonable accuracy. The calculation of $g_\parallel$ (or $g_\perp - g_\parallel$) was not performed during these preliminary experiments. It will be clear that in order to determine this value, it is necessary to record the curves with the greatest possible accuracy, in order to reduce the error on applying equation (5.20). Such an accuracy could only be obtained by systematic measurements of the values $g_\perp$ and $g_\parallel$ for different samples under identical conditions, and comparison with samples for which $g_\perp$ and $g_\parallel$ are known from other measurements.

§5.3

DETERMINATION OF THE TRUE LINE WIDTH FROM THE SHAPE OF THE ASYMMETRIC LINE

We will now look into the problem of the possibility of finding $\Delta B_{1/2}$ of the single line from the information obtained from a polycrystalline sample. We will first consider the case $\delta \gg 1$ and assume that the line has Gaussian shape.

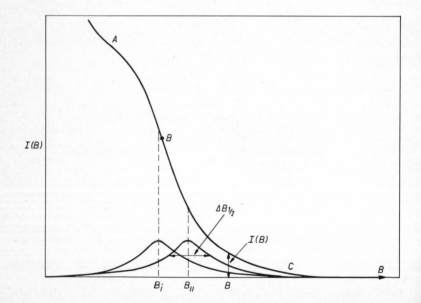

Fig. 5.8. Diagram of the edge of an asymmetric absorption line.

The principle of the calculation can be easily understood from Fig. 5.8 which shows the side ABC of the asymmetric absorption line in the vicinity of $B_\parallel$, and on which individual groups of lines are drawn, corresponding to equal intervals dB. As before, we will neglect the amplitude variation on the sloping edges (this is another assumption in our basic approach). The contribution of the line centred at B_i to the amplitude $I(B)$ at the point B is

$$d\mathscr{I}(B) = I_0\, e^{-(B-B_i)^2/0\cdot36(\Delta B_{1/2}^G)^2}\, dB_i$$

The total amplitude at point B, which consists of the contributions of all lines with $B_i < B_\parallel$ is equal to

$$\mathscr{I}(B) = I_0 \int\limits_{B_i = B_\parallel}^{B_i = B_\perp} e^{-(B-B_i)^2/0\cdot36(\Delta B_{1/2}^G)^2}\, dB_i$$

or if we introduce

$$z = \frac{B - B_i}{0\cdot6\,\Delta B_{1/2}^G}$$

$$\mathscr{I}(B) = 0\cdot6\,\Delta B_{1/2}^G\, I_0 \int\limits_{z_\parallel}^{z_\perp} e^{-z^2}\, dz \tag{5.23}$$

with

$$z_\parallel = \frac{B - B_\parallel}{0\cdot6\,\Delta B_{1/2}^G}$$

$$z_\perp = \frac{B - B_\perp}{0\cdot6\,\Delta B_{1/2}^G} \tag{5.24}$$

As $B - B_\parallel \ll B_\parallel - B_\perp$ for $\delta \gg 1$, then $z_\perp \gg z_\parallel$, and we can write

$$\mathscr{I}(B) \approx 0\cdot6\,\Delta B_{1/2}^G\, I_0 \int\limits_{z_\parallel}^{\infty} e^{-z^2}\, dz$$

$$= 0\cdot3\sqrt{\pi}\,\Delta B_{1/2}^G\, I_0 \left(1 - \frac{2}{\sqrt{\pi}} \int\limits_{0}^{z_\parallel} e^{-z^2}\, dz\right) \tag{5.25}$$

It should also be noted that $Z_\parallel = 0$ at the point $B = B_\parallel$, and from this, $\mathscr{I}(B) = 0\cdot3\sqrt{\pi}\,\Delta B_{1/2}^G I_0$. Thus it follows that for $B \geqslant B_\parallel$

$$\mathscr{I}(B) = \mathscr{I}(B_\parallel) \left(1 - \frac{2}{\sqrt{\pi}} \int\limits_{0}^{z_\parallel} e^{-z^2}\, dz\right) \tag{5.26}$$

We can now determine the value of $\Delta B_{1/2}^{G}$ in the following way. We choose a certain value of B on the side of the asymmetric line, for which $\mathscr{I}(B) < \mathscr{I}(B_{\parallel})$. From this we can find $1 - \mathscr{I}(B)/\mathscr{I}(B_{\parallel})$, which, by (5.26), has the following value:

$$\frac{2}{\sqrt{\pi}} \int_{0}^{z_{\parallel}} e^{-z^2} \, dz$$

From tables of the error integral we find the corresponding value of $Z_{\parallel}$, and from equation (5.24) we can determine $\Delta B_{1/2}^{G}$. If the values of $\Delta B_{1/2}^{G}$ agree for the different values of B, then this implies that the line shape really follows the Gaussian law. This solution can of course also be performed graphically.

We also want to consider how the above deductions change the individual lines in the case of the Lorentzian shape. We have already seen that the central part of the line is described by precisely the same numerical factors for both Gaussian and Lorentzian laws. The values of $g_{\perp}$ and $g_{\parallel}$ can also be determined by the methods described above. The only difference is in the determination of $\Delta B_{1/2}$ from the sides of the line. Here, equation (5.26) is modified as follows:

$$\mathscr{I}(B) = \mathscr{I}(B_{\parallel}) \left(1 - \frac{2}{\pi} \arctan \frac{B - B_{\parallel}}{0 \cdot 5 \, \Delta B_{1/2}^{L}} \right) \tag{5.27}$$

The calculation of $\Delta B_{1/2}^{L}$ from this equation does not present any difficulty.

However, we must also consider the fact that the edges of a Lorentzian line often change to the Gaussian shape (as discussed in Chapter 4). Since each ordinate of the edge of an asymmetric line is composed of different parts of individual lines, so equation (5.27) is, in general, only valid close to $B_{\parallel}$, so long as the main contribution to $\mathscr{I}(B)$ results from parts of lines which are of Lorentzian shape. From the above, it is clear that the anamorphosis method for the determination of ν_e from the sides of an asymmetric line (see Chapter 4) is not applicable in the general case. Nevertheless, one can calculate this transition region, if only approximately, by means of other suitable methods.

All of our calculations are related to the case of strong anisotropy (as has already been pointed out), for which $\delta = (B_{\parallel} - B_{\perp})/\Delta B_{1/2} \gg 1$. The above equations are not applicable to the analysis of lines with weak anisotropy, for which $\delta \leqslant 1$. However, these cases are of less interest to us, since the lineshape is approximately symmetrical. In principle one can formulate equations which allow analysis of lines with arbitrary δ, on the basis of the paper by Tschirkov and Kokin,[3] in which are given the values of the function $\mathscr{I}(B)$ for an asymmetric Lorentzian curve for various different parameters.†

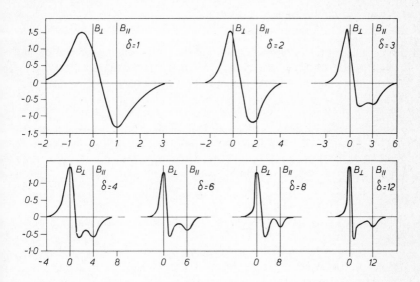

Fig. 5.9. Asymmetric E.S.R. line (computer calculations).

Using this method of calculation, Lebedev[6] has given a new method for the determination of the parameters of an asymmetric line for which the only available plot is in derivative form. He showed that the derivative of an asymmetric line can be characterized by three experimental parameters, ΔB^*, A and A', and he calculated curves which connect these parameters with $B_\parallel$, $B_\perp$ and $\Delta B_{1/2}$, the main characteristic values of an asymmetric line. By the use of these curves, he also calculated the characteristic data of the E.S.R. signal from a peroxide radical in irradiated Teflon (see Chapter 9).

† In the work cited, the calculations were also carried out for larger values of δ (up to $\delta = 24$), but as the calculations are rather complex, we considered it more useful to use the simpler method presented above.

To end this section, we would like to mention the calculations recently carried out by Lebedev at IPC, in which he used an electronic computer to determine the shapes of asymmetric E.S.R. lines for various values of δ. The curves shown in Fig. 5.9 demonstrate that for $\delta \geqslant 5$, the values of $g_\parallel$ and $g_\perp$ can be determined directly from the position of the maximum and minimum of the curve $\mathscr{I}(B)$, to within an accuracy of 5 to 10 per cent relative to Δg. If $g_\parallel$ and $g_\perp$ are calculated in this way, then $\Delta B_{1/2}$ can be calculated from the value of A (or A').

§5.4

LINE SHAPES OF PARTIALLY ORIENTED POLYCRYSTALS WITH AXIAL SYMMETRY

All that we have said so far has been concerned with polycrystals with completely random orientation of the symmetry axes of the individual crystals with respect to the external magnetic field. However, for the solution of many problems it is worthwhile to consider the case of partially oriented polycrystals, in which the axes of the individual anisotropic centres exhibit a preferred direction, but nevertheless without the degree of order of the single crystal being attained. In this case there is naturally a dependence of the spectrum shape on the orientation of the sample in the magnetic field.

A rigorous solution to this problem demands that we know the angular distribution of the orientations in equation (5.3). Thus the calculation becomes even more complex. For some particularly important cases of this type we can, however, apply a qualitative analysis of the E.S.R. lines without going into detailed calculations. Such an analysis has been carried out by Lebedev, Shidomirov and Zvetkov.[7] These authors considered the E.S.R. spectra of partially oriented chain molecules, with the paramagnetism arising from a free radical, the symmetry axes of which lie either parallel or perpendicular to the chain axes.

It may be assumed that the E.S.R. spectrum of such a sample does not differ appreciably from the hypothetical spectrum, which would give a mechanical mixture of a completely oriented and a completely disoriented phase. As it is presumably impossible to determine accurately the 'composition' of such a mixture, all the final results following from this model have a distinctly qualitative character. Nonetheless, as we shall now see, this model can be a great help in the analysis of the spectra.

We will consider a sample which consists of partially oriented chain molecules with paramagnetic centres, the axes of which ($\vec{\mu}$) lie perpendicular to the chain axis $(\vec{K})$. Let the preferred orientation of the chains $(\vec{L})$ be perpendicular to the direction of the constant magnetic field (B). In accordance with the above, we can represent the spectrum of such a sample as a superposition of E.S.R. lines of randomly oriented chains upon the E.S.R. of a 'single crystal' made up of chains accurately oriented in the preferred direction $(\vec{K} \parallel \vec{L})$. The E.S.R. line of the random phase is in this case the usual asymmetric line with its maximum close to $g_\perp$.

The oriented phase can be represented schematically in the following way:

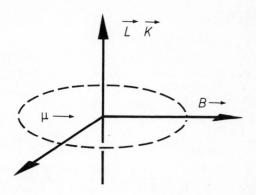

It can be seen quite clearly that in the given phase, orientations of $\vec{\mu}$ appear perpendicular as well as parallel to $\vec{B}$; whilst in the random phase all orientations are equally probable. The E.S.R. of the oriented phase is therefore symmetrical about its centre, and can easily be shown to have two maxima in the vicinity of the points $g_\perp$ and $g_\parallel$. In Fig. 5.10 are shown the integral and differential curves of the E.S.R. lines in the random (a) and oriented (b) phases.

Figure 5.11c shows the superposition of both these spectra (for an arbitrary choice of the ratio of oriented to random phase of approximately 1:1). It is not difficult to carry out such an analysis for other mutual orientations of $\vec{K}, \vec{\mu}$ and $\vec{B}$. The results of this analysis are shown in Fig. 5.11. As can be seen from this figure, very different lineshapes are possible with parallel oriented samples, varying from an almost completely symmetrical singlet to a doublet.

As an example we will consider the E.S.R. spectrum of a stretched sample of the polymer polytetrafluoroethylene (Teflon), which has been exposed to γ-irradiation in air. Under these conditions the peroxide radical ROȮ is formed (see Chapter 9).

Figure 5.12 shows the E.S.R. lines at room temperature of (*a*) a disoriented sample, (*b*) a sample oriented for $\vec{L} \perp \vec{B}$, and (*c*) a sample for which $\vec{L} \parallel \vec{B}$. From a comparison of Figs. 5.11 and 5.12, we can see that the experimental spectra agree with the theoretical spectra for $\vec{\mu} \parallel \vec{K}$. From this we come to the important conclusion, that at room temperature the axis of the peroxide radical in irradiated Teflon lies parallel to the axis of the polymer chain.

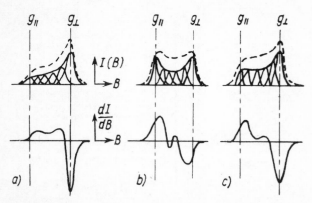

Fig. 5.10. Integral and differential curves of E.S.R. lines in the random (*a*) and oriented (*b*) phase for the case $\vec{K} \parallel \vec{L}$; (*c*) complete line for $a{:}b = 1{:}1$.

It has already been pointed out that the above arguments are only valid in the case of an axial symmetry for which the two limiting values of the *g*-factor are given by $g_x = g_y = g_\perp$ and $g_z = g_\parallel$. Many real samples come close to this ideal case. An example of a system in which all the three values of *g* differ greatly from each other, is that of $K_2\,Cu(SO_4)_2 \cdot 6D_2O$,[8] where

$$g_x = 2\cdot16 \qquad g_y = 2\cdot04 \qquad g_z = 2\cdot42$$

Other examples may be found in the monograph of S.A. Altschuler and B. M. Kozyrev.[9] The calculation of the function $\mathscr{I}(B)$ in the case of three different *g*-values was also carried out in the work of Tschirkov and Kokin.[3] The determination of g_x, g_y and g_z for single crystals can be carried out in the same way as described above, provided of course that one can rotate the sample independently about three mutually perpendicular axes.

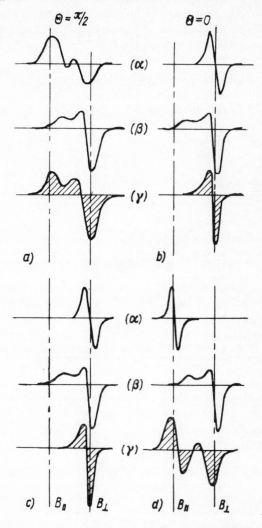

Fig. 5.11. Differential E.S.R. lineshapes for the oriented (α) and the random(β) phase, and the complete line (γ) for the cases:

$$(a)\ \vec{K} \perp \vec{\mu}, \vec{B} \qquad (b)\ \vec{K} \perp \vec{\mu}, \vec{K} \parallel \vec{B}$$
$$(c)\ \vec{K} \parallel \vec{\mu}, \vec{K} \perp \vec{B} \qquad (d)\ \vec{K} \parallel \vec{L}, \vec{B}$$

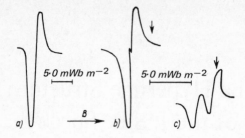

Fig. 5.12. E.S.R. spectra of the peroxide radicals in irradiated Teflon at room temperature

        (*a*) unstretched samples
        (*b*) samples stretched perpendicular to *B*
        (*c*) samples stretched parallel to *B*

The arrows indicate the positions of the absorption line of DPPH.

References

1. Low, W.: *Phys. Rev.,* **105** (1957), 801.
2. Bleaney, B., Bowers, K. D.: *Proc. Roy. Soc.,* **A 214** (1952), 451.
3. Tschirkov, W. K., Kokin, A. A.: *J. exp. theor. Phy.,* **39** (1960) 1381.
4. Sundaramma, K.: *Proc. Ind. Acad. Sci.,* **A 46** (1957), 232.
5. Molin, Ju. N., Zvetkov, Ju. D.: *J. phys. Chem., Moscow,* **33** (1959) 1668.
6. Lebedev, Ja. S., Zvetkov, Ju. D.: Shidomirow, G. M.: *Z. strukt. Chimii* **3** (1962), 21.
7. Lebedev, Ja. S.: *Ž. strukt. Chimii,* **3** (1962), 151.
8. Bleaney, B., Bowers, K. D., Ingram, D. J.: *Proc. roy. Soc.,* **A 228** (1955), 147.
9. Altschuler, S. A., Kosyrev, B. M.: *Paramagnetische Elektronenresonanz* (Electron Paramagnetic Resonance), Leipzig 1963.

Chapter 6

The Hyperfine Structure
of the E.S.R. Spectra

BASIC CHARACTERISTICS OF THE H.F.S. FORMED BY
INTERACTION WITH A MAGNETIC NUCLEUS

In Chapter 3 we considered the theoretical aspects of the origin of the
H.F.S. in E.S.R. spectra, which is caused by the interaction of the unpaired
electron with nuclear magnetic moments. In this chapter we propose to
give methods for the analysis of E.S.R. spectra with H.F.S., and we will
show, with concrete examples, what information a chemist can glean from
such an analysis. E.S.R. spectra with H.F.S. may be characterized by the
following four parameters: the number of components, their intensity
ratio, the magnitude of the splitting, and the width of the individual
components.

First, we will consider the simplest case, that in which the H.F.S. of the
E.S.R. spectrum is produced by radicals of one type. We will assume that
the individual H.F.S. components are completely symmetrical, and that
the measurements are carried out under conditions which are well below
saturation.

The simplest E.S.R. spectra to analyse are those in which the unpaired
electron is localized directly on the nucleus having the magnetic moment.
Fig. 6.1 shows the E.S.R. spectra of atomic hydrogen (*a*) and atomic
deuterium (*b*). As can be seen, the spectrum of the hydrogen atom consists
of two lines. For an understanding of this spectrum, we can limit ourselves
to a simple qualitative argument, which is quite adequate in interpreting
the E.S.R. spectra of not only the hydrogen atom, but also considerably
more complicated radicals. For this we need only consider the well-known
fact that the spin reversal time of a nucleus in a magnetic field is
considerably greater than the corresponding time for the electron. This
means that in observing the reversal process of the electron spin at absorp-

tion of the microwave quantum, the direction of the nuclear magnetic moment can be considered as fixed. The spin of the proton is known to be equal to $\frac{1}{2}$. Thus if we neglect the small correction caused by the Boltzmann factor, we can assume that 50 per cent of the nuclear magnetic moments are parallel to the external magnetic field, and 50 per cent are antiparallel to it.†

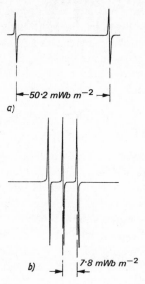

Fig. 6.1. E.S.R. spectrum of (*a*) the hydrogen atom, and (*b*) the deuterium atom.

The effective induction acting on the unpaired electron is in the first case equal to $B + \frac{1}{2}\Delta B$, and in the second case to $B - \frac{1}{2}\Delta B$. Here $\frac{1}{2}\Delta B$ is the additional induction caused by the magnetic moment of the proton. As the resonance transition of the electron occurs at the effective induction $B_0 = h\nu/g\beta$, this particular case leads to the observation of resonance for the first 50 per cent of the atoms at the external induction field $B_0 - \frac{1}{2}\Delta B$, and for the second 50 per cent at $B_0 + \frac{1}{2}\Delta B$.

The total E.S.R. spectrum of the hydrogen atom must therefore consist of a doublet with components of equal intensity which are equidistant from the E.S.R. line of the free electron. Thus it follows that the

† We may neglect the deviation of the distribution of the nuclear magnetic moment from the equilibrium state only in the case of E.S.R. spectra. For nuclear magnetic resonance, it is this very deviation which creates the spectra.

magnitude of the splitting ΔB_{HFS} is determined by the interaction between the magnetic moments of the nucleus and the electron, and is consequently not dependent on the strength of the external magnetic field, i.e. on the observation frequency.†

In a similar way, the analysis of the E.S.R. spectrum of atomic deuterium does not present any problems. The nuclear spin of deuterium is $I = 1$, and in an external magnetic field its magnetic moment has $2I + 1 = 3$ orientations, for which the projections of the moment in the direction of the magnetic field are equal to 1, 0 and -1. Since the statistical probabilities of all three states are the same, the spectrum consists of a triplet with equidistant components of equal intensity, the central line coinciding with the E.S.R. line of the free electron. The magnitude of the splitting, i.e. the separation between neighbouring components (ΔB_{HFS}) , is 50.2 mWb m^{-2} for hydrogen and 7.8 mWb m^{-2} for deuterium. These large values of ΔB arise from the fact that the unpaired electron in the hydrogen atom is described by a pure s-function and is localized at one single nucleus. From this it follows that ΔB_{HFS} is single-valued and determined by the magnetic moment of the nucleus. In full agreement with this, we get:

$$\frac{\Delta B_H}{\Delta B_D} = \frac{50.2}{7.8} = 6.44 \approx \frac{\gamma_H}{\gamma_D} = \frac{\mu_H}{I_H} : \frac{\mu_D}{I_D} = 2\frac{\mu_H}{\mu_D} = 2\frac{2.79}{0.86} = 6.48$$

where γ is the gyromagnetic ratio of the nuclei (analogous to the g-factor of the electrons).

The absolute value of the splitting for the hydrogen atom can be calculated theoretically on the basis of the equation for the contact interaction (see Chapter 3). Such calculations are in good agreement with experimental results. In no doublet other than that of the hydrogen atom is such a large value of the splitting observed. Therefore, the appearance of a doublet with $\Delta B_{HFS} \approx 50$ mWb m^{-2} in an E.S.R. spectrum may be considered as conclusive proof that atomic hydrogen is present in the system. The intensity of the E.S.R. line will give information on the concentration of the hydrogen atoms. This measurement is made even easier by the small width of the H.F.S. components, by their large separation (no overlapping) and by their symmetrical shape.

---

† This condition allows us to distinguish between spectra which originate from H.F.S. interaction and those which originate from anisotropic g-factor (see Chapter 5). In the latter case, Δg is constant and ΔB is not. Thus from measurements at different frequencies the separation between the maxima of the H.F.S. lines remains constant, whilst there is a change in the separation of lines, caused by the anisotropy of the g-factor.

Figure 6.2 shows the E.S.R. spectrum of the Mn^{2+} ion in dilute solution. There are six components, as would be expected from the Mn^{55} nucleus, the nuclear spin of which is $5/2$. The magnitude of the splitting is $\Delta B_{HFS} = 8.3$ mWb m^{-2}. In this case the theoretical calculation of ΔB_{HFS} is considerably more difficult. In reality the electronic configuration of the Mn^{2+} ion in its ground state corresponds to $1s^2 2s^2 2p^6 3s^2 3p^6 3d^5$, so no hyperfine structure could appear, as the unpaired electrons in this state are d-electrons, the wave functions of which are equal to zero at the site of the nucleus. If despite this a hyperfine structure is observed, then this shows that the ground state is actually a superimposition of the states $3s^2 3d^5$ and $3s 3d^5 4s$.

So far we have considered the interaction of the electron with a single nucleus, at which the electron is localized. In principle, a similar spectrum will be observed when the unpaired electron is not completely localized on the nucleus in question. The magnitude of the splitting will be determined by the contribution of the electron density at the given nucleus (for a particular value of the nuclear magnetic moment), and so will be smaller than in the completely localized examples given above.

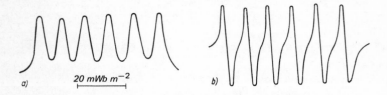

Fig. 6.2. E.S.R. spectrum of the Mn^{2+} ion.
    (*a*) absorption line
    (*b*) first derivative of the absorption line.

In the organic radical $R_1 - \overset{\bullet}{C}H - R_2$ the splitting due to the proton near the unpaired electron is 2.3 mWb m^{-2}. In the case of aromatic free radicals, for example the semiquinone ions in which the unpaired electron is distributed over a large number of centres, the splitting is even smaller (0.1 mWb m^{-2} and less). In the general case, the magnitude of the splitting due to a particular nucleus is determined by the electron density of the unpaired electron and by the effective contribution of the s-state. However, in some cases, as was shown in Chapter 3, electrons in p- and d-states can also influence the hyperfine structure, which leads to a broadening and anisotropy of the individual components.

§6.2

H.F.S. OF SEVERAL EQUIVALENT NUCLEI†

We will now consider the splitting observed when the unpaired electron interacts with several magnetic nuclei. For simplicity we will assume that the component widths are small compared to the magnitude of the splitting (i.e. well-resolved spectra). Our problem now is the deduction of the structure of the radical, from the number of components and their mutual separation.

We will begin with the simplest case of the interaction of the unpaired electron with identical nuclei in equivalent positions, for which $I = \frac{1}{2}$.

1. Two equivalent protons (radicals of the type $R-\dot{C}H_2$)

By arguments analogous to those used in the analysis of the E.S.R. spectra of H and D, it can be easily shown that all radicals can be divided into four classes, with respect to the orientation of the magnetic moments of the protons to each other, and also to the magnetic field. This is shown in Table 6.1.

Table 6.1

No.	Orientation of the nuclear spins with respect to B (for $I = \frac{1}{2}, n = 2$)	B_{eff}	B_{res}	Relative intensity
1	↑ ↑	$B + \Delta B$	$B_0 - \Delta B$	1
2	↓ ↑	B	B_0	} 2
3	↑ ↓	B	B_0	
4	↓ ↓	$B - \Delta B$	$B_0 + \Delta B$	1

This table also gives the corresponding values of B_{eff}, the effective induction at the unpaired electron, and B_{res}, the resonance induction. As in the previous case, ΔB_{HFS} is determined by the interaction of the magnetic moment of the unpaired electron and one of the protons. The states 2 and 3 are clearly indistinguishable as the protons are equivalent and B_{eff} and B_{res} are equal. So the spectrum of the radical $R-\dot{C}H_2$ consists of three equidistant lines with the intensity ratio 1:2:1 (the relative intensity is given in the last column of the table).

† *Calculations in this section are valid for cases in which the degeneracy of the SI-coupling is completely lifted, i.e. for the limiting case of the strong magnetic field. If the H.F.S. energy and the Zeeman energy are of the same order of magnitude, then additional lines appear which complicate the spectrum.[8]*

2. *Three equivalent protons* (*the radical* $\dot{C}H_3$)

Here, the states of alignment are all quite different (see Table 6.2, p. 149). Thus the spectrum of the radical CH_3 consists of four equidistant components with intensity ratio 1:3:3:1. This is shown in Fig. 6.3, which gives the spectrum of the methyl radical, obtained by U.V.-irradiation of polydimethylsiloxane.[1]

It follows that in the general case of an interaction of the unpaired electron with *n* equivalent nuclei of spin $I = \frac{1}{2}$, the spectrum is a multiplet of $2nI + 1 = n + 1$ equidistant components, the intensities of which follow the binomial coefficients. The intensity ratios for $n \leqslant 20$ are given in Table 1 of the appendix.†

The E.S.R. spectrum in the case of equivalent nuclei with spin $I = 1$ is somewhat more complicated. We will not go into great detail, but merely give tables of the H.F.S. components in the case of an interaction of the unpaired electron with two and three equivalent nuclei of this kind (Tables 6.3 and 6.4).

In both these cases the spectrum consists of a quintet with the intensity ratio 1:2:3:2:1, and a septet with the ratio 1:3:6:7:6:3:1.

It is also clear that for equivalent nuclei with $I = 1$, the number of components is still equal to $2nI + 1 = N$, which in this case is $N = 2n + 1$.

The calculation of the spectra for a large number of equivalent nuclei with $I = 1$ is very laborious if similar methods are used, so we recommend a better procedure, as follows.

If the intensity distribution in the case of $n - 1$ equivalent nuclei is known, $1:a:b:c:d:e$, we can obtain (for $I = 1$), the intensity distribution for *n* equivalent nuclei by a simple summation of three rows, each displaced one step:

1	a	b	c	d	e
	1	a	b	c	d
		1	a	b	c

$$1 : (a + 1) : (b + a + 1) : (c + b + a) : (d + c + b) : (e + d + c) \ldots$$

† The considerations above are only really applicable to the intensities of the integral of the (first derivative) line, rather than the line itself. Often the distribution of the maximum intensities is the same in both cases, but as pointed out in references 2 and 3, in the case of the H.F.S. of two or more α-protons near a carbon atom, the line widths of the various components can differ considerably from each other for different values of the projection of the total nuclear spin on the axis of the magnetic field. This leads to a change in the distribution of the maximum intensities (see also §3.8).

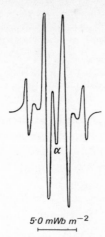

5·0 mWb m^{-2}

Fig. 6.3. E.S.R. spectrum of the methyl radical.
[The line in the centre of the spectrum (α) is caused by the radical $\overset{\cdot}{C}H_3$].

So the transition from $n = 2$ to $n = 3$ will give accordingly:

```
1  2  3  2  1
   1  2  3  2  1
      1  2  3  2  1
```
_____

$$1 : 3 : 6 : 7 : 6 : 3 : 1$$

which is in complete agreement with the results obtained previously. In Table 2 of Appendix 3 we have given the intensity distributions for equivalent nuclei with $I = 1$ for $n \leqslant 8$.

Table 6.2

No.	Orientation of the nuclear spins with respect to B (for $I = \frac{1}{2}$, $n = 3$)			B_{eff}	B_{res}	Relative intensity
1	↑	↑	↑	$B + \frac{3}{2}\Delta B$	$B_0 - \frac{3}{2}\Delta B$	1
2	↓	↑	↑			
3	↑	↓	↑	$B + \frac{1}{2}\Delta B$	$B_0 - \frac{1}{2}\Delta B$	3
4	↑	↑	↓			
5	↓	↓	↑			
6	↓	↑	↓	$B - \frac{1}{2}\Delta B$	$B_0 + \frac{1}{2}\Delta B$	3
7	↑	↓	↓			
8	↓	↓	↓	$B - \frac{3}{2}\Delta B$	$B_0 + \frac{3}{2}\Delta B$	1

Table 6.3

No.	Orientation of the nuclear spins with respect to B (for $I = 1$, $n = 2$)		B_{eff}	B_{res}	Relative intensity
1	↑	↑	$B + 2\Delta B$	$B_0 - 2\Delta B$	1
2	→	↑	} $B + \Delta B$	$B_0 - \Delta B$	2
3	↑	→			
4	↑	↓			
5	↓	↑	} B	B_0	3
6	→	→			
7	↓	→	} $B - \Delta B$	$B_0 + \Delta B$	2
8	→	↓			
9	↓	↓	$B - 2\Delta B$	$B_0 + 2\Delta B$	1

We will now very briefly consider the case of equivalent nuclei with spin $I = \frac{3}{2}$. In this case, there are four values of the projection onto the direction of the magnetic field: $+\frac{3}{2}$, $+\frac{1}{2}$, $-\frac{1}{2}$, $-\frac{3}{2}$. In the case of one single nucleus the spectrum consists of four equidistant components of equal intensity. In the case of two nuclei, we may obtain the spectrum by either of the two methods given above, and the resulting spectrum consists of seven components with intensity distribution 1:2:3:4:3:2:1. The calculation of the spectrum for an arbitrary number n of nuclei with $I = \frac{1}{2}$ is best made by the summation method, where, in this case, four shifted rows must be added each time. As before, the number of components is determined by the equation $N = 2nI + 1$; i.e. there are $3n + 1$ components. A table of the coefficients for $n \leqslant 8$ is also included in Appendix 3 (p. 319).

In concluding this section on the splitting caused by identical nuclei, we would like to consider the actual conditions which lead to such an interaction. It is known that the magnitude of the splitting is determined not only by the part of the electron density interacting with the nucleus in question, but also by the degree of s-hybridization of the atomic orbital at the nucleus. Equal or almost equal splitting will therefore only show the equality of the product

$$\rho_i \, | \, a_{si} \, |^2$$

where ρ_i is the density of the unpaired electron on nucleus i, and a_{si} the coefficient of the s-portion of the hybridized wave function at the i-th centre.

In some cases ρ_i and a_{si} must be equal for all centres, for reasons of

Table 6.4

No.	Orientation of the nuclear spins with respect to B (for $I = 1$, $n = 3$)			B_{eff}	B_{res}	Relative intensity
1	↑	↑	↑	$B + 3\Delta B$	$B_0 - 3\Delta B$	1
2	→	↑	↑			
3	↑	→	↑	$B + 2\Delta B$	$B_0 - 2\Delta B$	3
4	↑	↑	→			
5	↑	→	→			
6	→	↑	→			
7	→	→	↑			
8	↑	↑	↓	$B + \Delta B$	$B_0 - \Delta B$	6
9	↑	↓	↑			
10	↓	↑	↑			
11	↓	↑	→			
12	↓	→	↑			
13	→	↓	↑			
14	↑	↓	→	B	B_0	7
15	↑	→	↓			
16	→	↑	↓			
17	→	→	→			
18	↓	→	→			
19	→	↓	→			
20	→	→	↓			
21	↓	↓	↑	$B - \Delta B$	$B_0 + \Delta B$	6
22	↓	↑	↓			
23	↑	↓	↓			
24	→	↓	↓			
25	↓	→	↓	$B - 2\Delta B$	$B_0 + 2\Delta B$	3
26	↓	↓	→			
27	↓	↓	↓	$B - 3\Delta B$	$B_0 + 3\Delta B$	1

symmetry; as for example in the case of the symmetric semiquinones (see Chapter 8). In other systems, despite the fact that the E.S.R. spectra seem to indicate equivalence of the interaction, one cannot deduce that the values of ρ_i are equal (nor the values of a_{si}). So standard samples are used for calibration, the most widely used being the stable free radical diphenyl-picryl-hydrazyl (DPPH):

The E.S.R. spectrum of DPPH in solution consists of five equidistant components with an intensity ratio $1:2:3:2:1$, which shows the equality of the interactions of the unpaired electron with the two nitrogen nuclei α and β. However, from the structural formula it is clear that these two nitrogen atoms are structurally not equivalent. One must assume, therefore, that the degree of s-hybridization on nucleus β is considerably stronger than on nucleus α. It thus follows that ρ_i on nucleus α must be considerably larger than on β. An analogous compensation of the magnitudes of ρ_i and a_{si} is observed in many cases, where equal splittings are given by nuclei which themselves are non-equivalent and situated in different structural positions.

§6.3

H.F.S. OF NON-EQUIVALENT NUCLEI

We now consider the H.F.S. formed by interaction of the unpaired electron with non-equivalent nuclei. We will analyse the simplest example of two equal but structurally non-equivalent nuclei, 1 and 2, with spin $I = \frac{1}{2}$ and splitting constants $\Delta B_1 > \Delta B_2$. By deductions similar to those on p. 147, it can be shown that the spectrum consists of four components of equal intensity, which occur at the following values of the external magnetic field.

$$B_0 - \tfrac{1}{2}\Delta B_1 - \tfrac{1}{2}\Delta B_2 \qquad B_0 - \tfrac{1}{2}\Delta B_1 + \tfrac{1}{2}\Delta B_2$$

$$B_0 + \tfrac{1}{2}\Delta B_1 - \tfrac{1}{2}\Delta B_2 \qquad B_0 + \tfrac{1}{2}\Delta B_1 + \tfrac{1}{2}\Delta B_2$$

The same result can be obtained by successive construction of the E.S.R. lines produced by nuclei 1 and 2:

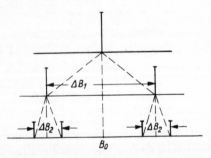

It can easily be seen that in the special case $\Delta B_1 = \Delta B_2$ the spectrum becomes a triplet with intensity ratio $1:2:1$, agreeing completely with the result obtained for two equivalent nuclei with $I = \frac{1}{2}$. By analogous reasoning for n non-equivalent nuclei, where all the values of ΔB are different from each other, and are not multiples of each other, one can show that the spectrum consists of 2^n components of equal intensity, the mutual separation of which is determined by the values of ΔB.

The picture of the splitting changes if the bond under investigation contains further groups of equivalent nuclei with $I = \frac{1}{2}$, which have differing values of ΔB. As an example of this we can consider the spectrum of the radical $\sim CF_2 - \dot{C}F - CF_2 \sim$. The H.F.S. of this radical arises from the interaction of the unpaired electron with a fluorine atom in an α-position and four equivalent atoms in a β-position. This is quite a complicated spectrum, but fortunately, as it is well-resolved, it can easily be split into two groups, each consisting of five equidistant lines. The intensities of the three outermost lines of each group are in the ratio 1:4:6, which strongly suggests they are components of a quintuplet arising from the interaction of the unpaired electron with four equivalent F^{19} nuclei. Even though the central components are not particularly well-resolved, they can easily be identified. From this spectrum one can easily obtain the values of ΔB_α and ΔB_β, which in this case are $9 \cdot 2 \pm 0 \cdot 2$ and $3 \cdot 4 \pm 0 \cdot 1$ mWb m^{-2} respectively. The spectrum may be synthesized from the theory, and this is shown at the bottom of Fig. 6.4.

We will not dwell further on more complicated cases. Suffice to say that the E.S.R. spectrum for groups of $n, p, m, \ldots$ equivalent nuclei with $I = \frac{1}{2}$, consists in the general case (no superimposition of lines) of $(n + 1)(p + 1)$ $(m + 1) \ldots$ lines. The spectrum will naturally appear very complex, but analysis is usually possible. If the values of ΔB for different groups are multiples of each other, then single lines may fall together, which leads to a change in the overall number of components. One should always bear this fact in mind, otherwise mistakes may be made in the interpretation of the spectrum. It will also be clear that if different nuclei with $s = \frac{1}{2}$ are both present in the system (e.g. H and F), then the spectrum will retain its shape. In the ideal picture under consideration (having no regard to line widths), the differences between the nuclei are shown only by the values of ΔB.

The analysis of the H.F.S. of E.S.R. spectra in systems with non-equivalent magnetic nuclei with $I = 1, \frac{3}{2}$ etc., and also in mixed cases where the system contains nuclei with different values of I, may be carried out in an analogous way. Spectra may naturally be very complex. Fig. 6.5 shows an example of this, the E.S.R. spectrum of the nitro-sofluoralkyl radical

$$\sim CF_2 - \underset{\underset{\displaystyle NO}{|}}{\dot{C}} - CF_2 \sim$$

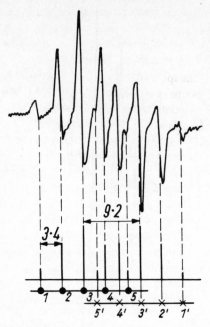

Fig. 6.4. E.S.R. spectrum of the radical ~CF$_2$–ĊF-CF$_2$~.

This spectrum consists of the superposition of a triplet of quintets. The splitting into five lines is produced by the four equivalent fluorine nuclei, and the triplet splitting by the nitrogen nucleus.

§6.4.

E.S.R. SPECTRA WITH POORLY RESOLVED H.F.S.: ANALYTICAL TREATMENT

The above discussions were concerned with the case of ideal resolution of the H.F.S. components, which is seldom obtained. More often than not spectra with complicated H.F.S. are not completely resolved.

The main causes of distortion in E.S.R. spectra containing poorly resolved H.F.S. are:

(a) The mutual overlapping of individual components.
(b) Different widths of individual components:

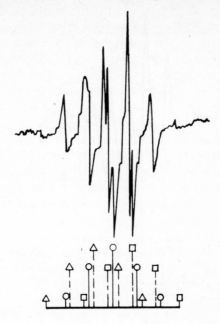

Fig. 6.5. E.S.R. spectrum of the radical $\sim CF_2 - \overset{\bullet}{\underset{|}{C}} - CF_2 \sim$
NO

(b_1) the broadening of the edge components relative to the central ones (see note on p. 89),

(b_2) the change in line width of components during the transition from low to high magnetic fields (see Chapter 3).

(c) The asymmetry of the individual components:

(c_1) due to anisotropy of the g-factors,

(c_2) due to saturation (see Chapter 2).

The problem of interpreting such poorly resolved spectra is a complex one, and there is no easy solution. The function of an analysis must be to obtain from the experimental spectrum the maximum amount of information (width, shape and intensity of the individual line, and the magnitude of the H.F.S. splitting).

We shall now consider some possibilities of interpreting a poorly resolved spectrum, based on a qualitative analysis of an equation which describes the overall spectrum. We will also demonstrate, by the simplest examples , how serious are the results of the distortions which occur for the reasons given above. Equations and procedures for analysis will be given, which apply to spectra of this type. These methods are simple, and in principle may be used for other more complicated spectra. The effort involved is, however, considerable. Thus, in the following section, we propose giving results obtained from a fast electronic computer.

We will now consider the quantitative characteristics of the poorly resolved spectra.

In the case of anisotropy of the g-factor (case c_1), the appearance of the spectrum is independent of the microwave power, and its shape is asymmetrical with respect to the centre of the spectrum. These same two characteristics also occur in the case of line broadening with increasing field (case b_2), i.e. independent of microwave power and an asymmetry of the total spectrum.

In the case c_2 the E.S.R. spectrum will alter with a change in the microwave power. If this occurs, then the microwave power must be reduced, and the measurement carried out at the lowest power consistent with detecting the spectrum.

We will now consider the case of spectra which result from super-imposition of symmetrical components. The simplest case occurs when all components are the same width. The analysis may be carried out in several ways, and many workers have suggested that a graph be constructed of the E.S.R. spectra of the assumed radicals for different values of the parameters

$$\alpha_1 = \frac{\Delta B_{HFS}^{(1)}}{\Delta B_i^{(1)}} \qquad \alpha_2 = \frac{\Delta B_{HFS}^{(2)}}{\Delta B_i^{(2)}} \quad \ldots$$

Here, $\Delta B_{HFS}^{(1)}$, $\Delta B_{HFS}^{(2)}$, . . . are the splittings for the corresponding line groups of the radical (e.g. for the H-atoms of the CH_2- and CH_3-groups of the radical CH_3CH_2), and $\Delta B_i^{(1)}$, $\Delta B_i^{(2)}$, . . . the corresponding individual line widths. The procedure is then to find out which theoretical spectra come closest to the experimental spectrum. It will be clear that this method is extremely difficult to apply in cases where complex radicals are involved, and particularly in cases where the true structure of the radicals cannot be predicted.

We will now consider a simple method which in some cases will permit us to carry out an analysis of the H.F.S., if the structure of the radical is known. This method is based on making certain approximations, which nevertheless allow us, in some cases, to make an accurate analysis of a poorly resolved H.F.S. The method involves the use of the ratios of the coordinates of the turning points of the curves $I(B)$ or $I'(B)$.

We will illustrate the value of this technique by some examples. For the sake of simplicity we will assume that all lines considered have Gaussian shape. The calculations are completely analogous in the case of a Lorentzian line shape.

1. For a 1:2:1 triplet, the analytical expressions for $I(x)$ and $I'(x)$ have the following form:

$$I(x) = I_0 \left[e^{-(\alpha+x)^2/2} + 2e^{-x^2/2} + e^{-(\alpha-x)^2/2} \right] \tag{6.1}$$

$$I'(x) = -I_0 \left[(\alpha+x) e^{-(\alpha+x)^2/2} + 2x e^{-x^2/2} + \right.$$
$$\left. + (x-\alpha) e^{-(\alpha-x)^2/2} \right] \tag{6.2}$$

where

$$x = 2 \frac{\Delta B}{\Delta B_i} \qquad \alpha = 2 \frac{\Delta B_{\text{HFS}}}{\Delta B_i} \qquad \Delta B = B - B_0$$

B_0 is the field value corresponding to the centre of the spectrum, ΔB_{HFS} the true separation between the H.F.S. components, and ΔB_i the separation between the points of maximum slope of the single lines (the line width).

The functions $I(x)$ and $I'(x)$ are shown in Fig. 6.6 for two values of α.

First we determine the value of α for which the maximum and the minimum of the absorption line for the first and third components disappear (Fig. 6.6 a, b). This condition may be written in the form $\alpha \leqslant \alpha_{\text{cr}}$, and α_{cr} is determined from the equations

$$I'(x, \alpha_{\text{cr}}) = 0, \qquad I''(x, \alpha_{\text{cr}}) = 0 \tag{6.3}$$

This relatively simple calculation in this case gives $\alpha_{\text{cr}} \approx 2 \cdot 7$. From this it may be concluded that in the case of a 1:2:1 triplet of Gaussian lines, a clear maximum is observed on the absorption curve [or the number of times $I'(x)$ cuts the zero line is greater than 1], when $\Delta B_{\text{HFS}}/\Delta B_i > 1 \cdot 35$.

When the value of α_{cr} is quite large, it follows that in all cases where the triplet spectrum is as in Fig. 6.6 a, i.e. $\alpha > \alpha_{\text{cr}}$, then over the range of the overlapping of the first and second components, the contribution of the third component is very small. The calculation of the coordinates and their ratios for extreme lines is thus considerably simplified. So for the abscissa of the first maximum on the absorption curve, we get the expression

$$x_{\max} = \alpha(1 - 2e^{-\alpha^2/2}) = F(\alpha) \tag{6.4}$$

The values of the quotients

$$x_{\max}/x_{\min} \qquad I_{\max}/I_{\min} \qquad I_{\max}/I_0$$

can be determined for different values of α. Table 6.5 shows such values for $2.8 < \alpha < 4.0$.

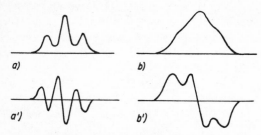

Fig. 6.6. Diagram of E.S.R. triplets with intensity ratio 1:2:1
(*a*) absorption line for $\alpha = 3.0$ (well resolved)
(*b*) absorption line for $\alpha = 1.5$ (poorly resolved)
(*a'*) and (*b'*) first derivative of the corresponding lines.

Table 6.5

α	2·8	3·0	3·3	3·6	4·0
$x_{\max}/x_{\min}$	1·40	1·56	1·65	1·72	1·79
$I_{\max}/I_{\min}$	1·06	1·18	1·44	1·83	2·93
$I_{\max}/I_0$	1·05	1·02	1·01	1·00	1·00

The analysis of a poorly resolved spectrum of the type (6.6*a*) is carried out in the following way. From the experimental value of the quotients $x_{\max}/x_{\min} = \Delta B_{\max}/\Delta B_{\min}$ (or $I_{\max}/I_{\min}$), we can find the value of α, either with the help of Table 6.5 or graphically. Since $x_{\max}/\alpha = F(\alpha)/\alpha = \Delta B_{\max}^{\exp}/B_{HFS}$ [$\Delta B_{\max}^{\exp}$ being the abscissa of the curve $I(B)$], by using α and the experimentally measured value $\Delta B_{\max}^{\exp}$, we can easily find ΔB_{HFS}, the true splitting constant. But as $\alpha = \Delta B_{HFS}/\Delta B_i$, we also obtain the line width ΔB_i. In this way both fundamental parameters ΔB_{HFS} and ΔB_i are determined.

The analysis is further simplified if we take into account that

$$\alpha \geqslant 3 \frac{\alpha - F(\alpha)}{\alpha} \leqslant 0.02$$

and hence $\Delta B_{max}^{exp} \approx \Delta B_{HFS}$. In this case x_{min} is a function of α, and ΔB_i, as before, is equal to $\Delta B_{HFS}/\alpha$.

The use of this analytical procedure can also be extended to spectra with a large number of components and with other ratios of intensity. In all cases we may ignore the more distant lines. The authors have made calculations, corresponding to the disappearance of the extreme wing components of an absorption line, for the multiplets with $n = 3$ (1:2:1), $n = 4$ (1:3:3:1), $n = 5, 7$ and 9. The corresponding values of α_{cr} were 2·7, 2·9, 3·0, 3·2 and 3·3 respectively. Since α_{cr} always increases with increasing n, the contributions of the more distant components for $n > 3$ will be even less than for the triplet.

Note that α_{cr} is smaller for pairs of lines at the centre than for pairs of lines at the edge of the multiplet, since the intensity ratios of neighbouring components in the central region are closer to unity than at the edge. Therefore, the resolution of the central components is better than at the edges of the spectrum.† For an analysis of a multiplet spectrum with $N > 3$ the position of the outermost maxima can always be described by an equation of the type

$$x_1^{max} = x_{1,0}^{max}(1 - 2e^{-\alpha^2/2}) \tag{6.5}$$

Here $x_{1,0}^{max} = [(n-1)/2]$ α is the abscissa of the maximum of the outermost component (in the case of an infinitely narrow line width, the true abscissa of the outermost component). Since if $\alpha \geqslant \alpha_{cr}$, then $2e^{-\alpha^2/2} \ll 1$, it follows from (6.5) that $x^{max} \approx x_{1,0}^{max}$.

The position of the other maximum is shifted by the same factor $(1 - 2e^{-\alpha^2/2})$, either to the right or to the left, and for an even greater accuracy the following equation may be used:

$$x_k^{max} \cong x_{k,0}^{max} = \frac{n+1-2k}{2}\alpha \qquad (k = 1, 2, \ldots, n) \tag{6.6}$$

It is clear from the above argument that within the entire spectrum, the separations between the maxima of the absorption curve (Fig. 6.8) $\Delta B_2 - \Delta B_3, \Delta B_3 - \Delta B_4$ etc. are exactly equal to the value ΔB_{HFS}. The value of $\Delta B_1 - \Delta B_2$ is at the most only 1 or 2 per cent smaller than ΔB_{HFS}. If we carry out the same calculation for large values of n, then from the values of $\alpha_{min}/\alpha_{max}$ or I_{max}/I_{min}, we arrive at the value of α for the given spectrum in the same way. The numerical values will of course vary, as they depend on the intensity of neighbouring lines.

† It should be noted that an improvement of resolution from the edge to the middle can also be brought about by a broadening, of the outside lines stronger than that of the central lines, through anisotropic interaction (see note to p. 89).

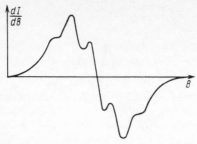

Fig. 6.7. E.S.R. spectrum with poorly resolved H.F.S. for an intensity ratio
1:6:15:20:15:6:1 at $\alpha = 1.5$

Until now we have limited our argument to the study of multiplets, in
which all maxima and minima of the absorption curve are separated from
each other. However, we can already see that a smearing-out of these
maxima can be observed at quite large values of α. How then can we
analyse a spectrum of the type shown in Fig. 6.6b and b'? One possibility
would be to carry out calculations analogous to the above methods, but
for the curve of the first derivative. Here, the calculations will become very
complicated. We will limit ourselves again to the 1:2:1 triplet. The
condition for the appearance of maxima on the curve $I'(x, \alpha)$ can again be
written in the following form:

$$\alpha \leqslant \alpha'_{cr}$$

where α'_{cr} is determined from the equations

$$I''(x, \alpha'_{cr}) = 0 \quad \text{and} \quad I'''(x, \alpha'_{cr}) = 0 \tag{6.7}$$

Even if we only consider two components in these equations, as we did
before (which in this case is generally less accurate, as α'_{cr} for the
derivative is smaller than α_{cr} for the absorption line), we can no longer
solve equation (6.7) analytically. By graphical solution we find that
$\alpha'_{cr} \approx 1.85$, i.e. the outside lines of the first derivative of a Gaussian 1:2:1
triplet disappear for $\Delta B_{HFS}/\Delta B_i \leqslant \alpha'_{cr}/2 = 0.93$. (Note: for the
absorption curve α_{cr} was 2.7).

Before closing this section on the superimposition of symmetrical lines
of equal width, we will also consider multiplet spectra with components of
equal intensity. In this case the accuracy is good for a large range of values
of α.

As we have seen above, we obtained the most information from the
curve $I'(x)$; so we will analyse this case in more detail. The simplest
example is a doublet (Fig. 6.9):

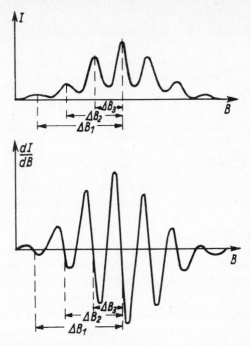

Fig. 6.8. Diagram of a multi-component E.S.R. spectrum with binomial intensity distribution (ΔB_1, ΔB_2, ... are the distances of the corresponding components from the centre of the spectrum.

$$\frac{I(x)}{I_0} = e^{-(x+\alpha/2)^2/2} + e^{-(x-\alpha/2)^2/2} \tag{6.8}$$

$$\frac{I'(x)}{I_0} = -\left[\left(x + \frac{\alpha}{2}\right) e^{-(x+\alpha/2)^2/2} + \left(x - \frac{\alpha}{2}\right) e^{-(x-\alpha/2)^2/2}\right] \tag{6.9}$$

with $x = 2\Delta B/\Delta B_i$ and $\alpha = 2\Delta B_{\mathrm{HFS}}/\Delta B_i$.

A direct calculation gives $h_2/h_1, x_{\max} = 2\Delta B_{\max}/\Delta B_i$ and $x_{\min} = 2\Delta B_{\min}/\Delta B_i$ as functions of $\Delta B_{\mathrm{HFS}}/\Delta B_i = \alpha/2$. The corresponding curves are shown in Fig. 6.10, and one can distinguish two ranges:

(1) $\Delta B_{\mathrm{HFS}}/\Delta B_i > 1$, with a clear minimum on the curve, and
(2) $\Delta B_{\mathrm{HFS}}/\Delta B_i < 1$, where the minimum has disappeared (Fig. 6.11).

In the first case ($\Delta B_{\mathrm{HFS}} > \Delta B_i$) Fig. 6.10 may be applied in the following manner:

Experimentally, we obtain h_2/h_1 and ΔB_{max} (or ΔB_{min}). From the curve of Fig. 6.10 and using h_2/h_1 we can find $\Delta B_{HFS}/\Delta B_i$. Also from the

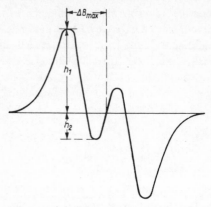

Fig. 6.9. Diagram of an E.S.R. spectrum with two components.

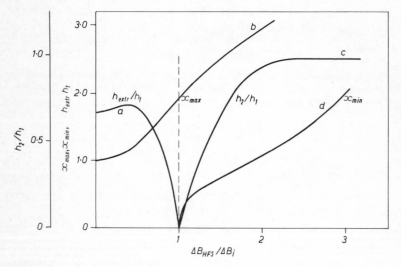

Fig. 6.10. Graphs for determining the values h_2/h_1, x_{max}, x_{min}, h_{extr}/h_1, for a spectrum with two components.

other curve of Fig. 6.10 we can find the corresponding values of x_{max} and x_{min}, and thus with the value of ΔB_{max} (or ΔB_{min}) we can calculate ΔB_i.

Within the useful range of the curves, not only can we determine the position of the maximum, but also the slope of the curve $I'(x)$ at the centre of the spectrum, or more conveniently, a parameter for the ratio h_{extr}/h_1 (see Fig. 6.11). The value h_{extr}/h_i in the range $\Delta B_{HFS} < \Delta B_i$ is also shown in Fig. 6.10. A qualitative analysis of the experimental results can be performed in the following manner (small inaccuracies being caused by errors in the determination of h_{extr}). From the value h_{extr}/h_1 we can determine $\Delta B_{HFS}/\Delta B_i$. By using $x_{max} = \Delta B_{max}/\Delta B_i$ and ΔB_{max} we find ΔB_i and thence ΔB_{HFS}. It is clear that such an analysis is only reliable if h_{extr}/h_1 for the doublet differs noticeably from the value for the single line (≈ 1.65). The above analysis is consequently only of practical value for

$$0.5 \leqslant B_{HFS}/B_i \leqslant 1$$

We will now consider a multiplet spectrum with six lines of equal intensity (Fig. 6.12). Analysis shows that in this case the curve $h_1/h_0 = f(\Delta B_{HFS}/\Delta B_i)$ coincides completely with that for the doublet (and it only makes sense to speak of h_1 for $\Delta B_{HFS} > \Delta B_i$). The curves $h_2/h_0, h_3/h_0$ etc. completely coincide with this curve for $\Delta B_{HFS}/\Delta B_i > 1.2$, and although $h_2/h_0 = h_3/h_0 = \ldots$ .the corresponding curve is shifted to the left with respect to the curve h_1/h_0. The different behaviour of the quotient h_1/h_0 signifies that for relatively small splittings of the outermost components, the contribution from the third component cannot now be neglected, since the components to the right and to the left no longer compensate for

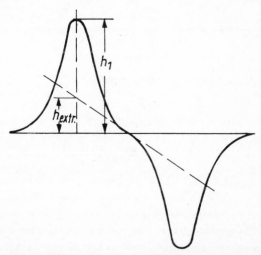

Fig. 6.11. Diagram of a poorly resolved E.S.R. spectrum with two components.

each other. Thus only if $\Delta B_{HFS}/\Delta B_i \geqslant 0\cdot79$, can ΔB_{HFS} be immediately determined from the separation of the centres of neighbouring lines of the experimental curve. The value of $\Delta B_{HFS}/B_i$ can be easily obtained from Fig. 6.13. Another example of a spectrum with $n = 6$ is shown in Fig. 6.14.

We will conclude this section by considering the triplet spectra 1:1:1 and 1:2:1, in which the outer lines are 10 per cent wider than the central line (Figs. 6.15 and 6.16), and $\Delta B_{HFS}/\Delta B_i = 1$ ($\alpha = 2$). The value of α was chosen so that for the 1:2:1 triplet, a weak minimum is still observed on the curve $I'(x)$. For purposes of comparison, we have also shown on the same

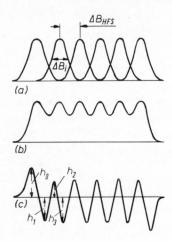

Fig. 6.12. Diagram of an E.S.R. spectrum consisting of six components of equal intensity
    (*a*) position of the individual components
    (*b*) envelope of absorption line
    (*c*) first derivative of absorption line envelope.

curves triplets with components of equal width. Calculation shows that in the case of the 1:1:1 triplet, the 10 per cent broadening of the outer components leads to an increase in the critical value $\alpha'_{cr} = 2(\Delta B_{HFS}/\Delta B_i)$ of from $1\cdot75$ to $1\cdot92$. Remember that for the 1:2:1 triplet α'_{cr} was $1\cdot85$. The 10 per cent increase in the width of the outer components thus leads to twice as much 'smearing-out' of the H.F.S. than does the doubling of the intensity of the central component. Poor resolution of a spectrum, particularly the steplike character of the first derivative of a symmetrical multicomponent spectrum, can therefore be caused by a superposition of individual components as well as by a change in their width.

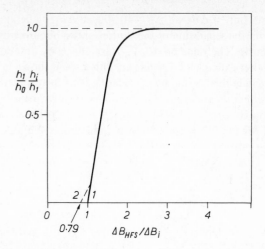

Fig. 6.13. Graph for the determination of h_1/h_0 and h_i/h_0 for an E.S.R. spectrum with six components of equal intensity
 (1) Curve for h_1/h_0
 (2) Curve for h_i/h_0 (i = 2, 3, 4, 5).

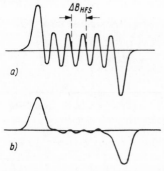

Fig. 6.14. Diagram of an E.S.R. spectrum with six components, for different values of $\Delta B_{HFS}/\Delta B_i$
 (a) $\Delta B_{HFS}/\Delta B_i$ = 1·2
 (b) $\Delta B_{HFS}/\Delta B_i$ = 0·9

We can now add a few final comments on the determination of the intensity of the individual components. In the examples considered so far, we have posed ourselves the problem of finding the parameters ΔB_{HFS} and ΔB_i for a spectrum of known shape.

In practice often one must solve a complicated problem, namely, that of determining from the spectrum the number and the intensity ratio of the

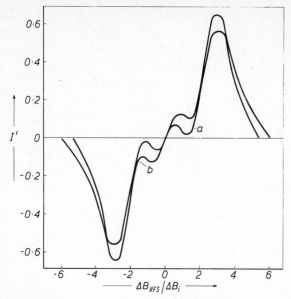

Fig. 6.15. Diagram of an E.S.R. spectrum with three components of equal intensity
($\alpha = 2$)

    (*a*) equal width of all components ($\Delta B_1 = \Delta B_2 = \Delta B_3$)

    (*b*) $\Delta B_1 = (1 \cdot 1)\Delta B_2 = \Delta B_3$

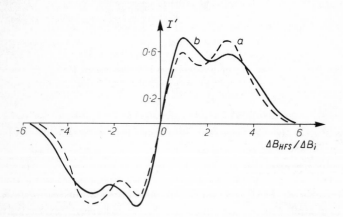

Fig. 6.16. Diagram of an E.S.R. spectrum with three components with intensity
ratio 1:2:1 ($\alpha = 2$)

    (*a*) $\Delta B_1 = \Delta B_2 = \Delta B_3$

    (*b*) $\Delta B_1 = (1.1)\Delta B_2 = \Delta B_3$

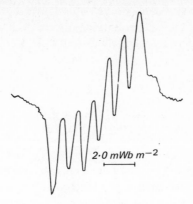

Fig. 6.17. 'Step-shaped' E.S.R. spectrum with many components [spectrum of the cyclic complex $(C_5H_5)_2TiH_2AlR_2$; see Fig. 8.12].

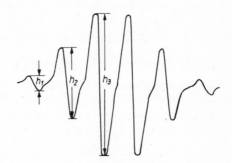

Fig. 6.18. Diagram of a multicomponent E.S.R. spectrum (first derivative).

individual components. There is no universal analytical procedure which will automatically give all the answers. For separated components of the absorption spectrum, the analysis does not present any particular difficulties, whereas the analysis of $I'(x)$ is somewhat more complicated. In this latter case one usually also uses the measurement of the ordinates of the maxima (e.g. h_1, h_2, h_3; see Fig. 6.18), where it is assumed in the first order approximation that the contributions of non-neighbouring components may be ignored (because $\alpha \gg \alpha_{cr}$), and thus h_i/h_k is approximately equal to the ratio of the corresponding coefficients a_i/a_k in the general expression $I(x) = \sum_{j=1}^{m} a_j f(x, \alpha_j)$. Such an analysis often gives very satisfactory results. However, we must keep in mind that these calculations assume that all components have equal widths. We have already seen how a small change in the width of the outer components can lead to considerable changes in $I'(x)$. Thus all results obtained by this method need to be carefully verified.

§6.5

E.S.R. SPECTRA WITH POORLY RESOLVED H.F.S.: ANALYSIS USING ELECTRONIC COMPUTERS

One possibility for the analysis of incompletely resolved E.S.R. spectra is to compare the experimental curves with others calculated theoretically. Papers have already been published in which the interpretation of the observed spectrum[4] and the calculation of the exact magnitude of the splittings[5] have been performed by comparison of the experimental spectra with the spectra calculated on electronic computers. However, both of these papers sought the answers to concrete individual problems, and their results cannot be generalized. So at the present time this method only becomes effective when assumptions may be made about the structure of the radical and calculations made for different values of the parameters. Only under these conditions could one try to determine the structure of an unknown spectrum, where one is not limited to either confirming a particular structure or replacing it with another one. Apart from this, we will also show that the real characteristic values of the spectrum under investigation can be calculated from the values of parameters obtained directly from the experimental data. It is clear that such calculations of the theoretical shape of E.S.R. lines with complicated H.F.S. are in most cases only possible with modern high-speed electronic computers.

The first step in this direction was made in 1961 on the electronic computer of the ICP.[6] The results of this program which included calculations on multi-component spectra with different intensity ratios for both Lorentzian and Gaussian line shape, were published in the form of a special atlas.[7] We will consider a few examples of the E.S.R. spectra obtained in this way. If the individual components are symmetrical, and their widths and the magnitude of the splitting are constant over the whole spectrum, then the appearance of the spectrum will depend only on one parameter, $\beta = \Delta B_i / \Delta B_{HFS}$ (Fig. 6.19).

Figure 6.20 shows (in first-derivative form) some theoretically computed spectra consisting of six Lorentzian lines of equal intensity.

β varies from 0·3 to 3, and the spectra are seen to range from completely resolved to completely unresolved. As one can see from Fig. 6.20, at the

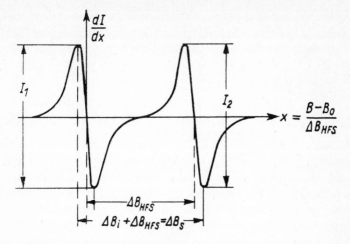

Fig. 6.19. Theoretical parameters of a spectrum with H.F.S.

B_0 centre line between the outer components

ΔB_i width of individual components, between points of maximum slope of the absorption line, i.e. turning points of the first derivative

ΔB_s total width of the spectrum

point of incomplete resolution ($\beta = 1$), the spectrum has a very specific shape, and an analysis with the usual methods would prove difficult. The consideration of theoretical spectra of this type shows that for components of equal intensity the splitting can be determined with reasonable accuracy from the separation between the central components, even in the case of poorly resolved spectra.

Figure 6.21 shows the theoretically computed spectra originating from five Lorentzian lines with binomial intensity ratio. Here, in the region $\beta \approx 1$, the sides lines begin to be swallowed up in the overall picture (see also p. 158). The experimental spectrum cannot therefore be interpreted with any certainty.

If a theoretical spectrum is found which agrees with the experimental one, then not only can we ascertain the structure of the latter, but we can also determine its parameters (ΔB_{HFS}, ΔB_i).

A very important result of these computations is the construction of special nomograms which relate the true values of the spectral parameters to the experimental values easily obtained from poorly resolved spectra. We produce examples of these nomograms in Figs. 6.22 and 6.23 for two of the structures which we have considered above. The nomograms permit

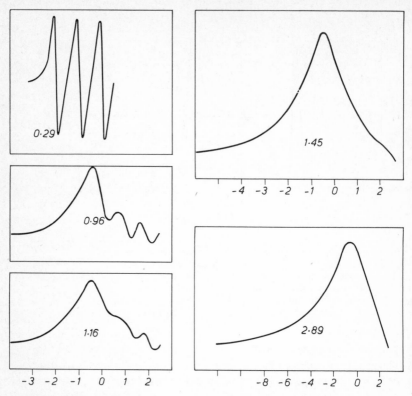

Fig. 6.20. Theoretical E.S.R. spectrum consisting of six H.F.S. components with equal intensity for a Lorentzian shape of the individual lines and different β (from 0·29 to 2·89)
Here, as in Fig. 6.21, only one half of the spectrum is shown, since the second half is a mirror image of the first.

rapid calculation of the spectral parameters. For example, with the nomogram of Fig. 6.23, individual line widths can be determined from the intensity ratio, if ΔB_{HFS} is known, a case commonly occurring in practice. In addition to this, the nomograms help to decipher spectra in cases where the theoretical spectra for different structures are similar to each other (this is often the case in components of weak H.F.S.). The use of theoretical spectra and the nomograms constructed from them open many new possibilities for the analysis of E.S.R. spectra.

It is clear that it will be impossible to match all experimental results with theoretical calculations. If, however, a choice of theoretical spectra is

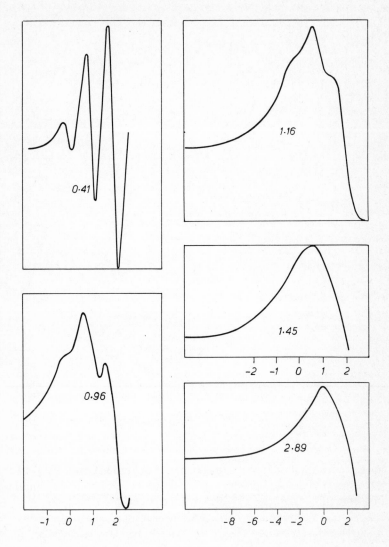

Fig. 6.21. Theoretical spectra of five H.F.S. components with intensity ratio 1:4:6:4:1 for Lorentzian shape of the individual lines, and with different values of β (from 0·41 to 2·89).

available, one can rapidly synthesize spectra of any required structure. The present theoretical computations also facilitate the direct analysis of the complex E.S.R. spectra with the help of universal or specialized electronic computers.

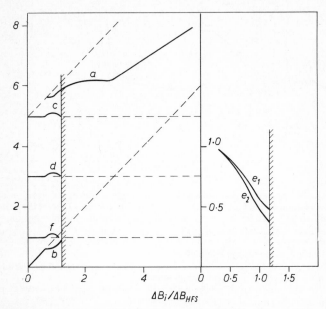

Fig. 6.22. Nomograms for the analysis of non-resolved E.S.R. spectra which consist of six components of equal intensity with Lorentzian shape.

(a) $\Delta B_s^*/\Delta B_{HFS}$, where ΔB_s^* is the separation between the maximum of the first and the minimum of the sixth components

(b) $\Delta B_i^*/\Delta B_{HFS}$, where ΔB_i^* is twice the separation between the maximum and the centre of the first components

(c) ΔB_{HFS}^* (1–6)/ΔB_{HFS}, where ΔB_{HFS}^* (1–6) is the separation between the centres of the first and sixth components

(d) ΔB_{HFS}^* (1–6)/ΔB_{HFS}, where ΔB_{HFS}^* (2–5) is the separation between the centres of the first and sixth components

(f) ΔB_{HFS}^* (3–4)/ΔB_{HFS}, where ΔB_{HFS}^* (3–4) is the separation between the centres of the third and fourth components

(e₁) I_2'/I_1' (e₁) I_3'/I_1', where I_1', I_2' and I_3' are the amplitudes of the derivatives of the corresponding components.

The material presented in this section will illustrate the many possibilities now open to us in the fields of automatic analysis. Advice on the use of the nomograms and spectral curves may be found in the atlas cited above,[7] and its forthcoming sections.

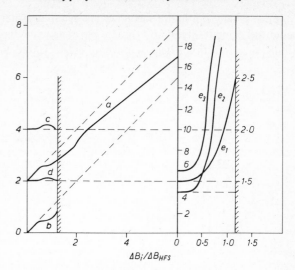

Fig. 6.23. Nomograms for the analysis of non-resolved E.S.R. spectra originating
from five components with binomial intensity distribution and Lorentzian line shape
(*a*) $\Delta B_s^*/\Delta B_{HFS}$, where ΔB_s^* is the separation between the maximum of the second
component and the minimum of the fourth component
(*b*) $\Delta B_i^*/\Delta B_{HFS}$, where ΔB_i^* is the separation between the maximum and the
minimum of the central component
(*c*) $\Delta B_{HFS}^*(1-5)/\Delta B_{HFS}$, where $\Delta B_{HFS}^*(1-5)$ is the separation between the
centres of the first and fifth components
(*d*) $\Delta B_{HFS}^*(2-4)/\Delta B_{HFS}$, where $\Delta B_{HFS}^*(2-4)$ is the separation between the
centres of the second and fourth components
(*e₁*) I_3'/I_2' (*e₂*) I_2'/I_1' (*e₃*) I_3'/I_1' where I_1', I_2', I_3' are the amplitudes of the
derivatives of the corresponding components. The vertical scale to the right
refers to the curve (*e₁*).

§6.6

E.S.R. SPECTRA WITH UN-RESOLVED H.F.S.

A case which is particularly difficult to analyse is that in which values of
$\Delta B_{HFS}/\Delta B_i$ are small, and the H.F.S. is completely smeared out, giving an
experimental curve which shows only the common envelope.

   An example of this is shown in Fig. 6.24, for the E.S.R. spectrum of
the anion of diphenylmethane in dimethylglycolether at 25°C and with a
concentration of the $(Ph)_2CH_2$ of (*a*) 10^{-4} M and (*b*) 2.10^{-2}. In the
case (*b*) we see one single line, which gives no information as to the
structure of the paramagnetic particle giving rise to the E.S.R. spectrum.
It has recently been shown, however, that such a spectrum can be very

useful in deciding on the degree of delocalization of the unpaired electron in a complex molecule. We can examine, one at a time, the H.F.S. of the E.S.R. spectra of a series of bonds in which the unpaired electron is delocalised on 1, 2, 3 etc. completely equivalent CH groups.

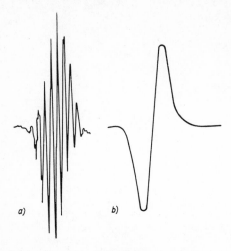

Fig. 6.24. Complete smearing-out of the H.F.S. in an E.S.R. spectrum
(a) E.S.R. spectrum of a 10^{-4} molar solution of the diphenylmethane anion in 1,2-dimethoxyethane
(b) the same spectrum for a 2.10^{-2} molar solution.

From the above, it follows that:

(1) the spectra consist of 2,3, 4, ... $n + 1$ equidistant components with binomial intensity distribution.
(2) the total spread of the spectrum is in all cases equal,
(3) the total intensity, obtained by summation over all components, is constant.

Figure 6.25 shows schematically some spectra of this type.

We see from Fig. 6.25 that as n increases, there is a large decrease in the total width of the line, which is shown by the envelope of all H.F.S. components of the spectrum. If, from the general binomial coefficients, we take a term with a sufficiently large n, then with the help of Stirling's equation we obtain the following expression for the envelope of the line:

$$f(n) = 2^n \sqrt{\left(\frac{2}{\pi n}\right)} \, e^{-(B-B_0)^2/[L/\sqrt{(2n)}]^2} \qquad (6.10)$$

where L is the magnitude of the splitting, which is characteristic for a CH-group of the type in question.

In cases where a smeared-out H.F.S. gives rise to a single line, this will be of Gaussian shape with the effective width†

$$\Delta B_{HFS} = 2\sqrt{(\ln 2)} \frac{L}{\sqrt{(2n)}} = 1 \cdot 18 \frac{L}{\sqrt{n}} \qquad (6.11)$$

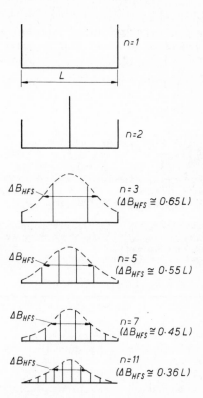

Fig. 6.25. Diagram showing the narrowing of a non-resolved E.S.R. line as a result of an increase in the number of H.F.S. components.

If we compare the value of $1 \cdot 18/\sqrt{n}$ with $\Delta B_{1/2}/L$, which is determined from the envelope of the H.F.S. lines, then we can show that equation (6.11) is applicable for $n \geqslant 3$. For cases in which ΔB_{HFS} is comparable

† Here, ΔB_{HFS} is the half-width value of the envelope of a line with smeared-out H.F.S.

with the width of the individual components ΔB_i, the effective experimentally observed line width (for Gaussian line shape of the individual components) is described by the following expression:

$$\Delta B_{eff} = \sqrt{(\Delta B_{HFS}^2 + \Delta B_i^2)} \qquad (6.12)$$

Knowing ΔB_{eff}, ΔB_i and L, then we may calculate n, i.e. the number of the equivalent CH-groups with which the unpaired electron interacts.

The above procedure for the determination of n is naturally only valid in cases where the line narrowing is caused by intensity distribution and not by exchange interaction. This is so if ΔB_{eff} is independent of concentration and if the line has Gaussian shape. In the case of exchange narrowing, $\Delta B_{eff} = f(c)$, and the line has Lorentzian shape.

References

1. Voevodski, V. V.: *Kinetika i Kataliz,* **1** (1960), 45.
2. Chochran, E. L., Adrian, F. I., Bowers, V. A.: *J. chem. Phys.,* **34** (1961), 1161.
3. Shidomirov, G. M., Molin, Ju. N.: *Ž. strukt. Chimii.*
4. Libby, D., Ormerod, M. S., Charlesby, A.: *Polymer,* **1** (1960), 212.
5. Chen, M., Sane, R. V., Walter, R. J., Weil, J. A.: *J. Phys. Chem.,* **65** (1961), 713.
6. Lebedev, Ja. S., Tschernikova, D. M., Tichomirova, N. N.: *Ž. strukt. Chimii,* **2** (1961), 6.
7. Voevodski, V. V., Lebedev, Ja. S.: *Atlas teoretičeski rasscitannych spektrov elektronnogo paramagnitnogo resonansa* (Atlas of Theoretically Calculated E.P.R. Spectra), Izd-vo AN SSSR 1962.
8* Heuer, K., Neubert, R., Sonneck, K. D.: *Exp. Techn. d. Phys.,* **13** (1965), 231.

PART II

THE APPLICATION OF E.S.R. TO THE SOLUTION OF CHEMICAL PROBLEMS

Most reviews on the application of E.S.R. to chemical problems are simple descriptions of the results of various authors, and make no attempt to summarize the material collected in the last five or ten years. Our objective in this part of the book is not so much a detailed commentary on the numerous published works, as a consideration of the role of E.S.R. in modern chemistry, and the many new uses of the technique.

As we are primarily interested in chemical processes, we will not bother to go into all the applications of E.S.R. to the solution of problems of structural chemistry; in particular we will completely leave out the problems appertaining to crystal chemistry, which are covered adequately by a series of monographs.[1,2] Our prime interest will be the new methods of investigating intermediate products and primary reactions which have been made possible by the discovery of E.S.R. We will consider a series of different problems, each aimed at a different chemical feature, and do not propose to enumerate all works relating to the problem in question, but only to consider one or two relevant papers. However, our final conclusions will, in most cases, apply to all problems in that particular area.

Chapter 7

Free Radicals in Chemical Reactions

The use of E.S.R. is obviously extremely important in the investigation of chemical processes which take place via the action of free radicals.

It is well known that free radicals were first discovered in the year 1900 by the American scientist Gomberg, who successfully investigated hexaphenylethane and proved the existence of the particle $(Ph)_3\dot{C}$ with trivalent carbon as a stable chemical bond.[3] The idea of the formation of free radicals with an unsaturated carbon atom makes it possible to explain a large number of chemical effects, such as the formation of dimerization products, and a series of kinetic peculiarities in complex processes, etc.

In 1918 Nernst[4] put forward the hypothesis that free radicals played a decisive role not only in reactions in the liquid phase, but also in all fast reactions in the gas phase. There was much indirect evidence for this hypothesis, but it was only in the late 'thirties that the first direct spectroscopic methods were used for the detection of radicals formed during chemical reactions, those of free hydroxyl in rarefied hydrogen and carbon-monoxide flames.[5]

After this, reactions in the gas phase were for a long time the focus of all investigations of the role of radicals as intermediate products in chemical reactions. Mass spectroscopy was also applied in this field,[6-9] in addition to absorption and emission spectroscopy. However, the question of the identification of free radicals in condensed phases (liquids and solids), and the investigation of their chemical properties, remained almost unsolved until the beginning of the 1950s. The only sources which gave us any ideas on the possible structure of these particles were indirect chemical data based on an analysis of the final products. Only in some cases—when the radicals were formed in concentrations of over 5 or 10 per cent of the concentrations of the original products—was it possible to use the direct method of measurement of the paramagnetic susceptibility.[10] Even then, this method gave scant information about the nature of the paramagnetic particles.

This state of affairs was changed with the discovery of electron spin resonance, which made it possible to study radicals in various media.

The sensitivity of E.S.R. is at present another limitation on the application of the technique to the investigation of the structure and reactions of free radicals. As we saw above (Chapter 2), reliable measurements can be carried out only for a static concentration above $1-5 \cdot 10^{14}$ cm^{-3}. However, the recombination time of free particles such as free atoms, the alkyl, alkoxy, alkylperoxide and many other radicals in the liquid and gaseous phase, is so large that the static concentrations in normal thermal and photochemical reactions are much smaller than this minimum value.

The detection of free atoms by means of E.S.R. has until now only been successful in one fast chemical process, namely, in the combustion of hydrogen in rarefied flames. For this measurement Panfilov[11] used a combination of the spectrometer EPR-2 with a very simple kinetic irradiation arrangement: inside the cavity was placed a quartz tube, through which flowed the detonation gas ($H_2 + O_2$) at a pressure of 3 to 20 torr, with a flow velocity of 10 to 20 cm s^{-1} (Fig. 7.1). The tube was enclosed in a small electrical furnace, which produced temperatures up to 600°C. When the combustion point was exceeded, a stationary flame burned in the tube, and the E.S.R. spectrum showed a clear doublet from the appearance of the hydrogen atoms (Fig. 7.2).† The calculation of the concentration of hydrogen atoms, by double integration of these lines, leads to values of 10^{15} to 10^{16} cm^{-3}, which is in good agreement with calculations made on the basis of the theory of branched chain reactions.

This technique has recently been applied by Panfilov, Asatian and Nalbandjan[12] in the detection of above-equilibrium concentrations of hydrogen atoms in carbon-monoxide flames with a small amount of molecular hydrogen added. Since, from the chemical mechanism of the CO combustion, it follows that in this flame large concentrations of oxygen atoms are produced, Asatian and Nalbandjan[13] undertook in addition the direct identification of oxygen atoms in the combustion zone. The results of these investigations also verified the results of the chain reaction theory.

Although the application of E.S.R. in the investigation of fast reactions in the gaseous phase is no doubt of great interest, the development of this

† The wide non-resolved line in the spectrum was obviously formed by stable radicals produced by the interaction of the hydrogen atoms with the potassium metaborate with which the walls of the tube were coated, which is known to act as a slowing-down agent for the heterogeneous recombination of the hydrogen atoms.

field is only in its early stages, and further results, which would for example allow comparison with mass spectrometry, have not yet been obtained.

The investigation of radicals formed by reactions in the liquid phase was actually instigated by the coming of E.S.R. and its applications, but, for the reasons mentioned above, the scope of application is in most cases limited to relatively few active radicals and radical ions. However, as is well known, the radicals can often be considered as completely stable products and can be examined by chemical methods or by simple magnetic weighing.

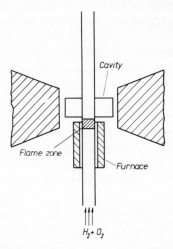

Fig. 7.1 Sketch of the arrangement for the measurement of the concentration of atoms in rarefied flames.

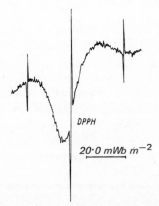

Fig. 7.2 Spectrum of hydrogen atoms in a hydrogen flame.

Nevertheless in these cases E.S.R. plays an indispensable role, since it permits an accurate determination of the actual structure of the radical (or radical ions). So this method enables us to acquire, for example, an accurate determination of the structure of the radical ions of different semiquinones,[14] positive and negative aromatic radical ions,[15] and many other less active paramagnetic centres.[16] We will now apply the results of these investigations to the problem of exactly how the spin density of the unpaired electron in complex paramagnetic centres is distributed (see Chapter 8).

In considering kinetic measurements in liquids, we propose to give an example which may be considered as a limiting case. The radical we wish to consider (triphenylmethyl) is so stable that its concentration reaches a few per cent of that of the hexaphenylethane. Information about its concentration and reaction rate were however until recently only obtainable on the basis of indirect chemical measurements. As triphenylmethyl has a characteristic and distinctive E.S.R. spectrum, it is a good subject for rigorous quantitative kinetic measurements. The work[17] carried out at ICP in 1958 by Diatschkovski, Bubnov and Schilov was based on the following problems:

1. Direct measurement of the equilibrium constant

$$(PH)_3C - C(PH)_3 \rightleftharpoons 2(Ph)_3\dot{C}$$

and the recombination rate of the triphenylmethyl radicals over a temperature interval which was usually large enough for the binding energy Q of the hexaphenylethane and the activation energy E of the recombination process to be accurately determined.

2. Direct proof of Semenov's hypothesis[18] on the possibility of radical formation from the bimolecular reaction

$$AB + CD \rightarrow \dot{A} + BC + \dot{D}$$

in cases where the bond B–C is essentially stronger than the bonds AB and CD. As an example of this, the following reaction was chosen:

$$(PH)_3CCl + LiC_2H_5 \rightarrow (Ph)_3\dot{C} + LiCl + \dot{C}_2H_5 \tag{I}$$

The course of this reaction may be followed through the formation of the stable radical $(Ph)_3\dot{C}$.

For the solution of the first problem, measurements were carried out on dilute solutions of hexaphenylethane in toluene immediately following its rapid cooling from room temperature to the temperature of investigation.

Figure 7.3 shows the kinetic recombination curves of the radical $(Ph)_3\dot{C}$ at two temperatures, $-50°C$ and $-64°C$. The measured points were completely in accordance with a kinetic law cf second order, which permits a determination of the rate constant, and, if the experiment is carried out at various temperatures, the activation energy:

$$k_{rec} = 3·9 . 10^7 \exp\left[\frac{-7000 \pm 500}{RT}\right] \text{l/mol s}$$

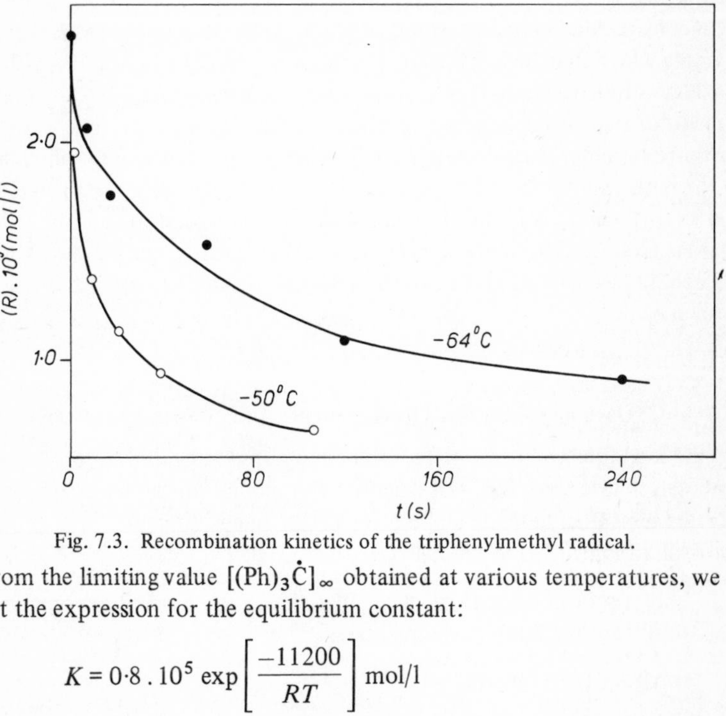

Fig. 7.3. Recombination kinetics of the triphenylmethyl radical.

From the limiting value $[(Ph)_3\dot{C}]_\infty$ obtained at various temperatures, we get the expression for the equilibrium constant:

$$K = 0·8 . 10^5 \exp\left[\frac{-11200}{RT}\right] \text{mol/l}$$

The values of E and Q obtained in this way agree very closely with the values calculated earlier from the chemical data.

Figure 7.4 shows some results obtained by Diatschkovski, Bubnov and Schilov[17] on their investigation of the reaction (I). As the two solutions [$(Ph)_3CCl$ and LiC_2H_5 in toluene] are mixed, there is a rapid increase in the concentration of the $(Ph)_3\dot{C}$, followed by a slow decrease as a result of the recombination process, until finally the equilibrium concentration $[(Ph)_3\dot{C}]_T$ at the given temperature is reached. It has been shown by direct measurement that the initial jump in the concentration is hardly at all dependent on the heating-up of the mixture by the reaction. From this it follows that this jump actually demonstrates the formation of an above-equilibrium concentration of the radicals as a result of the rapidity of the reaction (1).

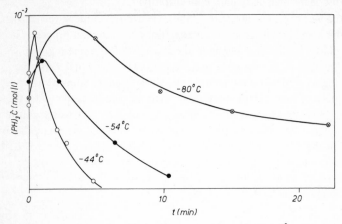

Fig. 7.4. Kinetic measurements of the concentration of the $(Ph)_3\dot{C}$ radical during the course of the reaction $(Ph)_3CCl + LiC_2H_5$.

These experiments did not succeed in detecting a spectrum of the radical C_2H_5. This is not really surprising, as even if this radical were formed, its concentration would be too small to enable detection. The authors assumed, for purely chemical reasons (the primary gaseous reaction products were ethane and ethylene, with butane almost entirely absent), that under the given conditions in general no free ethyl is formed, but a form of complicated metallo-organic complex, e.g.

$$C_2H_5 \ldots Li \ldots C_2H_5$$

which rearranges itself on the formation of C_2H_6 and C_2H_4 (see §8.5).

Despite the great interest in the use of E.S.R. in studies of radical reactions in the liquid phase, and in understanding the mechanism involved, so far as we know there have only been, until now, two systematic investigations in this direction. These are the work of the Americans Gardner and Fraenkel on the reactions in liquid sulphur,[19] and the work of Lebedev, Zepalov and Schliapintoch[20] on the identification of free radicals in the oxidation of cumene in the liquid phase.

In the first investigation, it was found that when liquid sulphur was heated, free radicals were formed as a result of the breaking of the

polymer chains. From the fact that these radicals are formed in
considerable concentrations, it follows that either their mobility in liquid
sulphur is very small, or that they form separate clusters, with the free
valence located inside the cluster, which would explain their low activity
and subsequent high stationary concentration.

In the work of Lebedev *et al.*,[20] the oxidation of cumene was chosen,
from the many detailed kinetic investigations of oxidation processes in the
liquid phase. In this case, owing to the strong sterical hindering, the
recombination of the peroxide radicals $PhC(CH_3)_2 O\dot{O}$ which form the
chain, is slowed down considerably, and the stationary concentration is
therefore very high. On the basis of accurate kinetic measurements, these
authors calculated the expected radical concentration during the course of
the reaction. The oxidation process was carried out in a special container
placed in the cavity of the spectrometer, with conditions ($T = 60–120°C$,
concentration of the prime components 10^{-1} M) such that a radical
concentration of the order of 10^{16} cm^{-3} was formed, i.e. many times the
minimum detectable concentration.

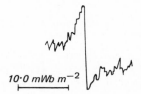

$10·0$ mWb m^{-2}

Fig. 7.5. E.S.R. spectrum of the radical $PhC(CH_3)_2 O\dot{O}$, formed by the oxidation of
cumene.

During the course of the stationary reaction the authors observed a
clear asymmetrical E.S.R. signal (Fig. 7.5) which was similar in shape to
that of other peroxide radicals. They obtained completely identical spectra
when different chemicals were used as the oxidation initiators, such as
azoisobutyronitril and dicyclohexylpercarbonate, or when the oxidation
was carried out catalytically in the presence of cobalt stearate.

The radical concentration agreed to within an accuracy of 50 per cent
with the calculated value, and the reaction rate of the oxidation process
was determined with the same accuracy. From this it follows that the
E.S.R. spectrum is really caused by the radical of the oxidation chain and
not by the influence of the added materials. It is very worth while to note
that no averaging-out of the anisotropy of the *g*-value as a result of the
rotation was observed, although it was measured in the liquid phase. The

reason for this could be that under these conditions the oxygen atoms of the peroxide group are so strongly bound intermolecularly, that the effective rotation frequency is considerably smaller than the magnitude $\Delta g(\beta/h)B$, which according to Fig. 7.5 is of the order of magnitude of 10^7 s^{-1}. It would be very interesting to investigate how the anisotropy changes when the temperature is increased and when the spectrum is observed at different frequencies. The fact that insufficient work has been carried out on the application of E.S.R. to the investigation of the mechanisms of chemical reactions, is clearly connected with the fact that until now, the applications of E.S.R. in chemistry were carried out mainly by physicists, who limited themselves to structural determination of the chemical samples, and were not particularly interested in kinetic problems. It is clear that this field will develop rapidly in the near future.

A series of results on the reaction rate of radicals formed by the interaction of ionizing radiation with solids, will be given later in Chapter 9.

References

1. Bleaney, B., Stevens, K. W. H.: *Rep. Progr. Phys.,* **16** (1953), 108.
2. Altschuler, S. A., Kosyrev, B. M.: *Paramagnetische Elektronenresonanz* (Electron Paramagnetic Resonance), Leipzig 1963.
3. Gomberg, M.: *JACS,* **22** (1900), 757
4. Nernst, M.: *Zs. Elektrochemie,* **24** (1918), 335.
5. Kondrat'ev, V. N.: *Svobodnyj gidroksil* (Free Hydroxyl), ONTI 1939.
6. Eltenton, G.: *J. Chem. Phys.,* **15** (1947), 455.
7. Lossing, F. P.: *Ann. N.Y. Acad. Sci.,* **67** (1957), 499.
8. Foner, S. N., Gudson, R. L.: *J. chem. Phys.,* **21** (1953), 1374, 1608.
9. Lavrovskaja, G. K., Skurat, V. T., Tal'roze, V. L., Tancyrev, T. D.: *C.C.R. Acad. Sci. U.R.S.S.,* **117** (1957), 641; Tal'roze, V. L. i dr.: *Prib. i Techn. Eksp.,* **6** (1960), 78.
10. Michaelis, L.: *Ann. N.Y. Acad. Sci.,* **40** (1940), 39; Michaelis, L., Granik, S.: *JACS,* **70** (1948), 624, 4275.
11. Panfilov, V. N., Cvetkov, Ju. D., Voevodskij, V. V.: *Kinetika i Kataliz,* **2** (1961), 295; **1** (1960) 333.
12. Asatjan, V. V., Panfilov, N. V., Nalbandjan, A. B.: *Kinetika i kataliz,* **2** (1961), 295.
13. Asatjan, V. V., Akopjan, L. A., Nalbandjan, A. B.: *C.C.R. Acad. Sci. U.R.S.S.,* **141** (1961) 1, 129.
14. Venkataraman, B., Fraenkel, G. K.: *JACS,* **77** (1955), 2707; *J. Chem. Phys.,* **23** (1955), 588.
15. Weissman, S., Townsend, J., Paul, D., Pake, G.: *J. chem. Phys.,* **21** (1953), 2227; Chu, T., Pake, G., Paul, D., Townsend, J., Weissman, S.: *J. Phys. Chem.,* **57** (1953), 504; Lipkin, D., Paul, D., Townsend, J., Weissman, S.: *Science.,* **117** (1953), 534; Weissman, S., de Boer, E., Conradi, J.: *J. chem. Phys.,* **25** (1956), 796.
16. Ingram, D. J. E.: *Free Radicals as Studied by Electron Spin Resonance,* London 1958.

17. Diatschkovski, F. S., Bubnov, N. N., Schilov, A. E.: *C. C. R. Acad. Sci. U.R.S.S.,* **122** (1958), 629; **123** (1958), 870.
18. Semenov, N. N.: *O nekotorych problemach chimičeskoj kinetiki i reakcionnoj sposobnosti* (On some Problems of Chemical Kinetics and Reaction Ability), Izd.-vo AN SSSR 1954.
19. Gardner, D., Fraenkel, G. K.: *JACS,* **78** (1956), 3279.
20. Lebedev, Ja. S., Zepalov, V. F., Schliapintoch, V. Ja.: *C.C.R. Acad. Sci. U.R.S.S.,* **139** (1961), 1409.

Chapter 8

The Application of E.S.R. in the Investigation of Electron Delocalization Phenomena

The idea of the possibility of a rapid displacement of the electrons in a complex molecule has been acknowledged for a long time by the majority of chemists, since only by its acceptance can we get a clear general picture of the many chemical reactions of complex molecules which contain a system of conjugated bonds, atoms with combined electron shells, etc. The same concept is basic to many quantum chemical calculations which help to establish our understanding of the structural character of complex molecules. In general, there is no doubt as to the correctness of this assumption, primarily because it is in agreement with the results of a wide variety of chemical experiments. Nevertheless, development in this direction, interesting though it may be, was delayed for a long time because there was no possibility of the study by direct methods of conjugation effects, which would allow us to clarify the various mechanisms which lead to their appearance and to investigate the quantitative character of the processes involved. Owing to the lack of such direct experimental methods, the only approach to this problem was by approximate quantum-mechanical calculations, the range of application of which could not, unfortunately, be precisely ascertained. Thus these methods, which were without doubt correct for a certain limited range of parameters, were taken as absolutely correct far beyond these limits. This incorrect application led to false results, and the whole concept of these quantum-mechanical calculations, which were based on the principle of delocalization, was placed in doubt.

E.S.R. was the first basic physical method which allowed direct detection of the presence of electron delocalization. But here we should also state that since E.S.R. is applicable only to paramagnetic centres, its range of application is considerably smaller than the range of the delocalization concept. It was shown in Chapter 3 that E.S.R. will measure only the delocalization of the spin density of an unpaired electron.

188

From the experimental results of the measurements of the spin distribution, it is not very far to a complete picture of the delocalization of all electrons of the molecule.

In addition to this, by virtue of the low energy of the quanta used and the wide range $(10^{10}-10^7 \text{ s}^{-1})$, E.S.R. is the only physical technique for the study of electron displacements which correspond to very small interaction energies. These are extremely important for an understanding of the kinetic character of complex reactions, particularly in catalytic and biological systems.

Thus we can truthfully say that the findings of E.S.R. can serve as an important resource, not only for the foundation of modern electron theory, but also for the formulation of the general basis of a theory of chemical processes which takes all possible electron displacements in the molecules into account.

§8.1

DELOCALIZATION OF UNPAIRED ELECTRONS IN STABLE RADICALS AND RADICAL IONS

An example of an unequivocal conclusion about delocalization is given by the analysis of the E.S.R. spectrum of α,α'-diphenyl-β-picrylhydrazyl (DPPH) (Fig. 8.1). The five equidistant lines with intensity ratio 1:2:3:2:1 signify that the spin of the unpaired electron is divided approximately in half between the α- and the β-nitrogen atoms (see Chapter 6). If we look at the valency diagram with the unpaired electron on the α-atom, we see that the partial localization of the unpaired electron on this atom requires it to have a positive charge. The nitrogen atom in this structure is therefore

$$\text{(I)}$$

represented by a tetravalent ion N^+. On the other hand, it follows from this that the radical DPPH must have a large electric dipole moment, e.g. in relation to the molecule of the diphenyl picryl hydrazine. Measurements of the dipole moments of these materials were carried out in 1930 by Wolf and co-workers, and later by Turkevitch and co-workers.[1] The latter found $D_M = 3.6$ Debye and $D_R = 4.9$ Debye, and on the basis of these measurements suggested an admixture of a resonance structure of the type (I). As we have seen, E.S.R. measurements carried out 20 years later

verified the truth of these qualitative pictures of the structure of the radical
DPPH.

More recently detailed information on the delocalization of the spin of
the unpaired electron in DPPH has been obtained. Measurements were made
in the liquid phase, and in the complete absence of oxygen;[2] the width of
the individual components was reduced sufficiently to allow each of the five
lines of the spectrum in Fig. 8.1 to split into a large number of finer lines
(Fig. 8.2). An analysis of the spectrum shows the presence of an interaction
of the unpaired electron with the protons of the phenyl ring (which is of
course smaller than the interaction with the α- and β-nitrogen atoms).

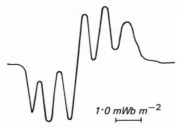

$1 \cdot 0 \, mWb \, m^{-2}$

Fig. 8.1. E.S.R. spectrum of the radical DPPH in benzene.

The technique in this measurement of completely removing the oxygen,
which often acts as a paramagnetic impurity and widens the individual
H.F.S. components, is a very important method for improving the
resolution of the H.F.S. of complex E.S.R. spectra.

*Recently a special technique has been developed for high resolution
E.S.R.[39]* The resolution was increased to 1 part in 10^6, and in order to
achieve this, some changes in the experimental technique were necessary.
The long relaxation times corresponding to the small line widths (§3.9)
required a reduction of the microwave power in order to prevent saturation.
The upper limit for the frequency of the magnetic field modulation was
10 kHz (§2.5). On the other hand the signal amplitudes are very small, as
one must work with a highly diluted sample in order to reduce the spin-spin
interaction, and also the sample volume must be kept small to avoid the

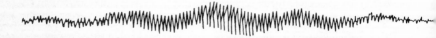

Fig. 8.2. E.S.R. spectrum of the radical DPPH in tetrahydrofuran in the absence of
oxygen.

inevitable inhomogeneity of the magnetic field. For these measurements one therefore uses the highest sensitivity superheterodyne spectrometer.*

A large amount of the experimental and theoretical work on the study of the delocalization of the spin density was carried out on the *p*-benzosemiquinone ion radical and its derivatives. Indeed, even for the simplest anion of this class one would expect the spin of the unpaired electron to be localized not only on the oxygen atom, as follows from the usual formula,

$$\dot{O}\!\!-\!\!\overset{H\ H}{\underset{H\ H}{\Big\langle\!\!\!\Big\rangle}}\!\!-\!\!\bar{O} \tag{II}$$

but also other structures of the type

$$\bar{O}\!\!-\!\!\overset{H\ H}{\underset{H\ H}{\Big\langle\!\!\!\Big\rangle}}\!\!-\!\!O \tag{III}$$

in which the unpaired spin is localized on one of the hydrogen atoms of the ring. E.S.R. measurements[3] showed (Fig. 8.3) that the spectrum of this anion radical in the liquid phase consists of five H.F.S. components with intensity distribution 1:4:6:4;1, which would suggest an interaction of the unpaired electron with the hydrogen atoms.

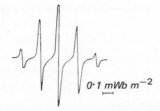

0·1 mWb m⁻²

Fig. 8.3. E.S.R. spectrum of the semiquinone ion radical $(O-C_6H_4-O)^-$.

Several problems arose during the theoretical analysis of these results connected with the fact that the unpaired electron of the anion radical must be a *p*-electron, and, according to current theory in the late 1940s, would not be able to produce an H.F.S. with the protons, since its density in the plane of the aromatic is equal to zero. This apparent contradiction arises not only in the case of the semiquinones, but also in the case of any free radical in which the unpaired electron is distributed over a system of conjugated bonds, and also in others of the same class as DPPH and triphenylmethyl, considered above. This problem was thoroughly investigated for the example of the semiquinones, since they were the first of this class to be extensively studied by E.S.R. McConnell[4] showed (see also Chapter 3) that in the fragment

$$\mathrm{>\overset{\cdot}{C}-H}$$

as a result of the interaction of the unpaired p-electron of the C-atom with both electrons of the σ-bond C—H, the final density of the unpaired electron at the proton must be in an s-state. According to the calculations of McConnell the H.F.S. splitting produced by this effect amounts to about $2 \cdot 25$ mWb m^{-2}. This result agrees very well with those obtained by measurements on the alkyl radicals produced by irradiation of organic solids and liquid ethane (see below). By comparison of these results with the E.S.R. spectra of the semiquinones, for which the magnitude of the H.F.S. splitting is approximately equal to $0 \cdot 24$ mWb m^{-2}, McConnell concluded that the spin density on each C—H group of the ring was approximately $0 \cdot 1$. This result is easy to understand. It means that the proportion of structures of type III in actual molecules is not larger than $0 \cdot 6$. In the case of substitution of one or more ring protons by chlorine, the number of H.F.S. components is reduced, since the splitting by these nuclei is not resolved. The corresponding spectra[5] consist of four, three, two and one lines (see Fig. 8.4). It is interesting to note that through partial substitution of H by Cl, the magnitude of the splitting by the remaining ring-protons changes slightly. For the example given above, the value of approximately $0 \cdot 24$ reduced to $0 \cdot 20$ mWb m^{-2} for the ion of 2,5-dichloro-p-benzosemiquinone. This can be associated with a redistribution of the spin density of the unpaired electron as a result of the redistribution of the charge density in the ion radical. If this is in fact so, then one would expect an even larger effect from the substitution of the protons by fluorine. Frank and Gutovski[6] showed in a later work that the introduction of two fluorine atoms into the ring reduced the splitting by two other protons to $0 \cdot 13$ mWb m^{-2}.

Stone and Maki[40] detected a noticeable influence of the solvent on the H.F.S. coupling constant of the semiquinones. In particular, the C^{13} H.F.S. coupling constants in (aprotic) solvents such as acetonitrile and dimethyl sulphoxide are larger than in (protic) solvents such as water and alcohol (see also §8.7).*

If the hydrogen is substituted by methyl groups, then it appears that although the hydrogen atoms of these groups are quite distant from the ring, the H.F.S. splitting produced by them comes close to the value of the splitting caused by the ring protons.[3] Thus the magnitude of the splitting in the tetramethyl-*p*-benzosemiquinone ion is 0.15 mWb^{-2} for all twelve protons of the four methyl groups, and the total splitting is almost

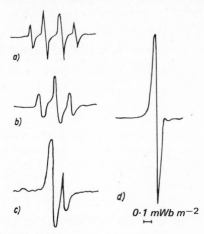

Fig. 8.4. E.S.R. spectra of chlorine-substituted semiquinones.

    (*a*) monochlorosemiquinone
    (*b*) 2,3-dichlorosemiquinone
    (*c*) trichlorosemiquinone
    (*d*) tetrachlorosemiquinone

2.3 mWb m^{-2}, i.e. almost as much as the splitting of a CH fragment, which has an unpaired electron. The original theory of McConnell implies that the interaction of the unpaired electron with the proton in the fragment C–C–H should be considerably smaller than in the fragment C–H, so the above result could be considered as evidence that to the ground state of the ion $[0–C_6(CH_3)_4–0]^-$ we should ascribe a structure like

$$[C_6(CH_3)_3O_2]^- \ldots CH_3$$

However, such a conclusion is in complete contradiction with the chemical features of these ions. It is also clear that in these ions, the structure in which the unpaired electron is localized on the oxygen atoms occurs in considerable proportions, and this also tends to contradict the above explanation. Therefore, such a structure for this radical ion should not be taken seriously. Apart from this, experimental results have shown that in some organic radicals, which have only aromatic and methyl-CH bonds (perinaphthene (IV),[7] demesitylmethyl (V)[8]), a total splitting is observed which is considerably larger than the maximum value ΔB_Σ = 2·3 mWb m^{-2} obtained by McConnell for a CH fragment [in (IV), ΔB_Σ = 4·9 mWb m^{-2}, and in (V), 4·8 mWb m^{-2}]. In all of these cases, the theory presented above is obviously inadequate. It was necessary to seek some other explanation for these large values of the total splitting.

At this stage it would appear useful to give a brief outline of the chemical interpretation of the theoretical calculations for the fragments $\dot{C}H$ (1),[4] and $\dot{C}$–C–H (2),[9] since with the help of a qualitative picture the data which will be given later can be more easily understood.

A simplified spin-model of the fragment (1) has the following form:

$$\underset{1\ 2\ 3}{\overset{\uparrow\uparrow\!\downarrow}{>C-H}} \tag{1}$$

Here 1 is the symbol for the spin of the unpaired electron, 2 and 3 are the symbols for the electron spins of the C–H bond. By the interaction of spins 1 and 2, the bond of 2 and 3 on the radical is weakened slightly, and a certain density of the unpaired spin 3 appears on the nucleus H. If 1 corresponds to a complete electron, then according to the calculations of McConnell the H.F.S. splitting due to the hydrogen nucleus is 2·25 mWb m^{-2}.†

In the case of the fragment (2),

$$>\underset{\downarrow}{\dot{C}}-\overset{\big|}{\underset{\big|\,\uparrow\!\downarrow}{C}}-H \tag{2}$$

the interaction has a completely different character. The theory of McConnell is by its very nature equivalent to the well known rule in free radical chemistry, that a C–H bond which is in the β-position to a free valence is very much weaker than a common C–H bond, as the separation of the corresponding atom simultaneously results in the formation of a double bond. In other words, the β-hydrogen atom of the fragment (2) is essentially more mobile than one in an α-position. It is therefore to be expected that without any external influence, an appreciable density of the unpaired electron also exists on the H nucleus in question. This condition

_____

† McConnell predicted theoretically that the spin density on the hydrogen nucleus in the CH fragment must exhibit negative polarization, i.e. that the corresponding magnetic moment is antiparallel to the moment of the unpaired electron. This prediction has since been proved directly by nuclear resonance and double resonance techniques.

can be expressed by using the method of the valence model, in a formula of the type:

$$>C\!=\!\!\overset{|}{\underset{|}{C}}\cdots\dot{H} \tag{2'}$$

The proportion of this structure present can be determined sufficiently well from the experimental data: for a free hydrogen atom the H.F.S. constant is equal to 50.0 mWb m^{-2}, and for the CH_3 group in the ethyl radical it is approximately 2.7 mWb m^{-2}. From this it follows that the statistical weight of the structure $(2')$ in the case of fragment (2) is approximately equal to 0.05. McConnell's calculations, which were performed before the publication of the E.S.R. measurement of the ethyl radical, give, with corresponding assumptions, a value of the splitting constant which are very close to the real values. A reasonable solution was thus obtained for the problem of the magnitude of the total splitting in tetramethyl-p-benzosemiquinone and in dimesitylmethyl.

However the question of the magnitude of the splitting in perinaphthene remained confused, as in this sample there are no β-hydrogen atoms, and the total splitting, as in dimesitylmethyl, is considerably larger than the maximum value of approximately 2.3 mWb m^{-2} for a CH fragment.

In order to explain this state of affairs, McConnell had to extend the theory.[10] This extension proved itself to be essential in explaining a multitude of very different spectra. The addition to the theory was that in considering a conjugated system with delocalized unpaired electrons, one cannot assume that one is always dealing with an unpaired electron.

We will consider this general situation for the very simple example of the allyl radical $\dot{C}_3H_5$. From the ideas presented here, it follows that the true structure of this radical can be presented, to a first approximation, by a superposition of the two following structures:

$$\dot{C}H_2-CH=CH_2 \qquad CH_2=CH-\dot{C}H_2$$
$$\;(1)\quad\;(2)\quad\;(3)\qquad\quad (1)\quad\;(2)\quad\;(3)$$

If this description were sufficiently close to the true structure, then the E.S.R. spectrum of the allyl radical would consist of five lines (or more precisely, five poorly resolved doublets). The splitting between the five main components would be approximately equal to $0.5\ \Delta B_{CH} = 1.15$ mWb m^{-2}. Accurate measurements on different radicals of the allyl type give an actual splitting of 1.5 to 1.6 mWb m$^{-2} \approx \frac{2}{3}\Delta B_{CH}$ between the individual components,[11] and a total splitting considerably larger than ΔB_{CH}.

McConnell showed[10] that this result is understandable if one assumes that in certain systems with conjugated double bonds the unpaired electron has a perturbing effect on the π-electrons of the double bond, and whilst the total spin is conserved, these become effectively de-paired. As a very rough approximation, this leads us to the idea that, in addition to the distribution of the spin density corresponding to the usual structural picture,

$$\underset{1}{\uparrow\downarrow}\ \underset{2}{\uparrow}\ \underset{3}{}\qquad\qquad \underset{1}{\uparrow}\ \underset{2}{}\ \underset{3}{\uparrow\downarrow}$$

in a real radical we must also consider the arrangement of the spin density

$$\underset{1}{\uparrow}\ \underset{2}{\downarrow}\ \underset{3}{\uparrow}$$

This picture represents a system with three unpaired electrons, which however interact with themselves so strongly that the total spin remains equal to $\frac{1}{2}$.

If we assume, for the sake of simplicity, that all three models are of equal statistical weight, then we find that the density of the unpaired electron on atoms 1 and 3 has the value of $\frac{2}{3}$, and for the middle atom the value $\frac{1}{3}$. According to the foregoing argument, the total density of the unpaired electron on the whole particle, normalized to unity, is

$$\tfrac{2}{3} + \tfrac{2}{3} - \tfrac{1}{3} = 1$$

The total splitting is however proportional to the sum of the absolute values of the densities on the different atoms:

$$\tfrac{2}{3} + \tfrac{2}{3} + \tfrac{1}{3} = \tfrac{5}{3}$$

In other words,

$$\Delta B_{\Sigma} \approx \tfrac{5}{3}\Delta B_{CH} \approx 4{\cdot}0 \text{ mWb m}^{-2}$$

and

$$\Delta B_{HFS} = \tfrac{2}{3}\Delta B_{CH} = 1{\cdot}5 \text{ mWb m}^{-2}$$

which agree with the experimental results.

In the general case of the delocalization of the unpaired electron in a strongly conjugated system, a partial additional de-pairing of the electrons of the system can thus occur, as a result of which the projection of the effective electron spin along the field axis has a different sign for different atoms, or, as it is normally expressed, there are different polarizations. For this very reason, the total splitting is not determined by the usual summation,

$$\sum_i \rho_i \, |a_{si}|^2$$

but by the more general summation,

$$\sum_i |\rho_i| \, . \, |a_{si}|^2$$

which admits the possibility of a negative ρ_i. Here we must naturally fulfill the normalization condition,

$$\sum_i \rho_i = 1$$

which takes into account that the total spin of the particle is caused by an unpaired electron.†

§8.2

SPIN DELOCALIZATION IN CONNECTION WITH MULTI-ELECTRON BONDS

The interesting results which we have so far obtained on the E.S.R. investigation of the delocalization of the unpaired electron in a complex molecule, illustrated above by the examples of DPPH and the various derivatives of p-benzosemiquinone, pose the question as to whether it is possible to use this method for the study of particles with a so-called deficiency structure, i.e. of particles in which the sum total of the bond is considerably more than half of the participating electrons. Unfortunately the majority of the stable bonds of this kind are diamagnetic,‡ e.g. the boranes and metallo-carbonyls, and in addition to this, the ions of these bonds are very unstable; for these reasons, until recently E.S.R. could not be used to examine the character of these multi-electron bonds.

During the last few years a completely new class of materials with multi-electron bonds has been studied in the U.S.S.R. and in other countries, and these can also in a sense be described as deficiency structures. These are the so-called 'sandwich' complexes, in which one metal ion is situated between two parallel cyclopentadienyl or benzene rings.[13] Examples of this are dicyclopentadienylferrum (ferrocene) and dibenzolchrome.

In the first example, it can be deduced that initially there are 10 Fe–C bonds and 10 aromatic C–C ring bonds formed by 18 electrons (8 electrons

† The question of negative spin density was considered in Chapter 3 within the framework of the molecular orbital method.

‡ More recently a paramagnetic carbonyl has been discovered.[12] The E.S.R. spectrum of this substance has, until now, not been investigated.

from the Fe-atom and 10 electrons from the two cyclopentadienyl rings),
and in the second example, 12 Cr–C bonds and 12 aromatic bonds of the
benzene rings are formed by 18 electrons (6 electrons from the chromium
and 12 electrons from the benzene rings). However, electron deficiency
bonds of this type are sometimes extremely stable. Thus the ferrocene
evaporates without decomposing.

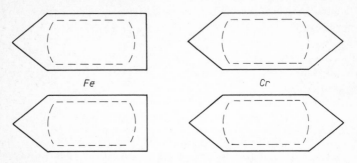

This high stability is obviously connected with the fact that all electrons
of this complex molecule are bound in a similar fashion to, for example, the
six π-electrons of the benzene molecule. This effect is so great that, unlike
the rather unstable deficiency structures which decompose following
ionization, the ions of the 'sandwich' bonds are sometimes very stable. On
the other hand a number of neutral molecules of this type are paramagnetic.
Thus it follows that after the discovery of these bonds, the real possibility
arose of using E.S.R. to examine molecular systems with deficiency
multi-electron bonds.

The paramagnetic ions of chromebenzol $[Cr(C_6H_6)_2]^+$ and its derivatives
have been well studied chemically.[14] As we can see from the spectra of
$[Cr(C_6H_6)_2]^+$ as well as its derivatives, shown in Fig. 8.5, the dilute
solutions ($\leqslant 10^{-3}$ M) give more-or-less well resolved hyperfine structures,
which can be attributed to the H.F.S. interaction with the protons of the
two benzene rings neighbouring the chromium. The truth of this statement
follows primarily from the analysis of the number of H.F.S. components.
We can clearly detect 11 components in the spectrum of the $[Cr(C_6H_6)_2]^+$
ion. (If all ring protons were taken into account, then the number of
components would be equal to 13, but from the binomial law it follows that
the first and thirteenth components are twelve times weaker than the
second and the twelfth; thus the extreme edge components can only be
detected with great difficulty.) On the substitution of the protons by phenyl
and alkyl groups, the number of components decreases, in accordance with our

assumptions. So in the case of $[Cr(C_6H_5-C_6H_5)_2]^+$ the number of components is equal to 9, i.e. two less than in the spectrum of $[Cr(C_6H_6)_2]^+$. In the case of the introduction of a substituent in only one ring $[Cr(C_6H_6)(C_6H_5-C_6H_5)]^+$, the symmetry of the spectrum clearly changes, again proving the assumption that the H.F.S. is caused by the protons of both benzene rings neighbouring the chromium.

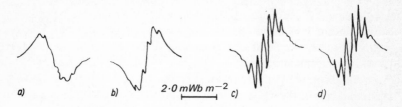

Fig. 8.5. E.S.R. spectra of the dibenzolchrome cation and its derivatives.
(a) $[(C_6H_6)_2 Cr]^+$, (b) $[(C_6H_5 - C_6H_{11})_2 Cr]^+$;
(c) $[(C_6H_6)(C_6H_5 - C_6H_5) Cr]^+$; (d) $[(C_6H_5 - C_6H_5)_2 Cr]^+$

It is interesting that, in most of the bonds examined, the magnitude of the splitting was independent of the type of substituent, of the number of protons in the rings, of the nature of the solvent and of the temperature, and was always constant and equal to

$$\Delta B'_{Cr(ArH)_2^+} = 0.37 \pm 0.05 \text{ mWb m}^{-2}$$

On the basis of this result we can assume that the collective interaction of the electrons in the system $[Cr(C_6H_6)_2]^+$ is so strong that it cannot be destroyed even by the introduction of such substituents as R or Ph, and also that the magnitude of ΔB is not sensitive to substitution. In the system $[Cr(C_6H_6)_2]^+$ the unpaired electron of the chromium is always so strongly localized in the benzene rings that it brings out the H.F.S. splitting. For a qualitative comparison of the experimental measurement of ΔB with the theoretical calculation, a standard of reference must be given. It was natural for such a measure to choose the value $\Delta B_{CH} = 2.25$ mWb m^{-2} found by McConnell,[4] which as we have seen represented a correct value for the calculation of ΔB in the fragment C–H of the p-benzosemiquinones and the allyl radicals. However, the analysis of the experimental results using this simple idea leads to a very strange result. Since $[Cr(C_6H_6)_2]^+$ has twelve equivalent hydrogen atoms and $\Delta B' \approx 0.37$ mWb m^{-2}, the total splitting obtained is

$$\Delta B_\Sigma = 12 \Delta B' = 4.45 \text{ mWb m}^{-2} = 1.98\Delta B_{CH}$$

On the other hand it follows from purely magnetic measurements that each ion of the chromebenzol contains only one unpaired electron. As there is complete symmetry, the possibility of a change in sign of the spin density in the rings must in this case be excluded. Quite apart from this, an alternating sign was not observed in the ions $(ArH)^-$ and $(ArH)^+$.

There are two possible explanations for this inconsistency. One can assume that in these molecules, for some unknown reason, the value of ΔB_{CH} found by McConnell must be doubled. If this explanation were correct, then it would result in some very unpleasant consequences for the theory, since here a quantitative comparison of the splitting due to the C—H fragments of different molecules would not be possible. The other explanation consists of the application of McConnell's hypothesis on the alternating sign of the whole molecule. In fact, one assumes that in the two rings there are, on the average, 0·99 spins with equal polarization, and on the chromium atom 0·98 spins with the opposite polarization, so giving a completely satisfactory explanation of the experimental data.

Thus the formal spin-model of the system can be represented in the following way (with the approximation $0·98 \approx 0·99 \approx 1$):

$$[C_6H_6 \: Cr \: C_6H_6]^+$$
$$\uparrow \quad \downarrow \quad \uparrow$$

Such an interpretation of the experimental data seems at first sight to be very unnatural, and the applied method of analysis very subjective. However, further investigations have confirmed, in a most convincing way, this picture, which appeared initially to be so unlikely. If the suggested spin-model does in fact correspond to the real distribution of the spin density, then the spin density on the chromium atom must be approximately equal to one. This deduction may be verified directly. In the naturally occurring isotope mixture of chromium, the Cr^{53} isotope is 9 per cent abundant; it has a considerable nuclear magnetic moment, and a nuclear spin of $\frac{3}{2}$. From the work of Manenkov and Prochorov[15] it is known that the H.F.S. splitting for Cr^{53} in $Cr_2O_3 . nAl_2O_3$ is equal to $1·84$ mWb m^{-2}. For a solution to the present problem the H.F.S. splitting due to the Cr^{53} dibenzolchrome ion was required. This was obtained by measurement of the E.S.R. spectrum of the bisdiphenylchrome cation, under recording conditions of maximum sensitivity and best possible resolution. One can see in the spectrum, shown in Fig. 8.6, on both sides of the main group of lines, two more groups which exhibit a clear H.F.S. with the same splitting and intensity distribution as the main group. The intensity of the satellites is about 50 times smaller than the intensity of the main

lines. This agrees well with the intensity ratio to be expected,
$0.25 \times 0.09 = 0.023$, which is calculated from the consideration that the
E.S.R. line of the ions of the Cr^{53} is split into four components of equal
intensity.

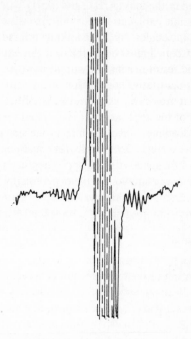

Fig. 8.6. E.S.R. spectrum of $[Cr(C_6H_5 - C_6H_5)_2]^+$ with Cr^{53}-H.F.S.

We consider the above example to be extremely important, firstly
because the actual result itself is direct proof of such an unusual picture of
the distribution of the spin density in a complex molecule, and secondly
because the H.F.S. splitting of an isotope of small abundance was used for
the quantitative analysis of the E.S.R. data. This procedure can be very
important for the investigation of complicated systems by means of E.S.R.
Recently Stschegolev and Karimov[16] showed, in a nuclear resonance study
of $[CR(C_6H_6)_2]^+$ and $[Cr(C_6H_5 . CH_3)_2]^+$ ions at $4°K$, that the shifts of
the proton lines for the ring protons and the α-protons of the alkyl groups
have opposite signs. This result shows undisputably that the H.F.S. of the
E.S.R. spectrum is actually caused by the presence of an unpaired electron
in the π-system of the benzene ring. These results can thus be considered as

independent proof, on the basis of the analysis of the E.S.R. data,† of the picture of the spin density distribution given above.

§8.3
ON THE POSSIBILITY OF 'BLOCKING' THE DELOCALIZATION

Until now we have considered only systems in which the delocalization of the unpaired electron manifests itself in the form of a specific distribution of the spin density on the molecule, a distribution which could be measured directly by the magnitude of the H.F.S. splitting produced by the atoms at various positions in the molecule. Since in reality the spin of the electron is not divisible, such an argument is possible only in cases in which the molecular displacement frequency of the spin is considerably larger than the frequency of measurement. The measurement of the electron displacement by means of the H.F.S. already proves the presence of a multicomponent spectrum which originates from delocalization of the spin on two or more atoms, and that the delocalization rate, i.e. the frequency of the transition of the spins from one position to another, is considerably larger than the separation of the H.F.S. components, expressed in frequency units.

We have already pointed out that this value, which can be regarded as the characteristic frequency of the technique, is usually very small. For example, in the case of the benzosemiquinone ions

$$\Delta B = 0{\cdot}2\text{--}0{\cdot}3 \text{ mWbm}^{-2}$$

which corresponds to a frequency $\nu_{HFS} \approx 5\text{--}10$ MHz or to an energy $\Delta E_{HFS} \approx 10^{-3}$ cal/mol.

Since the displacement frequency of the spins in the phenyl structure $-(C_6H_4)-$, which is equal to $10^{14}\text{--}10^{15}$ Hz ($10\text{--}100$ kcal/mol), is many orders of magnitude larger than the above, the model of the 'smeared-out' spin proves itself a very good fit.

The situation is changed completely when we examine systems in which, for some reason or another, the displacement is markedly slowed down. Here, in cases in which we can assume, on the basis of other considerations, that displacements with the usual energies of approxi-

---

† In the meantime Stschegolev and Karimov have shown that the ring protons are polarized positively relative to the total spin of the molecule. This result contradicts the distribution diagram of the spin density which we have postulated. For an interpretation of all the experimental facts one can assume a somewhat more complicated diagram, $[C_6H_6(\downarrow)Cr(\uparrow\,\uparrow\,\uparrow)C_6H_6(\downarrow)]^+$, which naturally requires additional proof.

mately 5–20 kcal/mol barely appear, the confirmation of a corresponding H.F.S. will signify that nevertheless such displacements will take place, but with frequencies lying in the interval $10^{14} > \nu > 10^6$ Hz.

If, however, an H.F.S. is absent, which corresponds to a displacement of the spin over the entire system, then this means that a potentially available displacement will result with a frequency smaller than 10^6 Hz.

As an example of measurements of this type, we should mention the work carried out recently at ICP by Solodovnikov on the H.F.S. of the E.S.R. spectra of aromatic anion radicals.

About ten years ago[7] it was discovered that the alkali metals react easily with condensed aromatic bonds such as naphthalene, anthracene etc. These reactions represent an electron transfer process from the metal atom on the aromatic molecule by the formation of a negative ion radical $(ArH)^-$.

More recently it has been found that under certain conditions (volatile solvent, reduced temperature) not only condensed aromatic bonds act in this way, but also bonds such as benzene and its alkyl derivatives. The aromatic anion radicals are produced in sufficiently high concentration to be examined by the techniques of E.S.R.[17] In the case of the benzene anion the E.S.R. spectrum consists of seven components (see Fig. 8.7). This indicates that the localization of the spin is equally probable on each of the carbon atoms of the benzene ring. In the case of toluene, ethyl benzene and other monoalkyl derivatives, the spectrum consists of

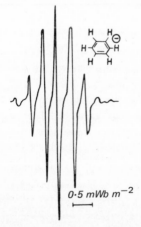

0·5 mWb m^{-2}

Fig. 8.7. E.S.R. spectrum of the ion radical $C_6H_6^-$.

five main components (see Fig. 8.8) which are formed by the interaction of the spin with the four equivalent protons. The spin density on the carbon atom in the para-position is also very small. The conclusion that only the hydrogen atom in the para-position does not participate in the basic H.F.S. splitting is verified by the fact that the E.S.R. spectrum of the p-xylol ion consists of the same five components as in the case of the monoalkyl-substituted benzene. The question of the reason for the 'blocking' of the para-position is very interesting theoretically. McConnell has considered this problem in some of his more recent papers.[18] For

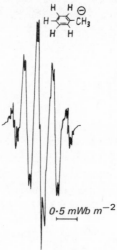

Fig. 8.8. E.S.R. spectrum of the ion radical $(C_6H_5CH_3)^-$.

present purposes, we need only accept the essential fact that in the ion radicals $(R . C_6H_5)^-$ only four protons of the phenyl ring participate in the basic H.F.S.

In one of Solodovnikov's papers,[19] he posed the question of how one may take advantage of the above-mentioned features of the spectra of the aromatic ion radicals, in order to investigate the displacement frequency of the electron in a complex molecule. In an attempt to do this, investiga-- tions were started on the E.S.R. spectra of the ion radicals of the aromatic bonds in which two phenyl rings are connected together by a more-or-less complex saturated carbon 'bridge'. The idea behind the experiment is as follows.

If after the electron interacts with the molecule, the displacement frequency of the electron between the two rings is larger than the frequency of the method, which in the present case is determined from the H.F.S. splitting of 0·3 mWb m^{-2} to be approximately 10^7 Hz, then we will observe in the E.S.R. spectrum of the ion radical an H.F.S. splitting which is caused by the protons of both rings, i.e. a spectrum of nine lines with binomial intensity distribution. If on the other hand $\nu_{disp} < \nu_{HFS}$, then we will observe an E.S.R. spectrum which is caused only by one phenyl ring, i.e. a spectrum of five lines, analogous to the spectrum of the ions of the type $(R . Ph)^-$.

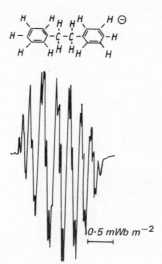

Fig. 8.9. E.S.R. spectrum of the ion radical $(C_6H_5-CH_2-CH_2-C_6H_5)^-$.

The experiments showed that in the case of the ion radicals of the diphenyls, the diphenylmethanes and the 1,2-diphenylethanes (dibenzyls), the E.S.R. spectrum consists of nine lines with binomial intensity distribution. In the case of the latter two ions one observes a small additional splitting due to the protons of the carbon-hydrogen 'bridge' (Fig. 8.9). Thus in all the three bonds considered, the electron transition between the rings takes place with a frequency greater than 10^7 Hz.

This result is exceptionally important in theoretical chemistry, insofar as it makes necessary a clearer understanding of the idea of 'conjugation'. Until now, it has been assumed in chemistry, that a conjugation, i.e. a strong interaction between multiple and aromatic bonds, results only via a σ-bond, as for example in butadiene or styrol. From the viewpoint of classical chemistry, the possibility of an interaction via two σ-bonds (diphenyl-methane) or even via three (dibenzyl) was considered extremely unlikely. However, one should not think that the results obtained are in any way contradictory to the previous experimentally confirmed ideas. Even so, the quantitative understanding of conjugation must be supplemented by present ideas. In the case of interaction via one σ-bond, the delocalization frequency is so large ($10^{14}-10^{15}$ Hz) that this effect leads to a noticeable lowering of the energy state of the molecule ($\approx 5-50$ kcal/mol). In the case of more complicated 'weaker conducting' bridges ($-CH_2-$, $-CH_2-CH_2-$, etc.) an interaction will also be present, but with considerably lower interaction energy, and accordingly the displacement frequency will be lower than the maximum value given above. This interaction has virtually no effect on the energy of the ground-state of the molecule, but it can exercise a large effect on the reactive behaviour of the molecule.

For an explanation of this we will assume that the interaction velocity of an aromatic ion radical with a reagent X in the condensed phase is deter-mined by the time τ_X during which the molecule is linked together with the ion, or is in the same 'cell'. In the event that $1/\tau_X = \nu_X$ is larger than ν_{Del}, and if the ion in question is a complex one with several aromatic rings, X will react only under the condition that the molecule will be in a 'cell' with the particular ring on which the electron is directly localized. If on the other hand $\nu_X < \nu_{Del}$ then the molecule reacts with an arbitrary ring of the ion radical. This effect can be extremely important in the case of high molecular bonds, where a weak interaction, which has virtually no influence on the energy of the system, can extend over a large distance across saturated bonds, or across a system of intermolecular bonds of the hydrogen-bridge type, etc.

Thus since the usual concept of conjugation is not applicable in the case of a weak conjugation, such effects must be characterized by a very small energy value, or better still by the displacement frequency of the electrons in the given system.

So far, all our conclusions have been based on results which allow us to calculate a lower limit of the displacement frequency, which in the systems that we have examined is represented by the value $\nu_{HFS} \approx 10^7$ Hz. It would be interesting to know actually how far ν_{Del} differs from this lower limit in these systems. It is our opinion that in dibenzyl, ν_{Del} does not exceed the lower limit by more than a factor of 10 to 100. This follows from the fact that if, in the ion radical p-$CH_3C_6H_4 . CH_2 . Ch(C_7H_{15})$. $CH_2 . C_6H_4 . p . CH_3$ we extend the bridge by another link, then the spectrum consists only of five lines. So in this case, ν_{Del} is already lower than ν_{HFS}. One may observe a similar spectrum with five H.F.S. components, indicating that the inequality $\nu_{Displ} < \nu_{HFS}$ holds, on the substitution of two hydrogen atoms of the C_2H_4 group of the dibenzyl by methyl groups. Since such a substitution can obviously not make any substantial change to the character of the conjugation, we must assume that in the dibenzyl ion, ν_{Del} is not much larger than ν_{HFS}.

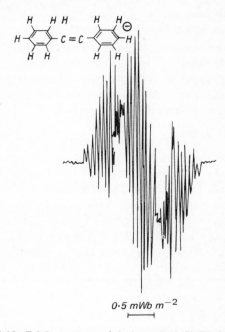

$0 \cdot 5 \ mWb \ m^{-2}$

Fig. 8.10. E.S.R. spectrum of the ion radical $(PhCH=CHPh)^-$.

If on the other hand one goes from the ion of the dibenzyl to the anion of the stilbene, in which ν_{Del} must come close to the maximum value given above $(10^{13}-10^{14}$ Hz), then the appearance of the spectrum changes completely. One can see from Fig. 8.10 that the density of the unpaired electron is localized mainly on the atoms of the bridge, and, apart from this, the phenyl-hydrogen atoms in the ortho-, meta- and para-positions are completely nonequivalent. From this it follows that ν_{Del}(dibenzyl) $\ll 10^{14}$ Hz, which again strengthens the argument that this value is only slightly larger than $\nu_{HFS} \approx 10^7$Hz.

The question of the change in the spectrum due to a change in ν_{Del} has recently been investigated in more detail by the theoretician Burschtein,[20] and independently by Alexandrov.[21] The basis of the first of these calculations is that the magnitude ν_{HFS}, which is constant for the class of compounds considered, is decided by the energy Q_{si} of the H.F.S. interaction of the unpaired electron spin with the nuclear moments of the protons of the aromatic ring, according to the relation:

$$\nu_{HFS} = \frac{Q_{si}}{h}$$

The delocalization frequency ν_{Del} is determined from ΔE, the energy difference between the energy levels, which originates as a result of the degeneracy of the system $[Ph-(CH_2)n-Ph]^-$. Thus we get, from the transition (delocalization) of the electrons between the two possible localization states which have the same energy E_0,

$$Ph^--(CH_2)_n-Ph \tag{I}$$

and

$$Ph-(CH_2)_n-Ph^- \tag{II}$$

which are two new energy levels with the energies $E_0 + \Delta E/2$ and $E_0 - \Delta E/2$.

In systems similar to the dibenzyl, where there is weak configuration, $\Delta E \ll kT \approx 10^{13}-10^{17}$ Hz. It can easily be shown that Q_{si} is also always considerably smaller than kT.

Under these conditions the shape of the spectrum depends on the value of the ratio $\Delta E/Q_{si} = \Theta$. For $\Theta \gg 1$ the spectrum is produced by the complete set of levels of both rings. For $\Theta \ll 1$ both structures (I) and (II) exist independently within the time interval $\tau_{HFS} = h/Q_{si}$. In this case the E.S.R. spectrum is produced by the levels of one ring and coincides with the spectrum of the monoalkylphenyl anion. In the case of $\Theta \approx 1$ the spectrum becomes complicated compared to the two limiting cases, as Burschtein has shown. This behaviour can be illustrated by the example of the E.S.R. spectrum of a very simple system $A \ldots A^-$. Here, it is assumed that each one of the two groups A contains only one proton, which interacts with the unpaired electron to give an H.F.S. One may see from Fig. 8.11, that apart from the known spectra, consisting of the two components ($\Theta \ll 1$) and three components ($\Theta \gg 1$), a spectrum of five components ($\Theta \approx 1$) can also be observed in systems of this type. In the systems which have been investigated experimentally, $[Ph-(CH_2)_n-Ph]^-$

had an even more complex character in the transition region $\Theta \approx 1$, since in each phenyl ring four protons interacted with the unpaired electron.

In a system with strong conjugation, $\Delta E \geqslant kT$, the spectrum can, in principle, change considerably, as all the molecules are concentrated in the lower level with $E_0 - \Delta E/2$, and the spectrum is determined by only one half of the system. However, it can be shown that in a system with two nuclei $(A)_2^-$, the E.S.R. spectrum coincides with that corresponding to the condition $\Delta E \gg Q_{si}$ ($\Theta \gg 1$). A more complicated picture, is observed in

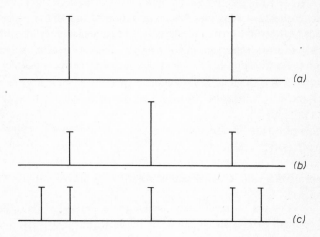

Fig. 8.11. Diagram of the E.S.R. spectrum of a hypothetical ion $(A \ldots A)^-$.

    (a) $\Delta E \ll Q_{si}$

    (b) $\Delta E \gg Q_{si}$

    (c) $\Delta E \approx Q_{si}$

the case of a system with a larger number of nuclei, e.g. $(A)_3^-$, $(A)_4^-$ etc., but as we know of no experimental investigations of such systems, we will not spend any more time on them.

In closing, a few more words should be said about the possible causes of such an interaction over a large number of saturated σ-bonds. This question is extremely interesting as we shall meet such a 'conductivity' of saturated hydrocarbon chains when we consider the energy transfer in the irradiation of solid hydrocarbons (see Chapter 9). Although until now there is no precise theory to explain these effects, it would appear to us that the ideas of McConnell[22] merit considerable attention, according to which an interaction over large distances can be caused by very small contributions from higher levels in addition to the ground state of the chain atoms. Thus according to his calculations, the contribution of the 3d-state of the carbon atom can lead to an exchange interaction which corresponds to a frequency of approximately 10^{11} Hz, although this state lies very high. This frequency is indeed very high in comparison with the frequencies which we have been dealing with, but it corresponds to an energy which contains only one per cent of the thermal energy, and has practically no influence on the energy of the molecule. Moreover, this condition can prove to be extremely important on turning from an examination of structure to an examination of the reactions in which the molecule in question takes part. The explanation of this ability to transfer charge (or energy) across saturated bonds over large distances can play an essential role in the understanding of complex chemical reactions. It is for this very reason that the study of analogous systems with completely different bridges is of great importance, particularly when hetero-atoms (Si, S, O, etc.), for which the contributions of higher states can be quite pronounced, play a part.

Another direction for these investigations is the study of systems with a large number of delocalization centres, which enable a charge-transfer to take place over large distances. In the next chapter we will consider some problems relating to this, which can be solved with the help of E.S.R.

§8.4

ELECTRON DELOCALIZATION IN HIGH MOLECULAR BONDS

E.S.R. can also be applied to the detection and study of displacement effects of the unpaired electron in those cases where as a result of these effects, only one single line with an indistinct H.F.S. is observed in the spectrum. In the cases of interest to us, such an indistinct or smeared-out spectrum can be explained by a strong delocalization in which the electron spin interacts with a very large number of nuclei. As a result, we obtain a spectrum with many H.F.S. components, and the mutual overlapping produces the observed picture. In Chapter 6 we described how one may calculate the total number of H.F.S. components from the effective line width. Assuming that the electron is in interaction with n equivalent protons, then there are $n + 1$ components, and the width of the line with the smeared-out H.F.S. (for components of equal shape and of line width ΔB_i) is

$$\Delta B_{\text{eff}} = \sqrt{\left((\Delta B_i)^2 + \frac{(\Delta B_0)^2}{n - 1} \right)} \tag{8.1}$$

where ΔB_0 is the splitting which corresponds to the interaction of an unpaired electron with a nucleus. (For the interaction of a p-electron in the CH-fragment with a proton, $B_0 = Q = 2 \cdot 25$ mWb m^{-2}.)

If ΔB_{eff} (the separation between points of maximum slope) is measured experimentally, then for a known ΔB_0 and an estimated ΔB_i, the value of n, i.e. the spread of the delocalization range, can be calculated. If on the other hand n is known, then ΔB_i can be more or less accurately determined from ΔB_{eff}. Solodovnikov[23] has applied this method in the analysis of the E.S.R. spectra of the anions of polymers, containing phenyl rings.

Polymers with conjugated double bonds

1. The anion of polyphenylacetylenes (PPA):

$$\left(\begin{array}{c} -C=CH- \\ | \\ Ph \end{array} \right)_n^{-}$$

In this case, in the molecular weight range of 700 to 1500, the spectrum consists of nine H.F.S. components with a splitting of approximately $0 \cdot 23$ mWb m^{-2}. This means that in the polymer molecule the electron delocalization only takes place between the two phenyl rings, where the

$$-C=CH-C=CH-$$

interaction with the bridge proton is so weak, in contrast to stilbene, that the H.F.S. components are not noticeably split. If a transfer of the electrons on the other rings takes place at all, then it does so with a frequency below 10^7 Hz.

2. A strong effect is observed in the ion of the polyparaxylidenes (PPX):

$$(-C_6H_4-CH=CH-)_n^{-}$$

The spectrum of the PPX ion (molecular weight = 2000, i.e. approximately 20 links) consists of one single line with width $\Delta B_{eff} = 0 \cdot 5$ mWb m^{-2}. Putting ΔB_i equal to zero, for the lower limit for n we find

$$n \geqslant 1 + \left(\frac{\Delta B_0}{\Delta B_{eff}} \right)^2 = 21$$

Assuming that the spin density is localized essentially on the benzene rings, it follows that the range in which the delocalization occurs with a frequency above 10^7 Hz, consists of five rings. However, we may suppose, as in the case of stilbene, that the delocalization occurs mainly on the bridge —CH=CH—, so that each monomer link contributes only two protons. Thus the delocalization range covers ten links, i.e. its spread amounts to over 6 nm.

Polymers without conjugated bonds

1. The anion of the polystilbenes (PS):

$$\left(\begin{array}{c} \overset{Ph}{\underset{\,}{|}} \overset{H}{\underset{\,}{|}} \\ -C-C- \\ \overset{\,}{\underset{H}{|}} \,\, \overset{\,}{\underset{Ph}{|}} \end{array} \right)^{-}_{n}$$

In sample solutions of medium molecular weight, from 1000 to 1300, a weak H.F.S. of nine components is observed, which shows that in this polymer the delocalization range encloses only two phenyl rings, i.e. one monomer link. Investigation of samples with higher molecular weight (approximately 3000) show a completely smeared-out H.F.S., with ΔB_{eff} equal to 0·65 mWb m^{-2}. Using equation (8.1) we find that $n = 13$. Thus with the extension of the chains there is an increased probability that three or more phenyl groups will maintain such an orientation, and that electron exchange will result between them with a frequency $> 10^7$ Hz.

2. Anion of the poly-1,1-diphenylethylenes (PDPE):

$$\left(\begin{array}{c} \overset{Ph}{\underset{\,}{|}} \\ -C-CH_2- \\ \overset{\,}{\underset{Ph}{|}} \end{array} \right)^{-}_{n}$$

At a molecular weight of 2800 only one line is observed with $\Delta B_{eff} = 1·0$ mWb m^{-2}. For $\Delta B_i = 0$ this gives $n = 6$, which suggests that in this case the delocalization takes place over only one link, i.e. that $n = 8$. Assuming this value, then conversely from equation (8.1) we get

$$\Delta B_i \approx 0·53 \text{ mWb m}^{-2}$$

3. The conclusion that $n = 8$ for the group —C(Ph)$_2$— is strengthened by the example of the polytetraphenylethylene anion (PTPE):

$$\left(\begin{array}{c} \overset{Ph}{\underset{\,}{|}} \overset{Ph}{\underset{\,}{|}} \\ -C-C- \\ \overset{\,}{\underset{Ph}{|}} \,\, \overset{\,}{\underset{Ph}{|}} \end{array} \right)^{-}_{n}$$

In this spectrum (at a molecular weight of 80 000) an H.F.S. with nine components is likewise observed. Clearly the interaction in the group Ph–C–Ph is much stronger than over the bridge –C–C– (and even more so for the bridge –C–CH$_2$–C–), so that all remaining links influence only the relaxation behaviour, i.e. the width of the components and not their number. For this reason, in the very high molecular-weight PTPE the arrangement of the phenyl groups leads to such a considerable narrowing of the components [as is also observed in the ion of the bisdiphenylchromes (see §8.2)], that the H.F.S. can be resolved. In this case ΔB_i must be somewhat smaller than $\Delta B_{HFS} \approx 0.25$ mWb m^{-2}, i.e. less than half the value of ΔB_i for the PDPE.

It would be very interesting to extend these investigations to polymers of different structures and with variable molecular weight. Here one should have the possibility of determining ΔB_i independently, or of changing its value in a particular direction.

It still remains to be mentioned, as Solodovnikov has stated, that in some E.S.R. spectra of polymer anions (polystilbene, polystyrol) there appears on the background of the more-or-less well resolved spectra, a sharp, intense, single line, which is connected with the existence of large, ordered ranges with effective delocalization. Further investigations of this problem are very essential for the clarification of the configuration of polymer molecules of this type.

§8.5

CHEMICAL PROCESSES IN COMPLEX SYSTEMS WHICH ARE CONNECTED WITH ELECTRON TRANSFER AND DELOCALIZATION

The question of electron delocalization within a molecule is closely connected with that of the possibility of intermolecular electron transfer. Reactions of this type which have been well investigated are the multiple oxidation-reduction processes, and the mutual conversion of particles, which can be in different charge states. The electron charge processes can be divided into two important classes: (a) the interaction of chemically identical particles, which differ from each other in their charge, as for example:

$$Fe^{2+} + Fe^{3+} \rightarrow Fe^{3+} + Fe^{2+} \tag{1}$$

$$(C_{10}H_8)^- + C_{10}H_8 \rightarrow C_{10}H_8 + (C_{10}H_8)^- \tag{2}$$

and (b), redox processes, during the course of which new forms of either component are produced which previously were not present in the system. Examples of reactions of this type are

$$Fe^{2+} + Cu^{2+} \rightarrow Fe^{3+} + Cu^+ \tag{3}$$

and many others.

Reactions of the first class cannot be studied by simple chemical methods, and for this reason, in the last twenty years radio-active isotopes have been successfully used to obtain information on the speed of such processes. It has recently been shown that these reactions can now be studied by E.S.R. Ward and Weissman[24] carried out investigations on the E.S.R. spectrum of the naphthalene ion for different concentrations of naphthalene, and found that the resolution of the H.F.S. depended to a great extent on the concentration of the naphthalene molecule in the system. If the speed of process (2) becomes so great that the lifetime τ of an anion $(C_{10}H_8)^-$ up to the beginning of an electron transfer reaction is comparable with the reciprocal line width $(\Delta B_i)^{-1}$ of the individual H.F.S. components, then it can be shown that ΔB_i is related to τ by the following equation:

$$\Delta B_i = \Delta B_i^0 + \frac{a}{\tau}$$

where ΔB_i^0 is the line width in the absence of non-ionic naphthalene, $1/\tau = k[C_{10}H_8]$, k being the reaction-rate constant of the reaction (2), and a is a coefficient which takes the line shape into account and converts τ into units of magnetic induction.

In the work of Ward and Weissman it was not the width ΔB_i that was measured, but I, the intensity of the first derivative of the central component of the multi-line spectrum of the ion $(C_{10}H_8)^-$, as a function of $[C_{10}H_8]$. Since for a given concentration the following is valid (see Chapter 4),

$$I(\Delta B_i)^2 = I^0(\Delta B_i^0)^2 = \text{constant}$$

it follows that

$$\sqrt{\frac{I^0}{I}} = \frac{\Delta B_i}{\Delta B_i^0} = 1 + ak\frac{[C_{10}H_8]}{\Delta B_i^0}$$

and by plotting (I^0/I) as a function of $[C_{10}H_8]/\Delta B_i^0$, the authors obtained a straight line, from which k could be determined (for a Lorentzian line $a = 0.65 \times 10^{-11}$ Wb m^{-2}). In Table 8.1 are shown values obtained at 30°C for the reaction-rate constant of (2) with different cations in two solvents, dimethoxyethane (DME) and tetrahydrofuran (THF).

Table 8.1

Cation	Solvent	k [l/mol . s]
K^+	DME	$(7 \cdot 6 \pm 3) \cdot 10^7$
K^+	THF	$5 \cdot 7 \cdot 10^7$
Na^+	DME	$1 \cdot 3 \cdot 10^9$
Na^+	THF	$1 \cdot 3 \cdot 10^7$
Li^+	THF	$4 \cdot 8 \cdot 10^8$

These results are extremely important in modern chemistry, since they allow a quantitative assessment of the influence of the medium and the nature of the positive ions in certain primary chemical actions, under otherwise equal conditions. Although considerable errors may occur in calculating the constants, these errors are most unlikely to exceed 50 per cent. The conclusion that a change in either the medium or in the cation has considerable effect on the rate constant, is thus completely reliable.

Certain conclusions may be drawn from the fact that the influence of the naphthalene in DME is essentially larger for Na^+ than for K^+, and also from the result obtained by the authors, that with the simultaneous presence of K^+ and Na^+, the resolution of the spectrum is the same as with only K^+ present. The conclusion drawn from this was that in this solvent no isolated ions exist, but only ion-pairs, where the equilibrium

$$Na^+ \ldots C_{10}H_8^- + K^+ \rightleftarrows Na^+ + C_{10}H_8^- \ldots K^+ \qquad (*)$$

is shifted far to the right-hand side of the equation.† If one accepts this idea, then the process considered in this present investigation can no longer be considered as a simple electron transfer. It must clearly be written in the following way:

$$(C_{10}H_8)^- \ldots Me^+ + C_{10}H_8 \rightarrow C_{10}H_8 + Me^+ \ldots (C_{10}H_8)^-$$
$$\quad (1) \qquad\qquad\qquad (2) \qquad\quad (1) \qquad\qquad (2)$$

and during the course of the reaction, apart from the transfer of an electron from molecule (1) to molecule (2), there also results the transfer of a metal atom. It is therefore extremely important to choose particularly those cases in which the existence of isolated anions $(ArH)^-$, not bound in ion pairs, can be proved indisputably. The question of the temperature dependence of

† *Direct proof has since been obtained of the existence of ion-pairs[41]* by the observation of an H.F.S. splitting additional to that attributed to the alkali metal nuclei on the sample of the diphenyl ion with tetrahydrofuran as solvent.*

the reaction-rate constant was not considered in further detail in the above work. Accurate measurements at different temperatures could give a great deal of interesting information on the mechanism of this process.

The formation of an ion pair

$$Me^+ \ldots ArH^-$$

during the interaction of neutral metal atoms and molecules, is one of the many examples which demonstrates how the electron transfer leads to the formation of more or less stable complexes. Such an ion pair is a characteristic limiting case of a class of complexes which have recently been described as *charge transfer complexes*. These are formed when, on the interaction of two particles A and B, the difference between the ionization potential of one and the electron affinity of the other (i.e. either the difference $I_A - A_B$ or $I_B - A_A$) is not too large. Here, in the system AB a new distribution of energy density occurs, which leads to the appearance of a negative charge at the acceptor and a positive charge at the donor.

The formation of charge transfer complexes was first proved by the accurate analysis of the optical spectra of such systems. For example, it has been shown[25] that if molecular iodine is added to benzene, then the U.V. absorption bands of the benzene are shifted towards the longer wavelengths, which was explained by the formation of a complex

$$C_6H_6^{+\delta} \ldots I_2^{-\delta}$$

in which the molecule I_2 carried an additional negative charge which corresponded to approximately 0·03 electron charge. In this case we are dealing with a partial electron delocalization of one molecule on another. If this delocalization is very small, then the complex AB is naturally very unstable and readily decomposes into the original molecules A and B. If the interaction is very strong, then the new distribution of the electron density can lead to a complete electron transfer, where either an ion pair analogous to that given above, $Me^+ \ldots C_{10}H_8^-$, or two isolated particles A^+ and B^- are formed, which differ from the original particles by one unit of charge. These new particles will of course exhibit completely different chemical properties, particularly the reduction-oxidation properties.

It is clear that, depending on the properties of the particles A and B, and on the solvent, various intermediate states can occur within the sequence:

A + B	$A^{+\delta} \ldots B^{-\delta}$	$\rightarrow$	$[A^+ \ldots B^-]$	$\rightarrow (A^+) + (B^-)$
(non-interacting particles)	(charge transfer complex with weak bond)		(ion pair)	(isolated ions)

If the particles A and B are diamagnetic, in accordance with the increase in the delocalization of this sequence, which is concurrent with the redistribution of the charge, then the singlet and triplet levels of the electron pair of the system AB approach each other. As a result of this the magnetic properties of the system change, and for a sufficiently large separation of $A^+ \ldots B^+$, the system behaves as two free radicals.

As we have seen above, E.S.R. can be applied to the investigation of paramagnetic ions or ion pairs, in which one or both components are paramagnetic. However, it is not impossible that magnetic effects analogous to those observed in organic biradicals may also appear in complexes with charge transfer in which the degree of delocalization is not too large. A systematic examination of the magnetic properties of such complexes in different media can thus prove to be very essential in formulating laws valid for a large number of very important chemical processes.

The application of E.S.R. to the investigation of electron delocalization on the formation of a complex is not limited to the discovery of newly formed paramagnetic particles. In cases in which the delocalization is small, it can also be detected via its influence on the electron shell of the paramagnetic atoms. It can manifest itself most easily in the width of the H.F.S. components. This was found to be so in the investigation of the E.S.R. spectra of the derivatives of the diphenylchrome cation (see §8.2), where the resolution of the H.F.S. in the sequence $[Cr(C_6H_6)_2]^+$, $[Cr(C_6H_5)_2C_6H_6]^+$, $[Cr[(C_6H_5)_2]^+$ improved considerably (see Fig. 8.5). Clearly, a qualitative explanation of this effect lies in the fact that although the delocalization is so weak that the spin density in the aromatic ring neighbouring the chromium atom cannot change appreciably, nevertheless the relaxation properties of the system change so strongly that the width of the individual components considerably decreases. In order to prove this theory, Tschibrikin carried out specific experiments with the compound $[Cr(C_6H_5COOH)_2]^+$. The resolution of the H.F.S. changes completely in parallel with the increase in concentration of the materials, which with the acid group can form pseudo-aromatic ring complexes, through which the sphere of the electron displacement increases.

On the basis of the theory of McConnell[42] on the E.S.R. line width in solutions, there is also another explanation for the variable line widths of different substituted dibenzenechrome cations. According to this theory the line width depends to a high degree on the correlation time of the rotational motion of the particles, which for a spherical particle of radius a in a liquid with viscosity η, has the value $4\pi\eta\, a^3/3kT$. An example of this result is the known dependence of the line width on the viscosity of the solvent. Now, all substitutions of both benzene rings lead to an enlarging of the effective radius a of the particles, and through this to a large change in the correlation time, which can result in a decrease of the individual line widths.*

Another possible result of the electron delocalization is the lifting of anomalous broadening, or very large shifts in the g-factor (see Chapter 3), which would otherwise prevent the E.S.R. experiments from being carried out. An example of this has been given by Ziegler in the investigation of the magnetic properties of homogeneous catalytic agents for the polymerization of olefins at low temperatures; this work was carried out at ICP by Schilov *et al.* One of the commonest systems of this kind is a mixture of the different halides of tetra- and trivalent titanium with trialkylaluminium,

$$TiCl_4 + AlR_3 \tag{1}$$

and

$$TiCl_3 + AlR_3 \tag{2}$$

We may now consider it well proven that the combination of the original components in system (1) results in a reduction of the tetravalent titanium, and that in all cases system (2) is catalytically active. Until recently it was assumed that although the trivalent titanium is paramagnetic, from its odd number of electrons, its E.S.R. spectrum could only be investigated at low temperatures, at which the relaxation time would be large enough for measurements to be made. It was shown in the first paper of Schilov and Bubnov,[26] however, that the precipitate formed on mixing the solutions of $TiCl_4$ and $Al(C_4H_9)_3$ in octane at room temperature, to which the catalytic activity is normally attributed, gives a perfectly recognizable E.S.R. signal with $g \approx 2$. Since the only paramagnetic atom in the system is the trivalent titanium, this result means that it is present in such a form that the above limitation is not valid. It was therefore of great interest to establish the structure of this compound. With this purpose in view, Schilov, Sefirova and Tichomirova[27] substituted $TiCl_4$ by $TiCl_2(C_5H_4)_2$. The catalytic activity in this case was not so large; however the system remained homogeneous on mixing, and thus E.S.R. could be used to better advantage. The results of this investigation were extremely interesting. On mixing the $TiCl_2(C_5H_5)_2$ with a surplus of AlR_3, a spectrum with a clear H.F.S. was obtained (Fig. 8.12). Since the middle six components of the spectrum had approximately equal intensity, it was clear that the unpaired electron of the paramagnetic titanium atom was to a certain extent interacting with the aluminium atom, as the Al was the only atom in the system with the nuclear spin I of 5/2 necessary to account for the formation of these six H.F.S. components.

For an explanation of the two outer components, it had to be assumed that each of the six H.F.S. components was split additionally into a triplet with intensity ratio 1:2:1, where the magnitude of the splitting was approximately the same as the basic splitting. Under these conditions a spectrum would be expected with eight components with an intensity ratio 1:3:4:4: 4:4:3:1, which agrees well with the experimental results. It was not possible to explain this splitting by considering the α-protons of the ethyl groups, as a substitution of $-C_2H_2$ by $-CH_3$ and iso-C_3H_7 did not change the spectrum.

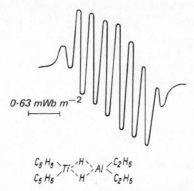

Fig. 8.12. E.S.R. spectrum of the cyclic complex $(C_5H_5)_2TiH_2Al(C_2H_5)_2$.

By a careful analysis of the initial substances the authors found that in the trialkylaluminium there was always present a certain number of molecules in which R was partially substituted by hydrogen. On the basis of this, it was assumed that the paramagnetic complex which caused the spectrum in Fig. 8.12 was a bridge structure in which two TiH and two AlH bonds were acted upon by a total of four electrons:

$$C_5H_5 \diagdown Ti \cdots \overset{\cdots H \cdots}{\underset{\cdots H \cdots}{}} Al \diagup_R^R \qquad (\alpha)$$

At about the same time as this, Schilov *et al.* also carried out an analysis on the basis of the detailed X-ray structure,[28] and suggested an analogous bridge structure for the Ziegler complexes, which was good supporting evidence for the H.F.S. analysis of the E.S.R. The proof of the formation of a complex of type (α) and the investigation of the distribution of the electron density within the structure shows some of the new possibilities which are opened by E.S.R.

In our opinion, a conclusion which is important for chemistry is that whilst investigating active particles which participate in the homogeneous catalytic processes above, one has to free oneself from the classical conception, which incidentally is what Ziegler himself did. Later investigations showed that the relatively stable complexes (α) appear only in the final stage of the interaction; the catalytic activity is connected with even more unstable forms, which represent intermediate stages between the original molecule and the complex (α). Investigations on the structure of this intermediate stage are still being carried out. It is clear that without the inquiry into the system (α) there would have been virtually no approach to the question of the nature of the catalytically active particles in the Ziegler process.

From the point of view of structure chemistry, the compound (α) must be considered as a complex of compounds of trivalent titanium and trivalent aluminium. The bond is affected by the delocalization of the unpaired electron of the titanium in the ring:

$$\diagdown \text{Ti} \underset{\cdot\cdot\text{H}\cdot}{\overset{\cdot\cdot\text{H}\cdot\cdot}{\cdots}} \text{Al} \diagup$$

Moreover, it is an important fact that a weak delocalization also leads to a lifting of the line-broadening characteristics of the Ti^{3+}-salts, and as a result of this the E.S.R. spectrum of the trivalent titanium can be observed at room temperature. In other words, in the compound (α) the trivalent titanium is placed in a crystalline field of changed symmetry, and this in itself enables the E.S.R. effect to be observed.* The spectrum of Ti^{3+} in an approximately cubic crystalline field can be observed only at liquid helium temperatures. On the other hand, in the strongly axial field of $KTi(C_2O_4)_2 \cdot 2H_2O$ an observation is already possible at liquid air temperature.*[43*] As we have seen in Chapter 3, the delocalization actually acts on the electronic levels of the paramagnetic atom in exactly the same way as an electric field of lower symmetry. It is therefore to be expected that the E.S.R. characteristics of the ion will undergo considerable change.

§8.6

ELECTRON TRANSFER UNDER THE INFLUENCE OF LIGHT

So far we have considered electron displacement processes by delocalization or by irreversible chemical reactions. Such processes are naturally limited by the difficulties of energy supply and activation. One of the ways to deal with this in chemistry, as is well known, is through the action of radiation energy in one form or another, such as U.V. light, X-rays, fast electrons, etc. A large number of different disturbing effects are induced in the primary molecule by the action of ionizing radiation, and so it is not normally possible to isolate just the electron transfer process. We will consider the chemical results of ionizing radiation in more detail in Chapter 9, which is devoted to the study of free radicals formed by such processes. However, it is to be expected that by the action of softer radiation, e.g. U.V. light, it is possible to produce electron transfer processes under somewhat easier conditions.

During the mid-1930s, Weiss[30] built up a hypothesis on the formation of molecular hydrogen by the irradiation of H_2SO_4 in a water solution containing Fe^{2+}, as a result of the formation of atomic hydrogen by the following reaction:

$$Fe^{2+} + H_2O + h\nu \rightarrow Fe^{3+} + OH^- + H \tag{1}$$

Dain and his co-workers[31] showed that this mechanism was also the basis for the photo-reduction of water solutions of Cr^{2+}. It has more recently been shown that for reactions of type (1), cations such as V^{2+}, Mn^{2+}, Co^{2+} as well as the anions SO_3^{2-}, I^-, SH^-, etc.[32] may also participate, as well as the Fe^{2+} and Cr^{2+}. The reaction suggested by Weiss,

$$M + H_2O + h\nu \rightarrow M^+ + OH^- + H \tag{2}$$

has been adopted by most authors. In the paper of Dainton *et al.*[33] it was shown that process (2) can initiate the polymerization of vinyl compounds. By carrying out the reaction in D_2O, Dainton showed that a D-atom can actually be detected in the end group of the polymer. This is a very good argument in favour of reaction (2).

After E.S.R. had been developed as a technique, the question was raised as to whether it would now be possible to detect directly the hydrogen atoms formed in reaction (2). During photolysis in the liquid phase, it is clearly impossible to detect the H-atoms, since their steady concentration will always be much smaller than the sensitivity limit of modern spectrometers. Therefore, Schelimov *et al.*[34] carried out reaction (2) in the solid phase, in order to stabilize the H-atoms formed and allow them to accumulate sufficiently for direct detection by E.S.R. It is known that at approximately liquid helium temperatures, the H-atom in an aqueous medium loses its mobility and becomes unable to react.[35] To obtain a lattice stable enough to permit complete stability of the H-atoms at higher temperatures, e.g. $77°K$, aqueous acid solutions (H_2SO_4, H_3PO_4, $HClO_4$) must be used instead of water. In these media, hydrogen atoms produced by X-irradiation at 77°K do not recombine for several hours.[36] This medium is also suitable for many photo-chemical experiments, as the aqueous acids, when cooled, give a transparent glass, whereas the solidification of pure water into a transparent body has not been successful. The authors[34] found that in both the systems

$$Fe^{2+} + H_2SO_4 + H_2O \quad \text{and} \quad I^- + H_2SO_4 + H_2O$$

on irradiation at 77°K with U.V. light at a wavelength of $\lambda = 253.7$ nm, an H-atom doublet was formed, which was identical with the doublet formed by X-irradiation. When the experiment was carried out with heavy water, in addition to the H-atom doublet, the triplet of the deuterium was also observed (Fig. 8.13). The quantitative measurements carried out by

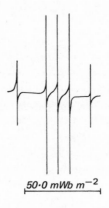

50·0 mWb m^{-2}

Fig. 8.13. E.S.R. spectrum of H- and D-atoms in the system $Fe^{2+} + D_2O + H_2SO_4$ after U.V. irradiation at 77° K.

Schelimov and Schuklaya allowed a determination of the quantum yield of the electron transfer from Fe^{2+} to H_2O. They obtained the following values:

CH₂SO₄	6·3 m	9·4 m	12·5 m
Φ(H)	0·06	0·11	0·07

It is interesting to note that under the same conditions of U.V. irradiation, the system $(C_6H_6 + H_2O + H_2SO_4)$ also gave an intense H-doublet (Fig. 8.14). This demonstrates that even the C_6H_6 molecule can take part in the photo-transfer reaction in this medium, in which the ionization energy in the gas phase is considerably larger than the energy of the

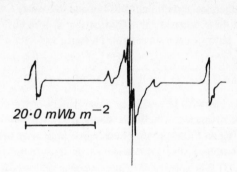

Fig. 8.14. E.S.R. spectrum of the system C_6H_6 + H_2O + H_2SO_4 after U.V. irradiation at $77°$ K.

absorbed U.V. quantum. In the central region of this spectrum a complicated H.F.S., clearly formed by three different radicals, is observed. Although this spectrum is rather complex, in the central region a relatively well-resolved quadruplet with a total splitting of approximately $2 \cdot 4$ mWb m^{-2} and an intensity ratio of 1:3:3:1 (Fig. 8.15a) can be seen. When the sample is heated, an irreversible change in the spectrum is observed: the H-atom doublet disappears, and the central region can be described as a superposition of a triplet of quadruplets, with splittings $\Delta B_{Tr} \approx 4 \cdot 5$ mWb m^{-2}

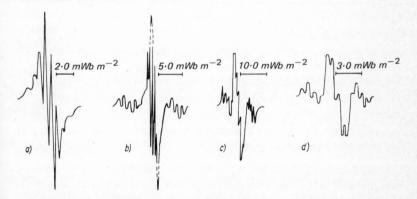

Fig. 8.15. (*a*) Central region of the spectrum shown in Fig. 8.14; (*b*) same after partial melting; (*c*) same after complete melting; (*d*) spectrum of C_6H_6 irradiated with fast electrons at $220°$ K.

and $\Delta B_{Qua} \approx 1 \cdot 0$ mWbm^{-2} on top of the original quadruplet (see Fig. 8.15b). On further heating the central quadruplet disappears, and a practically undistorted triplet of quadruplets is seen (see Fig. 8.15c). This spectrum is very similar to that of an irradiated sample of solid benzene (see Fig. 8.15d). It will later be shown (see §9.2) that this form of spectrum is produced by the overlapping of the spectra of the radicals $\overset{\bullet}{C_6}H_5$ and $\overset{\bullet}{C_6}H_7$, which are formed by the interaction of the hydrogen atoms with the benzene.

Although it is difficult to interpret accurately the spectra formed by U.V. irradiation of benzene-type solutions, we will give the following hypothetical interpretation of the observed spectra, which will at least give us a qualitative explanation of part of the experimental results. It is assumed that the photo-ionization of the benzene leads initially to the formation of a hydrogen atom and the ion pair $C_6H_6^+ \dots OH^-$:

$$C_6H_6 + H_2O + h\nu \rightarrow C_6H_6^+ \dots OH^- + H$$

Since in the ion-pair the positive charge is localized on the OH$^-$ closest to the carbon atom of the $C_6H_6^+$ ion, we can assume that essentially the unpaired electron interacts with only three protons, corresponding to the three most probable valence diagrams:

If this is in fact so, then in the first approximation the spectrum of the ion-pair is a quadruplet of three equivalent hydrogen atoms. The total spread of the spectrum should correspond approximately to the total splitting in the spectrum of the aromatic positive ion $C_6H_6^+$. This value is known to be about $3 \cdot 0$ mWb m^{-2} for complex aromatic ions,[37] and this is in reasonably good agreement with the value of $2 \cdot 4$ mWb m^{-2} which we get from Fig. 8.15a.

On the application of heat, the hydrogen atoms first bond themselves to the benzene, forming the C_6H_7 radical, and this produces the appearance in the spectrum of the triplet of quadruplets with ΔB_{Tr} and ΔB_{Qua}. On a further rise in the temperature, the ion pair can react under proton transfer.†

$$C_6H_6^+ + OH^- \rightarrow C_6H_5 + H_2O$$

† This representation can be compared with the hypothesis of Lewis and Lipkin,[38] according to which the reactions of the positive diphenylamin-ion also result from the splitting of a proton.

As a result, two types of radicals are formed in the system, C_6H_7 and C_6H_5, i.e. precisely the same two radicals postulated in connection with the radiolysis of solid C_6H_6. Thus the close similarity of the spectra shown in Fig. 8.15c and d is now explicable.

The experimental results presented in this chapter naturally cannot claim to cover completely the large number of results which have been obtained. We have set ourselves the goal, on the basis of new work, carried out mostly in the Soviet Union, of showing the many new applications now open to us, thanks to this technique, in a very important field of theoretical chemistry— the study of delocalization and electron transfer processes.

§8.7*
PRODUCTION OF FREE RADICALS

In the earlier sections of this chapter, we have shown, by examples taken from widely varying fields, how information can be gained on the structure of the components of organic free radicals from the E.S.R. spectra. The application of E.S.R. is however limited to paramagnetic materials, and the majority of organic compounds are diamagnetic. So if we wish to apply E.S.R. to organic chemical investigations, we will need, in addition to a good spectrometer, methods by which the materials of interest can be made paramagnetic. In Chapter 9 we will learn how this is done by high energy irradiation (X-rays, γ-rays, electron beams). Apart from a few exceptions (such as liquid C_2H_6; see p. 233), this technique is limited to solids, where in general low temperatures are necessary. A method which is applicable to liquids and at room temperatures, is the production of negative molecule ions by the reaction with free alkali metals (see §8.3 and §8.5). However, this also entails considerable experimental difficulties.

An elegant procedure of general application is the electrolytic production of free ion radicals. This was first used in 1959 by Maki and Geske.[44]* In the years since then a large number of organic compounds have been studied.†

The electrolytic production of free ion radicals may originate from reduction of the cathode (or oxidation of the anode):

$$R + e^- \rightarrow \dot{R}^- \tag{1a}$$

$$\dot{R}^- + e^- \rightarrow R^{2-} \tag{1b}$$

---

† The importance of this technique has been increased by the fact that the companies Varian Associates and JEOL offer electrolytic cells as an accessory to their spectrometers.

The electrolytic potential may be adjusted so that only reaction (1a) occurs, and a sufficient quantity of R^- radicals will be formed, with lifetimes suitable for E.S.R. studies. This potential may be determined polarographically; i.e. this procedure may also be regarded as supplementary to polarography, but having a more advanced starting point since E.S.R. already gives us detailed information about the nature of the radicals formed. A sketch of such an electrolytic cell is shown in Fig. 8.16*. A platinum wire or a drop of mercury is generally used as a cathode, and the anode takes the form of a saturated mercurous chloride electrode. The cathode is placed directly in the spectrometer cavity, so that even radicals with relatively short lifetimes may be studied. The cell is flushed with an inert gas (N_2) in order to exclude air-oxygen, which would otherwise have a harmful effect. Furthermore, in order to ensure sufficient conductivity at the beginning of the reaction (the materials usually investigated being non-electrolytic), a conducting salt is added, the decomposition voltage of which should lie as high as possible, so that the usable potential range is large. This is generally done by introducing quaternary propylammonium perchlorate $[(C_3H_7)_4N] ClO_4$. In choosing the solvent the following fact has to be taken into consideration: many usable polar solvents (H_2O, C_2H_5OH) are partially dissociated, and this causes the appearance of H^+ ions. As a result of this, the reduction at the cathode will be:

$$R \xrightarrow{e^-} \dot{R}^- \xrightarrow{H^+} \dot{R}H \xrightarrow{e^-} RH^- \xrightarrow{H^+} RH_2$$

The original radical ions $\dot{R}^-$ thus accept two protons and are immediately further reduced to the diamagnetic dihydrate RH_2. An example of this is the reduction of quinones (or the oxidation of hydroquinones) in alcoholic or aqueous solutions, which only give a reasonable concentration of semiquinone in an alcoholic medium in which the H^+ concentration is sufficiently small. Solvents which do not allow the dissociation of H^+ ions are described as *aprotic*. The most useful solvents of this type are acetonitrile $CH_3 . CN$, dimethylformamide $(CH_3)_2N . CHO$, and dimethylsulphoxide $(CH_3)_2SO$.

Having described the method, we would now like to give some examples of its application, which in part gives results analogous to those described in other sections of this book. Ludwig and Adams[45]* have studied the negative benzonitrile ion $(C_6H_5 . CN)^-$ in dimethylformamide (DMF). Depending on the concentration of the non-ionized benzonitrile, the spectrum undergoes a transition from a well-resolved spectrum of 54 single lines for a 2.5×10^{-3} molar solution, to a non-resolved single line at a

molar concentration of 0·65. A value was obtained for the rate constant of
the exchange reaction, which was in approximate agreement with that
found in naphthalene. An accurate determination is difficult as the
solution grows continually weaker in the vicinity of the electrode where
most of the ions are located.

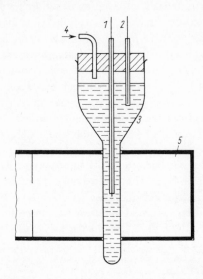

Fig. 8.16* Electrolytic cell for the production of free radicals.

1. working electrode   4. gas inlet
2. other electrode   5. resonant cavity for measurement
3. electrolytic container

The spectrum of the negative ion of 1,4-dinitrotetromethylbenzene in
DMF was observed by Freed and Fraenkel.[46*] The spectrum consisted of
five line groups, corresponding to a system with two equivalent nuclei with
$I = 1$. However, the intensity ratio deviates from the theoretical value of
1:2:3:2:1. The central and two outside lines are further split as a result of
interaction with the proton moments, whilst the two remaining lines are
not split. The authors explain this by a correlation of the hindered
rotation of both nitro-groups, as a result of the steric hindering due to the
methyl groups. The dependence of the N-coupling constant on the angle of
the nitro-group to the plane of the benzene ring thus leads to a considerable broadening of the individual components. An analogous effect was
also observed by the same authors on *m*-dinitrobenzene.[47*]

Stone and Maki[40]* studied the spectra of different semiquinones in dimethylsulphoxide and acetonitrile, and found noticeable differences in the coupling constants with respect to the values for aqueous and alcoholic solutions (see also p. 192).

References

1. Turkevitch, J., Oesper, P., Smyth, C.: *JACS,* **64** (1942), 1179.
2. Deguchi, Y.: *J. Chem. Phys.,* **32** (1960), 1584.
3. Venkataraman, B., Fraenkel, G. K.: *JACS,* **17**(1955), 2707, *J. Chem. Phys.,* **23** (1955), 587.
4. McConnell, H.: *J. Chem. Phys.,* **24** (1956), 632, 764; *Proc. Nat. Acad. Sci. V. S.,* **43** (1957), 721; Bersohn, R.: *J. Chem. Phys.,* **24** (1956), 1066.
5. Wertz, J., Vivo, I.: *J. Chem. Phys.,* **23** (1955), 2441.
6. Ingram, D. J. E.: *Free Radicals as Studied by Electron Spin Resonance,* London 1958, p. 156.
7. Sogo, P., Nakazavi, M., Calvin, M.: *J. Chem. Phys.,* **26** (1957), 1343.
8. Jarret, H., Sloan, G.: *J. Chem. Phys.,* **22** (1954), 1783.
9. Chesnut, D. B.: *J. Chem. Phys.,* **29** (1958), 43; McLachlan, A. D.: *Mol. Phys.,* **1** (1958), 233.
10. McConnell, H., Chesnut, D.: *J. Chem. Phys.,* **27** (1957), 984; **28** (1958), 107; Fujimoto, M., Ingram, D. J. E.: *Trans. Far. Soc.,* **53** (1958), 1304.
11. Molin, Ju. N., Korizki, A. T., Schamschew, W. N., Buben, N. Ja.: *Vysokomolekuljarnye soedinenija,* **11** (1962), 690; Kisseljow, A. G., Makulski, M. A., Lasurkin, Ju. S.: *Vysokomolekuljarnye soedinenija,* **8** (1960), 1678.
12. Ercoli, R., Calderazzo, F., Alberola, A.: *JACS,* **82** (1960), 2966.
13. Siehe Z. B. Nesmejanow, A. N., Perewalowa, E. G.: *Uspechi Chimii,* **27** (1958), 3; Pauling, L.: *The Nature of the Chemical Bond,* New York 1960.
14. Voevodski, V. V., Molin, Ju. N., Tschibrikin, W. M.: *Optika i Spektroskopija,* **5** (1958), 90; Bubnov, N. N., Solodovnikov, S. P., Sorokin, Ju. A., Tschibrikin, W. M.: *Bull. Acad. Sci. U.R.S.S.,* **23** (1959), 1263; Bubnov, N. N., Tschibrikin, W. M.: *J. phys. Chem., Moscow,* **33** (1959), 1891; Wettschinkin, S. I., Solodovnikov, S. P., Tschibrikin, W. M.: *Optika i Spektroskopija,* **8** (1960), 137.
15. Manenkov, A. A., Prochorov, A. M.: *J. exp. theor. Phys.,* **28** (1955), 755.
16. Stschegolev, I. F., Karimov, Ju. S.: *J. exp. theor. Phys.*
17. Tuttle, T., Weissman, S.: *JACS,* **80** (1958), 5342.
18. McConnell, H. M., McLachlan, A. D.: *J. Chem. Phys.,* **34** (1961), 1.
19. Voevodski, V. V., Solodovnikov, S. P., Tschibrikin, W. M.: *C.C.R. Acad. Sci. U.R.S.S.,* **129** (1959), 1082; Solodovnikov, S. P.: *Z. Strukt. Chimii,* **2** (1961), 282.
20. Burschtein, A. I.: *C.C.R. Acad. Sci. U.R.S.S.,* **135** (1960), 886.
21. Alexandrov, I. W.: *Optika i Spektroskopija,* **9** (1960), 679.
22. McConnell, H. M.: *J. Chem. Phys.,* **35** (1961), 508.
23. Solodovnikov, S. P., Voevodski, V. V.: *Optika i Spektroskopija,* **12** (1962), 32.
24. Ward, R. L., Weissman, S.: *JACS,* **76** (1954), 3612; **79** (1957), 2086.
25. Terenin, A. N.: *Uspechi Chimii,* **24** (1955), 121.
26. Schilov, A. Je., Bubnov, N. N.: *Bull. Acad. Sci. U.R.S.S. ser. chim.,* (1958) 384.
27. Sefirova, A. K., Tichomirova, N. N., Schilov, A. Je.: *C.C.R. Acad. Sci. U.R.S.S.,* **132** (1960), 1082.
28. Natta, G., Coradini, P., Bassi, J.: *JACS,* **80** (1958), 755.
29. Sefirov, A. K., Schilov, A. Je.: *C.C.R. Acad. Sci. U.R.S.S.,* **136** (1961), 599.

30. Weiss, J.: *Nature*, 136 (1935), 794.
31. Dain, B. Ja., Liberson, E. A.: *C.C.R. Acad. Sci. U.R.S.S.*, 28 (1940), 228; *Acta Physicochimica URSS*, 19 (1944), 410.
32. Uri, N.: *Chem. Rev.*, 50 (1952), 375.
33. Dainton, F. S., James, D.: *Trans. Far. Soc.*, 54 (1957), 649.
34. Schelimov, B. H., Fok, N. W., Bubnov, N. N., Voevodski, V. V.: *C.C.R. Acad. Sci. U.R.S.S.*, 134 (1960), 145; *Optika i Spektroskopija*, 11 (1961), 78.
35. Siegel, S., Flournoy, J. M., Baum, L. N.: *J. Chem. Phys.*, 34 (1961), 1782.
36. Livingston, R., Zeldes, H., Taylor, E.: *Disc. Far. Soc.*, 19 (1955), 166.
37. Weissman, S., de Boer, E., Conradi, J. J.: *J. Chem. Phys.*, 26 (1957), 963; Yokazava, Y., Miyoshita, I.: *J. Chem. Phys.*, 25 (1956), 796.
38. Lewis, G. N., Lipkin, D.: *JACS*, 64 (1942), 2801.
39* Hausser, K. H.: *Compte rendu du 11. Colloque Ampère 1962*, 421.
40* Stone, E. W., Maki, A. H.: *J. Chem. Phys.*, 36 (1962), 1944.
41* Nishiguchi, H., Nakai, Y., Nakamura, K., Ishizu, K., Deguchi, Y., Takaki, H.: *J. Chem. Phys.*, 40 (1964), 241.
42* McConnell, H. M.: *J. Chem. Phys.*, 25 (1956), 709.
43* Altschuler, S. A., Kosyrev, B. M.: *Paramagnetische Elektronenresonanz* (Electron Paramagnetic Resonance), Leipzig 1963, Tab. 4.2.
44* Maki, A. H., Geske, D. H.: *J. Chem. Phys.*, 30 (1959), 1356; Geske, D. H., Maki, A. H.: *JACS*, 82 (1960), 2671; *J. Chem. Phys.*, 33 (1960), 825.
45* Ludwig, P., Adams, R. N.: *J. Chem. Phys.*, 37 (1962), 828.
46* Freed, J. H., Fraenkel, G. K.: *J. Chem. Phys.*, 37 (1962), 1156.
47* Freed, J. H., Rieger, P. H., Fraenkel, G. K.: *J. Chem. Phys.*, 37 (1962), 1881.

Chapter 9

The Application of E.S.R. to the Study of Processes which take place via the Radiolysis of Solids

The main research problem in radiation chemistry, as in every other field of chemistry, is to understand the mechanism and direction of the process, and to assess and understand its effectiveness. In radiation chemistry, the measure of the effectiveness is the radiation yield G_R, which is usually expressed as the number of molecules of the product of interest formed per 100 eV of absorbed energy. The two aspects of the problem are very closely connected, since factors which have a strong influence on the course (the chemical mechanism) of the process, usually also have a considerable effect on the radiation yield. Out of the very large number of studies of the effects of radiation on matter, we will limit ourselves to those in which the application of E.S.R. has led to essentially new and interesting results which increase our chemical understanding of the subject. We will try very hard not to repeat data published in D. J. E. Ingram's monograph *Free Radicals as studied by Electron Spin Resonance*.

As we shall see below, one of the most important results and primary effects of ionizing radiation on matter is that the chemical bond is disturbed, which leads to the formation of molecular fragments—radicals. As a result of the large chemical activity of these particles, their stationary concentration in the liquid and gaseous phase is so small that it is usually impossible to measure it, even with such a sensitive technique as E.S.R. For this reason, the majority of E.S.R. investigations on the structure of radicals formed by irradiation are carried out on solids. In these, owing to the low mobility of the radicals, a considerable amount may accumulate.† The primary dissociation effect is often masked by secondary reactions, so

† Until recently, only one investigation[1] was known in which free radicals were observed during the radiolysis of liquids, and this was in the E.S.R. spectrum formed by the irradiation of liquid ethane at 135°K (see the next footnote).

making the measurement difficult, but these secondary effects may be prevented by the use of low or very low temperatures. In this way it is even possible to stabilize such active radicals as atomic hydrogen. Most of the work on the stabilization of radicals has been performed on irradiated organic solids of various structures.

§9.1

THE INVESTIGATION OF RADICALS FORMED BY IRRADIATION OF ORGANIC MATERIALS: GENERAL REMARKS ON THE CAPABILITIES OF E.S.R. IN THIS FIELD

The use of E.S.R. has given us a definite answer to the question: with what abundance are free radicals formed as a result of irradiation? In all known cases of the application of E.S.R. to the study of the action of ionizing radiation on organic solids, free radicals have been detected.† The mere fact of the formation of radicals by radiolysis does not, by itself, serve as a proof that the radical mechanism is predominant. To prove this, one must show that the amount of radicals formed is comparable with the total amount of molecules which would otherwise have been formed under the same conditions. Unfortunately, such comparisons are made extremely difficult by the shortcomings of chemical analysis in determining the stable products of the radiolysis. Strictly speaking, no data are available on such comparisons under comparable conditions.

Qualitative statements as to what part the radical components play in the overall mechanism can be obtained if accurate measurements are made of the radical formation in the linear part of the accumulative curve (at relatively small doses) and these values compared with the magnitudes of the radiation yield of the final product, e.g. of the hydrogen, also in the linear region, but at considerably higher doses. If the two values differ very little from each other, i.e. if the total yield of the molecular products G_M does not exceed the rate of radical formation by more than two or three times, then one can assume that the radical component is sufficiently large. One may sometimes draw quantitative conclusions in such cases where G_M and G_R are determined at different temperatures, since G_M is usually not strongly temperature-dependent.

On the basis of all available results, we can state that even if the radical mechanism of radiolysis is not the only possibility, in many cases it

---

† If the experiments are carried out at sufficiently low temperatures, the secondary reactions of the radicals, especially their recombination, can be avoided.

obviously does play an essential role. Thus the study of radicals by radiolysis no doubt throws light on its most essential processes, in some, if not all, cases.

First and foremost we should mention the most important procedures which may be applied to the study of the radical components of radiolysis by means of E.S.R.

The radiation yield G_R is usually determined as the number of radicals formed per 100 eV of absorbed energy. As we have already mentioned, these measurements are only of value if they are carried out in a clearly recognizable linear part of the dependence $[\dot{R}] = f(D)$, and not just at one or two points. Here, $[\dot{R}]$ is the radical concentration, and D the dose of absorbed energy. The absolute accuracy in the measurement of G_R by E.S.R. techniques is not particularly good, because of a multitude of uncertainties, and is equal to ± 40 per cent. If G_R is determined for several materials under identical conditions, then the accuracy improves and may reach ± 20 per cent. One must also keep in mind that the radiation yield is sometimes strongly dependent on the lattice structure. For example, frozen cyclohexane was irradiated under various experimental conditions, and values of G_R were obtained which were grouped around the values 1·6 and 4·0.[2,3] It has been shown at the Laboratory of Physical Sciences in the University of Paris, and independently at the Institute of Chemical Physics in Moscow, that these differences are a result of the way that the sample was frozen before irradiation. In the case of C_6H_{12} the change in G_R came about as a result of obtaining the H.F.S. of the spectrum. In other cases, the change in G_R due to differences in lattice structure is accompanied by an essential change in the spectrum.

In determining G_R one must also take into account that the recombination processes do not in all cases follow the usual kinetic laws of the first and second order. In some systems,[4,5,6] on warming the sample, which was irradiated at 77°K, in certain temperature ranges, a 'step-like' recombination was observed. If the sample is studied at progressively higher temperatures, then radical recombination occurs at temperatures up to a certain limit only (Fig. 9.1). We will not go into a detailed explanation of this effect, which is clearly caused by the characteristics of the frozen medium or by the distribution of defects formed by the irradiation. We will only make the following comment: if the experiments to determine radiation yield in the above systems are carried out in the temperature range within which a step-like recombination is observed, and not during the radiation but after a certain time lapse, then the values of G_R determined from the linear part of the dependence $[\dot{R}] = f(D)$ can be shown to be considerably lowered, since each time only a certain fraction $(n(T)/n_0)$ of the original radical is measured (see Fig. 9.1).

The identification of radicals formed by the irradiation of solids is even more complicated than the determination of G_R. This is particularly important in the case of an E.S.R. spectrum of a paramagnetic particle in a condensed medium, where the spectrum is determined not only by its chemical composition (i.e. the position of the atoms with respect to each other, the form and strength of the delocalization, etc.) but also by the

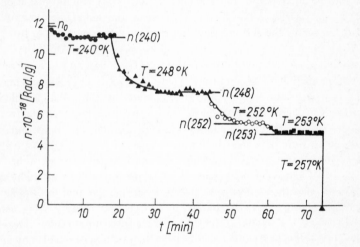

Fig. 9.1. Kinetics of the 'step-like' radical recombination in n-octylalcohol with increasing temperatures (irradiation of the sample at 95°K with D = 17 Mrd).

properties of the surrounding medium. An example of this may be seen in a comparison of the spectra of ethyl radicals, measured firstly in the liquid phase (Fig. 9.2a: irradiated ethane at 135°K, measured in a stream of high velocity electrons,)[1] and then again in a matrix of solid argon (Fig. 9.2b: photolysis of C_2H_5I at 4·2°K.[7] From this comparison it is found that, although the number of components and their relative position is the same in both cases, the line shape of the spectrum obtained at the lower temperature is so strongly distorted that only a detailed analysis can show that both spectra come from the same radical. In this case the change in the line shape arises from the 'freezing' of the rotation at the low temperature. A change in the crystal lattice can also lead to the same result. In this manner the

E.S.R. spectrum of irradiated Teflon, consisting of ten lines, smears out[8,9] (see Fig. 6.4) on cooling from 40 to 0°C, and then disappears completely,[10] which may be accounted for by the change-over of the lattice from triclinic to hexagon symmetry between 18 and 20°C. Thus further work is necessary if we wish to draw any conclusions on the structure of the radicals from the observed E.S.R. spectra of irradiated solids. The simplest procedure applicable is to investigate the temperature-dependence of the shape of the spectrum. In this case we must pay particular attention to whether the total

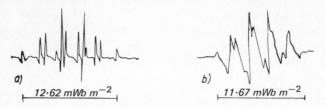

a)
$\vdash$ 12·62 mWb m^{-2} $\dashv$

b)
$\vdash$ 11·67 mWb m^{-2} $\dashv$

Fig. 9.2. E.S.R. spectra of ethyl radicals.
(*a*) In liquid ethane, at 135°K
(*b*) In a matrix of solid argon at 4·2°K

number of radicals remains the same at the different temperatures, and also whether the changes are reversible or not. If these changes, in the course of heating and subsequent cooling, are completely reversible, and if simultaneously the overall concentration is preserved (more or less), then we may conclude that the changes are produced exclusively by physical effects, e.g. the 'freezing-in' of the intermolecular movements, changes in the lattice structure of the surrounding matrix, etc. Since in this case both spectra—the original and the changed one—belong to the same radical, any conclusions from such data about the structure of the radicals are much more reliable than if only one spectrum had been available.

More detailed information on the structure of radicals formed by irradiation can be obtained from the study of single crystals. Since all radicals exhibit a preferred orientation with respect to the main axes of the crystal, we may take a whole series of different E.S.R. spectra with the single crystal in various orientations relative to the main magnetic field, and these will all refer to the same radical. If such results can be obtained, then it is possible to make a detailed comparison between all the various hypotheses on the structure of the radical, using the experimental results, and any conclusions drawn are usually quite unambiguous, even in spectra as complicated as succinic acid[11] or glycerine.[12]

Although this method is extremely accurate, its range of application is very limited, since it is not always possible to produce single crystals of the required size. On the other hand, the research worker is sometimes more interested in an incomplete molecular orientation, or even in the complete absence of orientation, rather than the irradiation effects in the crystalline state.

Recently, very interesting results have been obtained on polymers stretched prior to irradiation. Here, a preferred orientation occurs on the stretching axis, and the stretching of the sample in the magnetic field permits a study of the angular dependence of the E.S.R. spectrum. In this way a unique proof was obtained of the formation of allyl radicals by the irradiation of polymers such as polyethylene[13] and polypropylene,[17] and also interesting details on the structure of peroxide radicals in irradiated Teflon were obtained.[15]

Another very useful technique which permits identification of certain types of radicals by their E.S.R. spectra is the comparison of spectra obtained by irradiation of materials forming a homologous series, or differing from each other by replacement of atoms or isotopes by others of the same kind (e.g. substitution of H by D in certain positions of the original molecule).

The basic idea behind these methods is to gain information on the structure of the radical, not just on the basis of one spectrum, but from a variety of similar, but not identical, spectra. The differences between the spectra are created by known structural changes in the material under investigation. Naturally, care should be taken that such changes do not seriously affect the properties of the material, such as its form of crystal-lization, homogeneity, etc.

Conclusions on the structure of radicals in irradiated materials may also be drawn from a comparison of the E.S.R. spectrum obtained by irradiation at low temperatures, with the chemical structure of the stable radiolysis products of the same material at higher temperatures, or even in the liquid state.

So far we have only considered the case of the formation of one single type of radical as the result of irradiation. This in fact happens in the case of irradiation of linear polymers such as polyethylene or Teflon, or simple structures such as CH_4, C_2H_6, etc. However, in the case of polyvinyl-chloride the parallel formation of two radicals occurs,[8] as a result of irradiation. An even greater number of radicals may be expected from the irradiation of polymers with side chains, and from frozen low molecular organic materials with asymmetric structure.

The analysis of a spectrum caused by a number of different radicals, the relative concentrations of which are as yet unknown, presents a very difficult problem. In addition to the techniques already described, advantage may be taken of the fact that if the temperature is slowly increased, the mobility of the different radicals will change, and one may easily distinguish between them. In some cases, those radicals with a large mobility may even recombine. By comparing the changes in the shape of the spectrum and the total intensity, and applying the above procedures, the analysis of a complicated spectrum comprising a number of radicals may be carried out successfully.

One more case should be mentioned which facilitates the understanding of primary radicals formed by radiolysis. Although the primary excitation is evenly distributed over the mass of the material (proportional to the electron density), the chemical expression of this excitation, namely the primary disturbance of a chemical bond, is usually localized on a particular part of the molecular structure. We will deal more fully with this question below (see §9.2). Here, we are only interested in the case where, as a result of this effect, and even in materials with a complicated molecular structure, not all possible radicals are formed, but only a limited range of types. This considerably simplifies the analysis of the radical mechanism of the radiolysis.

§9.2

ON THE MECHANISM OF THE RADIOLYSIS OF ORGANIC SOLIDS

The number of papers published on the detailed analysis of the E.S.R. spectra of irradiated organic solids is unusually large, and it is quite impossible to consider here all these results, or even the majority of them. We would however like to note that in most cases the E.S.R. spectra obtained by different authors under identical conditions agree, usually even in the smallest details. Differences in the spectra of the same irradiated materials are usually produced by secondary reactions, the influence of which depends very strongly on the experimental conditions or on the techniques of cooling the sample. The latter can lead to a different basic configuration of the molecule of the irradiated material and this often causes very large differences in the H.F.S. and in the radiation yield, as we shall see below. As an example of the influence of the structure of the medium on the radical spectrum, we would like to go back to our comments on the radical $\dot{C}_2H_5$ in the liquid and solid phase (see p. 233). We said that the irradiation of C_2H_6 adsorbed on a solid surface forms the radical $(\dot{C}_2H_5)_{ads}$, the spectrum of which differs essentially from the spectrum shown in Fig. 9.2 (see §11.1).

For an example of the dependence of the shape of the spectrum on the configuration of the radical (the mutual positions of the bonds), we may take results obtained by the irradiation of linear and cyclic hydrocarbons. Fig. 9.3 shows spectra which were observed by irradiation of frozen organic

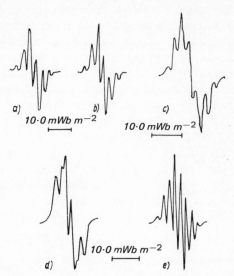

Fig. 9.3. E.S.R. spectrum of the radical $\sim CH_2 - \dot{C}H - CH_2 -$ by irradiation of (a) low pressure polyethylene, (b) paraffin (commercial), (c) $C_{12}H_{26}$, (d) cyclo-C_6H_{12}, (e) cyclo-C_5H_{10}.

materials: polyethylene,[13] high molecular paraffin,[16] the hydrocarbon $C_{12}H_{26}$,[17] cyclohexane[17] and cyclopentane.[17] With the exception of the first two, the spectra differ quite considerably from each other. Nevertheless, they all have the same structural formula:

$$\sim CH_2 - \dot{C}H - CH_2 \sim \qquad (I)$$

The differences in the H.F.S. of these radicals are essentially a result of differences in configuration. In the polyethylene and in the crystalline high molecular paraffin, it is known that the chains have a planar configuration (Fig. 9.4a), and as a result of this, all four protons of the two CH_2 groups connected to the CH group are completely equivalent so far as the interaction with the free valence is concerned. As the magnitude of the splitting for the α- and β-protons is approximately equal (see Chapter 6), we can expect a spectrum of six lines with a total splitting of approximately $5\Delta B_{spl} + \Delta B_i$ (ΔB_{spl}, the magnitude of the splitting, $\approx 3\cdot0$ mWb m^{-2}, and ΔB_i, the width of one component, $\approx 1\cdot0-1\cdot5$ mWb m^{-2}). The total splitting is approximately $16\cdot0-16\cdot5$ mWb m^{-2}, and agrees with the calculation.

In the case of the low molecular paraffin ($C_{12}H_{26}$), arbitrary orientations of the individual segments of the chain with respect to each other are possible, and for this reason, in addition to the planar configuration, the broken configuration is possible (see Fig. 9.4b), in which one proton of each CH_2 group has virtually no interaction with the free valence. In practice, in addition to the structures (a) and (b), the low molecular paraffin also gives an intermediate structure with a folded CH_2 group. The complete spectrum thus consists of a superposition of spectra with 6, 4 and 5 lines. This also explains the appearance of an additional line in the centre of the spectrum,

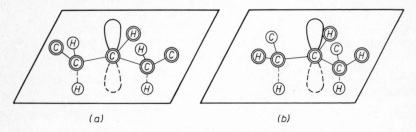

(a) (b)

Fig. 9.4. Sketch of the configuration of the hydrocarbon chain.

(a) planar (4 equivalent β-protons)

(b) broken (2 + 2 equivalent β-protons)

Atoms in one plane are shown with double circles.

which is shown in Fig. 9.3c. In the cyclohexane, because of the specific geometry of the ring, only the configuration shown in Fig. 9.4b is possible, and for this reason the total splitting is reduced to $12\cdot0$ mWb m^{-2} and the spectrum becomes more straightforward. In fact, the two effective β-protons are no longer equivalent to the proton in the α-position, which leads to a six-line spectrum. This non-equivalency clearly originates from the fact that in the radical $\dot{C}_6H_{11}$ the angle

cannot be straightened out to $120°$ because of the rigidity of the ring. The carbon atom can not then go over into the sp^2-state, as occurs in the linear hydrocarbons. Clearly the same situation also occurs in the case of the cyclopentane. Here we are dealing with five protons from the almost planar configuration, and the total splitting is approximately 16·0 to 16·5 mWb m^{-2}. However, in this case too, the angle

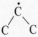

cannot be 120°, and so the protons of the CH_2 groups are not equivalent. The spectrum was interpreted by making the assumption[18] that the protons 1, 3 and 4 (Fig. 9.5) give only half as large a splitting as the protons 2 and 5.

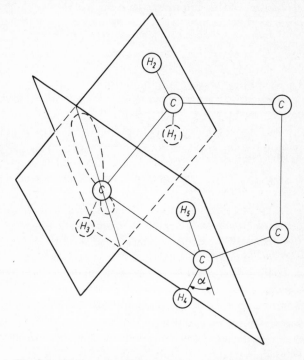

Fig. 9.5. Configuration diagram of the cyclopentyl radical.

We have carried out this short comparison of the different spectra of radical (I) in order to show the relatively large changes in the H.F.S. which can be produced by relatively small differences in the configuration. As the anlysis of the E.S.R. spectrum of each new radical requires a very detailed study, we will not consider any further examples of this type.

We will now try to show how E.S.R. may help in understanding the mechanism of the radiation effect.

As already mentioned, the essential questions in radiation chemistry are directed towards the primary reaction and the magnitude of the radiation yield. By far the greater proportion of the results obtained by the use of E.S.R. in the radiation chemistry of organic solids, have led to the conclusion that the primary chemical action of the radiolysis is the separation of a hydrogen atom. This follows directly from the result that where it is possible to stabilize the formation of the primary radical, under conditions in which no secondary reaction occurs, then the structure of these primary radicals agrees with the basic primary process:

$$RH + h\nu \rightarrow \dot{R} + \dot{H} \tag{1}$$

An example of this reasoning is given by the study of radicals (I).

In order to strengthen these conclusions it is also necessary to show that whilst $\dot{R}$ is being formed, simultaneously there occurs the formation of an equivalent amount of atomic hydrogen. This proves to be quite a difficult problem, as under the usual experimental conditions (temperatures of $77°K$ and higher, in a hydrocarbon medium) the hydrogen atoms have such a high mobility and recombine so rapidly, that direct detection becomes extremely difficult. However, at temperatures around those of liquid helium the hydrocarbon lattice becomes so rigid that even hydrogen atoms can be stabilized in it. Using this technique, Matheson and Smaller[19] investigated the E.S.R. spectrum of solid methane, γ-irradiated at $4 \cdot 2°K$, in the temperature range $4 \cdot 2 - 20°K$, and showed that methyl radicals and hydrogen atoms were formed with approximately the same yield. So we can consider the basic process (1) as proven. At higher temperatures, one may sometimes verify reaction (1) by considering the secondary reactions of the hydrogen atoms. We have recently obtained some very interesting results along these lines at ICP, by the irradiation of solid benzene.

From the irradiation of C_6H_6 at $141°K$ a spectrum was observed which consisted of a singlet superimposed on a triplet of quadruplets (Fig. 9.6a).[20] With slow heating to $220°K$, the intensity of the central singlet decreased quite considerably (evidently because of the recombination of the respective radicals), with a corresponding increase in the resolution of the multi-component spectrum. Here, each line was additionally split into three components (see Fig. 9.6b). On the basis of an analysis of the number of components, their intensity and the total splitting, it was concluded[21] that the spectrum shown in Fig. 9.6 was not produced by the radical $\dot{C}_6H_5$, as was originally assumed,[20] but evidently corresponds to the radical $\dot{C}_6H_7$,

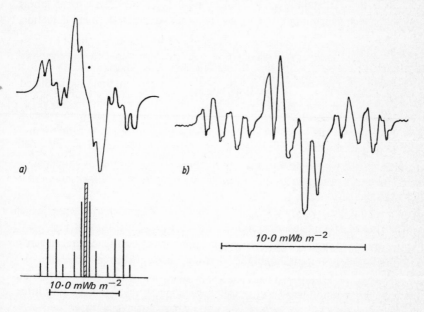

which is formed by the uniting of a hydrogen atom with a benzene molecule,

$$H + C_6H_6 \rightarrow \dot{C}_6H_7$$

The triplet with the splitting $\Delta B_{Tr} = 4\cdot5$ mWb m^{-2} originates from the interaction of the unpaired electron with the CH$_2$ group, the quadruplet with $\Delta B_{Qu} = 1\cdot0$ mWb m^{-2} is due to the interaction with the two ortho-protons and the one para-proton. The additional triplet splitting with

a)

10·0 mWb m^{-2}

b)

10·0 mWb m^{-2}

Fig. 9.6. E.S.R. spectrum of benzene.
(*a*) after irradiation by high energy electrons at 141°K
(*b*) after heating to 220°K

$\Delta B'_{Tr} = 0.35$ mWb m^{-2} arises, according to this analysis, from the two protons in the meta-position.†

As additional proof of the validity of this hypothesis as to the structure of the radical products from the radiolysis of solid benzene, we quote the results of detailed chemical analysis of the fraction C_{12} from the radiolysis products of liquid benzene.[22] According to this, the fraction C_{12} contained, in addition to diphenyl, the products phenylcyclohexadiene-2,5 and phenylcyclohexadiene-2,4. It can easily be shown that it is just these products which would be formed by the interaction of phenyl radicals with the radical $\dot{C}_6H_7$ of the given structure.

The assumption that, of the primary reactions in the radiolysis of solid hydrocarbons, the disturbance of a C—H bond is by far the most dominant, is in agreement with the cell principle suggested in 1934 by Frank and Rabinovitsch for photochemical reactions.[23] According to this principle, the probability of the recombination of two radicals formed in the condensed phase in the immediate vicinity of each other is considerably greater than the probability of the separation of the pair by emigration of one radical from the 'cell' of the molecule of the medium surrounding the pair. It is clear that the hydrogen atom has the best opportunity of escaping from such a 'cell'.

In the paper cited above[1] on the study of free radicals formed by the irradiation of liquid ethane, it was shown that, under the conditions described by the authors, the concentration ratio $(\dot{C}_2H_5)/(\dot{C}H_3)$ is approximately 20. This result proves that even in the liquid phase the primary separation of a hydrogen atom is essentially more probable than the disrupting of a C—C bond. In the solid phase the probability of disrupting a CH bond is even greater.

From all this, it follows that the principle of Frank and Rabinovitsch can be considered as a theoretical proof of the conclusions arrived at from a large amount of experimental data, i.e. that primarily a CH bond is broken.

However, in some cases the structure of the primary radicals which may be ascertained does not assume that the preferred primary reaction will be the disruption of a CH bond. Actually, if the molecule has several different kinds of non-equivalent CH bonds, then from the above arguments it cannot be predicted which bonds will be disrupted and which will not. A solution to this problem may be found if only one single radical type is formed by the radiolysis of the molecule in question. This

† Since this analysis, Fischer[81] has analysed the E.S.R. spectrum of the radical C_6H_7 in exactly the same way.

condition obtains in many cases. Molin *et al.*[24] have shown that if dicar-bonic acids, COOH . $(CH_2)_n$. COOH, are irradiated with high velocity electrons, at low temperatures $(- 130°C)$ where one may assume that the E.S.R. spectrum arises from the primary radicals formed by the radiolysis, then the spectra are very similar to each other in all irradiated systems from $n = 2$ to $n = 8$ (Fig. 9.7), but differ from the radical spectrum at $n = 1$ (Fig. 9.8).†

From this it follows that in COOH–$(CH_2)_2$–COOH (1), as in COOH–$(CH_2)_8$–COOH (2), the same radicals are formed by the primary reaction,

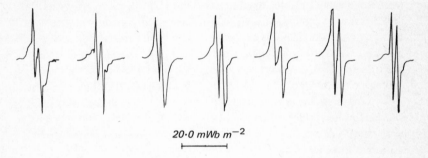

20·0 mWb m^{-2}

Fig. 9.7. E.S.R. spectra of dicarbonic acids irradiated at 143°K.

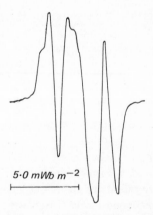

5·0 mWb m^{-2}

Fig. 9.8. E.S.R. spectra of irradiated malonic acid.

† The doublet spectra (Fig. 9.7) of the acids $(COOH)_2 (CH_2)n$, irradiated at $- 130°C$, cannot be compared directly with the spectra which originate by irradia-tion of these materials at room temperature.[35] In reference 24 it was shown that these more complicated spectra are caused by secondary radicals, which are also formed if the system irradiated at $- 130°C$ is heated.

and evidently represent the result of the separation of one H-atom from
the group CH_2-COOH.

According to the usual theories, the primary centres of electronic
excitation of the molecule, preceding the initial rupturing of the molecule,
are proportional to the mean electron density, i.e. approximately evenly
distributed through the material. Thus in the case of molecule (2) the
probability of primary excitation in one of the six central CH_2-groups
must be the same as the probability that it will occur in one of the
$-(CH_2COOH)-$ groups.

From the above results, obtained with the help of E.S.R., it follows
that the primary chemical damage takes place essentially only in these
final groups. To explain this contradiction one must assume that in the
systems considered, following the initial excitation, the excitation passes
along the $-(CH_2)_n-$ chain to the (CH_2COOH) group, in which, for
reasons not yet understood, the CH bond is very easily disturbed.

We now see that the continued application of E.S.R. in the study of
radicals formed by the radiolysis of complex organic compounds leads us
to a completely new effect, namely, energy transfer. These processes were
studied in more detail at ICP on the radiolysis of compounds with
phenyl-substituents.[26] Three compounds were investigated:

$$\begin{matrix} Ph \\ & \diagdown \\ & \quad CH-C_{11}H_{23} \\ Ph & \diagup \end{matrix} \qquad\qquad (A)$$

$$\begin{matrix} Ph \\ & \diagdown \\ & \quad CH-C_{11}H_{23} \\ cyclo\text{-}C_6H_{11} & \diagup \end{matrix} \qquad\qquad (B)$$

$$\begin{matrix} cyclo\text{-}C_6H_{11} \\ & \diagdown \\ & \quad CH-C_{11}H_{23} \\ cyclo\text{-}C_6H_{11} & \diagup \end{matrix} \qquad\qquad (C)$$

The samples were irradiated at $150°K$ with high velocity electrons (1·6
MeV). Apart from the investigation of the spectra of the primary radicals,
exact measurements on the radiation yield were undertaken. The E.S.R.
spectra of the samples A, B and an equimolar mixture of A + C (Fig. 9.9)
were very similar to each other, and came very close to the E.S.R. spectrum
of irradiated solid benzene. As we have already seen, the benzene triplet is
caused by the radical $\dot{C}_6H_7$, and so we have every reason to assume that in
the example considered by us the triplet is also produced by a radical
formed by the capture of a hydrogen atom by a phenyl ring. This triplet was
naturally not observed after irradiation in sample C.

We can therefore make certain statements about the fate of the hydrogen
in the systems A, B and A + C and show that they are formed by the

primary action. The question of the location of the primary rupture remains unsolved. On the basis of the results of the studies,[26] we can show that the hydrogen atoms are exchanged either only on the phenyl rings or in their immediate vicinity. In fact, if the primary separation of the hydrogen atom did result in the cyclohexyl group (in the case of B or A + C) then 50 per cent of the intensity of the spectrum would be produced by the corresponding radical, the total line width of which is $1 \cdot 0 - 1 \cdot 5$ mWb m^{-2} larger than the width of the benzene triplet. This would then be easily noticed in the corresponding spectrum.

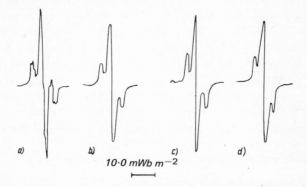

$10 \cdot 0$ mWb m^{-2}

Fig. 9.9. E.S.R. spectra observed after the irradiation of the following materials at 150°K:

(a) Benzene
(b) $(Ph)_2CHC_{11}H_{23}$ (A)
(c) $Ph(C_6H_{11})CH-C_{11}H_{23}$ (B)
(d) a mixture of 50% (A) and 50% $(C_6H_{11})CHC_{11}H_{23}$ (C)

As the total width of the spectra of the alkyl-radicals of type (I) is even larger ($16 \cdot 5$ mWb m^{-2}; see above), the lack of side lines in the spectrum of Fig. 9.9 allows us to conclude that the formation of primary radicals by the disturbance of a CH bond in the $C_{11}H_{23}$ group is also extremely unlikely. An analysis of the spectrum leads us to the conclusion that in the case considered the primary rupture of a hydrogen atom can take place either in the phenyl ring or possibly in the tertiary group.† Consideration of the table of radiation yields (Table 9.1) leads us to the same conclusions.

† As a result of very strong conjugation the E.S.R. spectrum of the radical Ph$\dot{C}$R′R″(RPh) can naturally differ very strongly from the spectrum of the usual radical R$\dot{C}$R′R″; therefore on the basis of the available data we cannot exclude the possibility that the irradiation of materials A and B creates a radical (RPh).

In saturated and alicyclic hydrocarbons the value of G_R is 4–6 (100 eV)$^{-1}$ compared to $G_R \approx 0.2$ for benzene and even smaller G_R-values for stronger conjugated systems (see Table 9.3). If therefore the radicals in the compounds A and B were formed in the saturated part of the molecule, then we would expect G_R-values of several (100 eV)$^{-1}$, as is also the case in the pure C compound. The fact that G_R for the compounds A and B comes very close to the G_R-value for benzene is a very strong argument that the primary rupture is located in the vicinity of the phenyl rings.

Table 9.1

Compound		G_R [1/100 eV]
C_6H_5 >CH–$C_{11}H_{23}$ C_6H_5	(A)	0·42
C_6H_5 >CH–$C_{11}H_{23}$ C_6H_{11}	(B)	0·46
C_6H_{11} >CH–$C_{11}H_{23}$ C_6H_{11}	(C)	4·9
Mixture of A and C with the volume ratio 1:1		0·73
Benzene		0·23
Cyclohexane		1·6-4

In reality we assume that the distribution of the primary excitations is proportional to the electron contribution of the individual molecules and atom groups, so in the absence of a transfer of energy in the compounds considered, the following should be observed:

For the compound A: 50 per cent radicals from the C_6H_5 groups with $G_R = 0.2$–0.3 (100 eV)$^{-1}$, and 50 per cent radicals from the $C_{11}H_{23}$ groups with $G_R = 6$ (100 eV)$^{-1}$; i.e. the effective yield would be equal to $G_R^{eff} = (0.2 + 5)/2 = 2.6$ (100 eV)$^{-1}$.

For the compound B: 25 per cent radicals from the C_6H_5 with $G_R = 0.2$–0.3 (100 eV)$^{-1}$, 25 per cent radicals from the C_6H_{11} with $G_R = 4$ (100 eV)$^{-1}$, 50 per cent radicals from the $C_{11}H_{23}$ with $G_R = 5$–6 (100 eV)$^{-1}$ and $G_R^{eff} = (0.2 + 4)/4 + 5/2 = 3.5$ (100 eV)$^{-1}$.

The results of these primitive calculations are in such complete contradiction with the experimental results that the concept of some form of energy transfer mechanism, which removes this contradiction, is sufficiently well established.

With the objective of strengthening the concept of the possibility of an energy transfer along one saturated chain, a large number of compounds of the general character A–D have been investigated.[27] Here A signifies an atomic group which acts as an acceptor of the excitation energy, and D a donor group. The concept of the 'effectivity' α of the energy transfer was introduced; α is calculated from the deviation of the effective radiation yield from the value which would be observed if energy transfer were absent. The values of α for a series of compounds are compiled in Table 9.2 from the data given in reference 27. We see that α fluctuates between the limits 0·65 and 0·95, depending on the structure of the molecules studied. From this it follows that the destruction of the simple additivity of radiation action by the 'energy transfer' effect is a common and important phenomenon.†

Table 9.2

Compound	α
C_6H_5–cyclo-C_6H_{11}	0·87
$\begin{array}{c}C_6H_5\\ \diagdown\\ CH-C_{11}H_{23}\\ \diagup\\ C_6H_{11}\end{array}$	0·93
$\begin{array}{c}C_6H_5\\ \diagdown\\ CH-C_{11}H_{23}\\ \diagup\\ C_6H_5\end{array}$	0·92
C_6H_5–$(CH_2)_3Si(CH_3)_3$	0·90
C_6H_5–$(CH_2)_3Si(C_2H_5)_3$	0·77
C_6H_5–C_6H_4–C_8H_{17}	0·81
C_8H_{17}–C_6H_4–C_8H_{17}	0·76
C_6H_5–C_6H_4–$\underset{\underset{O}{\|\|}}{C}$–$C_7H_{15}$	0·83
CH_3–C_6H_4–C_6H_4–CH_3	0·95

Although we do not as yet know the mechanism of this energy transfer, the very existence of the effect is enough to make it important for an understanding of the different mechanisms of radiation protection, direct radiation action, etc.

It remains to be noted that even before the application of E.S.R. to the study of this problem, many interesting results were obtained which could

† More recently there have been attempts[28] to replace this hypothesis, that the distribution of the primary excitation is determined from the distribution of the electron density, by a theory that the different atomic groups have distinguishable energy absorption coefficients. This theory cannot however explain the details given above, nor many other known facts, without additional hypotheses. Consequently, we will not go further into this question.

be considered as an indication of the existence of an energy transfer during the radiolysis of organic solids. Alexander and Charlesby[29] obtained such results by investigating the influence of naphthyl substituents on the effectiveness of chaining paraffins under the influence of radiation, as did Porter and Chilton,[30] by the spectroscopic study of the formation of the radical $(PH)_3\dot{C}$ by γ-irradiation of a transparent solid solution of $(PH)_3CH$ in a mixture of methyl cyclohexane and isopentane. In the latter case it is not impossible that the effect ascribed to the energy transfer originates from the secondary reaction of hydrogen atoms, as has been indicated by Hammill.[31]

§9.3

DEPENDENCE OF THE RADIATION YIELD ON THE CHEMICAL STRUCTURE: 'HOT' HYDROGEN ATOMS

As we have shown in the last chapter, a systematic analysis of the results of the hypothesis that the primary reaction separates a hydrogen atom leads us to the conclusion that in many cases this separation takes place at a specific location. A detailed analysis of this effect leads us further to the concept of the transfer of excitation energy. In putting forward this concept, we use without further comment the well-known experimental result that there are large differences in the radiation yields of different organic molecules. Systematic measurements of G_R in the solid phase[27] show that the corresponding values for aromatic compounds are considerably smaller than for alkanes and olefins, and at the same time, the smaller the value, the larger the degree of conjugation. This is particularly clear in the variation of G_R for the series $C_6H_5-C_6H_{11}$, $C_6H_5-C_6H_9$, $C_6H_5-C_6H_7$ and $C_6H_5-C_6H_5$ (Table 9.3).

Table 9.3

Compound	G_R $(100 \text{ eV})^{-1}$
paraffin ⎫ polyethylene ⎭	5
cyclohexane	4
cyclohexylhexine ⎫ cyclohexylacetylene ⎭	4
benzene	$0 \cdot 23 \pm 0 \cdot 04$
phenylacetylene	$0 \cdot 09$
phenylcyclohexane	$0 \cdot 55$
phenylcyclohexene-1	$0 \cdot 2$
phenylcyclohexydiene-1,5	$0 \cdot 07$
diphenyl	$0 \cdot 045$
terphenyl	$0 \cdot 045$

Since the G_R for the primary separation of a hydrogen atom depends closely on the characteristics of the mechanism of this primary reaction, it was necessary to study the relationship between G_R and the structure of the irradiated molecule. Recently Molin[32] demonstrated a simple and original approach to this problem. The basis of this approach is the hypothesis of Terenin and Kasha,[33,34] according to which an aromatic molecule in an electronically excited state rapidly goes over in to the lowest excited state, and further transformations will occur essentially on molecules which are in this state (Fig. 9.10).

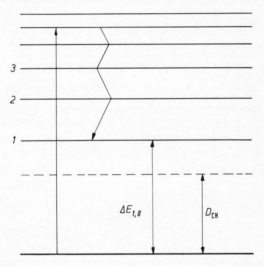

Fig. 9.10. Diagram of electron-levels and electron-transfer in a complex molecule.

As the lifetime in the lowest excited level can be quite large, we may assume that the separation of a hydrogen atom will also result preferentially from molecules in this state. If on the other hand we assume that for the disruption of a CH bond an energy of $D_{CH} = 4\text{--}4\cdot5$ eV is required, then it is to be expected that for molecules with $\Delta E_{1,0} > D_{CH}$ the separation of an H-atom results with a considerably larger yield than for molecules with $\Delta E_{1,0} < D_{CH}$. Since $\Delta E_{1,0}$ also becomes smaller with increasing degree of conjugation, the qualitative statement as to the decrease in G_R with an increase in the degree of conjugation is a natural result of the analysis. For a proof of this conclusion, Molin[32] compared the long-wavelength limit of the U.V. spectra of different aromatic hydrocarbons with the corresponding values of G_R (Table 9.4).

Table 9.4

Compound	$\Delta E_{1,0}$ [eV]	D_{CH} [eV]	$\Delta E_{1,0}-D_{CH}$ [eV]	G_R [1/100 eV]
saturated hydrocarbons		-4	6–3	4–6
alcohols		-4	≈ 3	3–12
carbonic acids		≈ 4	≈ 2	3–7
ethylene and acetyl-lene derivatives		3·3	≈ 2–4	4
benzene	4·7 [3]	4·5–4·3	≈ 0	0·23
phenylacetylene			≈ 0	0·09
diphenyl	4·2 [3]	4·5–4·3	< 0	0·045
terphenyl	4·2 (?)		< 0 (?)	0·045

Remarks:
1. E_{max} is the position of the long-wave absorption bands (orientation value): $\Delta E_{1,0}$ is the energy of the lowest excited electronic state; D_{CH} is the dissociation energy for the weakest CH bond.
2. Literature: [1] *Application of spectroscopy in chemistry*, ed. W. West, Moscow 1959: [2] A. Gilem and E. Stern, *Electron spectra of organic compounds*, Moscow 1957; [3] W. L. Bronde, E. A. Israilewitsch *et al.*, *Optika i Spektroskopija*, **5** (1958), 113; [4] N. N. Semjonov, *On some problems of chemical kinetics and reaction ability*, Moscow, 1958.

The values in this table are a convincing proof that the above qualitative explanation for the relationship between G_R and the structure of complex aromatic molecules is correct. It is however very probable that the range of application of this hypothesis is actually much wider and covers not only aromatic and pseudo-aromatic systems, but also systems with saturated bonds. In considering energy transfer along saturated chains, we come to the conclusion that in such chains, there must be excitation states which can rapidly be shifted from one position in the molecule to another, as is necessary to break a CH-bond in such an excited group. Since such a movement must not cause large losses, we can assume that it takes place with the participation of the lowest excited level of the saturated system. As saturated hydrocarbons are permeable up to almost 140 nm, we can assume that this level does not lie below 6 or 7 eV, and consequently that $\Delta E_{1,0}$ is in this case much larger than D_{CH} (see Fig. 9.10).

If the transition of a light quantum between the states 1 and 0 is forbidden (and we know that the luminescence yields from irradiated saturated organic materials are very small), then for a molecule in state 1 there are only two possibilities.† These are: (a) internal conversion, i.e. the transition

---

† Since we are here only considering paraffin chains with no additional links, then according to our reasoning an eventual energy transfer will not produce any changes. In the mechanism which we are considering, the resulting processes may occur equally in any part of the system.

1—0 by a simultaneous distribution of the total energy $\Delta E_{1,0}$ over the degrees of freedom of oscillation of the system, and (b) the dissociation of a CH bond, where the essentially smaller energy $(\Delta E_{1,0} - D_{CH})$ is distributed, so that a considerable part of the kinetic energy may be given to the lighter particle, the hydrogen atom. It is very clear that with increasing $\Delta E_{1,0}$ the second process will always become more probable, since the transition probability for internal conversion always becomes smaller. Evidently the large values of G_R for saturated hydrocarbons are also connected with this effect.

From this hypothetical interpretation of the reasons for large differences in the G_R-values of organic molecules, we come to an extremely important conclusion. During the radiolysis of saturated hydrocarbons, the hydrogen atoms separated, can at the instant of their separation have a kinetic energy of the order of magnitude of $\Delta E_{1,0} - D_{CH} = 3-4$ eV $= 75-100$ kcal/mol. These 'hot' atoms can differ essentially from the usual thermal atoms, which are in thermal equilibrium with the lattice, so far as their reaction ability goes. The difference is particularly noticeable at low temperatures, at which even low activation thresholds can almost completely stop the reaction of thermal atoms. 'Hot' atoms can affect the reaction in the following way:

$$H^* + RH \rightarrow H_2 + \dot{R}$$

leading to the formation of a large quantity of molecular hydrogen, which is always observed during the radiolysis of saturated hydrocarbons and corresponding polymers.

The hypothesis on the formation of 'hot' atoms has been discussed several times in the literature on the radiolysis of hydrocarbons in the solid and liquid phase. However, in these works it was introduced exclusively to explain the observed reactions between the different end products, particularly those of the molecular hydrogen. Recently a detailed study of this subject was published by Dewhurst,[35] who by means of this hypothesis explained the dependence of the hydrogen yield from the radiolysis of n-hexane in the liquid phase on the temperature and on the acceptor admixture. Independently of this, Molin[36] showed with the aid of this hypothesis that a quantitative connection can be obtained between the results of the radiolysis of liquid hydrocarbons and the reactions in frozen hydrocarbons. We can further assume that to a certain extent the reaction of the so-called 'molecular' formation of H_2 by the radiolysis also depends on the reactions of the 'hot' atoms. At the present time, we cannot really distinguish between the process

$$\sim CH_2-CH_2 \sim + h\nu \rightarrow \sim CH = CH \sim + H_2$$

and

$$\sim CH_2 - CH_2 \sim + h\nu \rightarrow \sim \overset{\bullet}{C}H - CH_2 \sim + H* \rightarrow CH = CH \sim + H_2$$

The idea presented above naturally requires some proof. There are, however, no definite statements in the literature which exclude such a hypothesis. Interesting conclusions on this question could be gained by a comparison of G_R for solid paraffin and compounds of the types A and C (see Table 9.1 and 9.3).

Basic objections to the hypothesis of the reaction of 'hot' hydrogen atoms in the radiolysis of hydrocarbons were always the results of the radiolysis of aromatic compounds and similar substances. In these cases the reaction yield of molecular hydrogen G_{H_2} was always very small,[22] and it was necessary to assume that for certain reasons the formation of 'hot' hydrogen atoms in these systems was not very probable. There were no general criteria to specify in which cases the reactions of 'hot' atoms were essential, and in which not.

It has been shown above that conclusions as to the possibility of the formation of 'hot' atoms cannot be obtained from either the composition of the product, or from the results of the subsequent analysis of the mechanism of the primary action of the radiolysis.

From this one can assume that 'hot' hydrogen atoms will only participate in such systems in the basic process of the radiolysis, when the difference $\delta = \Delta E_{1,0} - D_{CH}$ is sufficiently large. This difference can be determined independently by physical methods. On the other hand, one may come to some conclusions about the magnitude of this difference from the yield of the free radicals. the larger δ is, the larger is G_R and the more probable is the participation of 'hot' hydrogen atoms in the radiolysis.

To conclude, we can state that besides its importance in the identification of free radicals formed by radiolysis, and in the determination of a quantitative measure of the radiolysis—the yield of free radicals—E.S.R. also allows us for the first time to obtain direct experimental proof of an energy transfer, to explain the dependence of the radiation yield on the structure of the irradiated materials, and to investigate the question of the role 'hot' atoms play in the radiolysis of organic solids.

§9.4

FREE RADICALS FROM THE RADIOLYSIS OF BIOLOGICAL MATERIALS

With reference to the application of E.S.R. to the study of the radiolysis of organic materials, we will now consider the results obtained by the investigation of solid biological materials. The importance of such work is clear. E.S.R. allows the possibility of an accurate study of free radicals formed in biological materials under the influence of ionizing radiation. Of particular interest are the detection of free radicals, and the study of the kinetics of their accumulation and removal as a function of the radiation dose, the water content, the oxygen pressure, etc. From these studies we can come closer to an understanding of the working mechanism for materials for radiation protection.

In addition to this, the E.S.R. study of irradiated biological materials allows us to use the free radicals formed for detailed structural studies of compounds which are important biologically. In this case the ionizing radiation serves only as a means of introducing unpaired electrons into the system of interest, the E.S.R. spectrum of which throws light on the characteristics of the original structure.

Since the first work of Combrisson and Uebersfeld[37] on the E.S.R. spectra of amino-acids irradiated in a nuclear reactor, a large number of papers have been devoted to the study of free radicals formed by the action of ionizing radiation on important biological materials, cells and tissue of animal and plant origin. In this book we shall not dwell at great length on the numerous studies of the E.S.R. spectra of irradiated biologically-active low-molecular materials, such as the amino acids, di- and tripeptides, nucleotides, carbohydrates, sulphur-containing compounds, etc. The determination of the structure of the corresponding radicals from the E.S.R. spectra (particularly from the H.F.S. of the spectra) does not differ appreciably from the analogous problems of radiation chemistry. A complete structural determination is generally only possible through a careful analysis of the E.S.R. spectra of irradiated single crystals of the corresponding material, and for a correct interpretation it is often necessary to measure the E.S.R. spectra over a wide temperature range. As an example of a careful structural analysis by means of the E.S.R. spectra of irradiated single crystals of biologically active low molecular materials, we can turn to the excellent work of Whiffen.[38] Descriptions of E.S.R. spectra formed by the irradiation of biochemically active materials can be found in numerous other papers.[39-77]

We would like to try to formulate some general conclusions, on the basis of available experimental material, restricting ourselves to two important classes of biopolymers: proteins and nucleic acids. On irradiation of the amino-acids, which are the monomers from which the protein is formed, free radicals are formed which show a very characteristic spectra with a complicated H.F.S. Typical examples of such spectra are shown in Figs.

9.11 and 9.12. Generally speaking, irradiated amino-acids show a broad
E.S.R. spectrum with a spread-out H.F.S., resulting from the interaction of
the unpaired electron with the protons and perhaps with a N^{14} nucleus.
These features may be seen in the E.S.R. spectra of glycine, alanine, valine,
lysine, leucine, norleucine, glutamic acid, aspartic acid, serine, hystidine,
proline, arginine and theonine. As an example for structural interpretation,
we will consider the E.S.R. spectrum of irradiated alanine
$[CH_3CH(NH^+)COO^-$, Fig. 9.12].

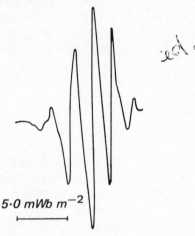

$5 \cdot 0 \ mWb \ m^{-2}$

Fig. 9.11. E.S.R. spectrum of γ-irradiated polycrystalline valine (aminoisovaleric acid)
at room temperature.

The spectrum of the irradiated polycrystalline powder shows a quintet of
equidistant components with intensity ratio 1:4:6:4:1. A small additional
splitting of each component may be observed. A study of a single crystal of
alanine at an arbitrary orientation in the magnetic field revealed a quintet
spectrum without additional splitting. A change in orientation leads to a
minor change in the g-factor. Thus the weak additional splitting in the
spectrum of the powder is caused by the anisotropy of the g-factor. The
main gaseous product of the radiolysis is ammonia. We can ascribe the
following structure to the radical which is formed:†

$$\begin{array}{c} H \\ \diagdown \\ H-C-\overset{\textstyle\cdot}{C}-COOH \\ \diagup \quad | \\ H \quad\ \ H \end{array}$$

† As in the radiolysis of polymethylmethacrylate (see §9.2), the radical considered
here is evidently also formed by a secondary reaction of the hydrogen atoms.

As a result of a sufficiently rapid rotation of the CH_3 group about the C–C bond, all the β-protons give equal H.F.S. constants. In this case, as also for the radical R–CH–R in polyethylene (see p. 237), the splittings due to the α- and β-protons are evidently equal. As the temperature is lowered, a

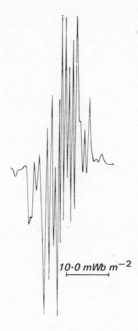

10·0 mWb m^{-2}

Fig. 9.12. E.S.R. spectrum of γ-irradiated polycrystalline alanine (α-aminopropionic acid) at room temperature.

distinct change in the spectrum results, and it becomes a symmetrical quintet with an intensity ratio 1:2:2:2:1 (see Fig. 9.13). It appears that the unpaired electron, after the freezing-in of the rotation of the CH_3 group, can interact only with three more protons (one α- and two β-protons), where the H.F.S. constant of the α-proton is twice as large as that of the β-proton. Under these conditions the E.S.R. spectrum becomes simply a quintet with an intensity ratio 1:2:2:2:1.

The radiation yield G_R of free radicals for amino-acids of this group is very high,† and according to the data of many different authors amounts to between one and ten radicals per 100 eV of absorbed energy.

In irradiated aromatic amino-acids (tyrosine, tryptophan) one observes, as expected, considerably narrower E.S.R. singlets and essentially lower yields, in agreement with the statements made above on the radiation yield of aromatic compounds. Amino-acids containing sulphur (cystein, cystine) after irradiation give a characteristic E.S.R. signal with a spread-out anisotropy of the g-factor. The average value of the g-factor (for polycrystalline samples) is larger than the free electron value and equals 2·025.

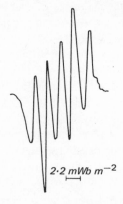

$2 \cdot 2 \; mWb \; m^{-2}$

Fig. 9.13. E.S.R. spectrum of γ-irradiated polycrystalline alanine at 77° K.

In the spectra of irradiated proteins, which represent polymers of amino-acids, one would expect an additive superimposition of the individual spectra. Experiments show, however, that all irradiated protein spectra conform to three possible types: a small asymmetric singlet of 0·5—1·0 mWb m^{-2} width, a symmetric doublet with $\Delta B_{HFS} = 1 \cdot 5 - 1 \cdot 6$ mWb m^{-2} (in both cases with g-factors which closely coincide with that of the free electron), or an asymmetric displaced 'cystein-type' signal (this last is usually observed in samples of protein with high cystein or cystine content). The yield of free radicals is as a rule one or two orders of magnitude smaller than for the majority of amino-acids.[71,76,78]

---

† Unfortunately exact accumulation curves of the radicals formed by irradiation are available for only a few substances. In the majority of cases either no quantitative data are given, or only for very large doses ($\approx 10^7$ R).

Analogous effects may be seen in irradiated natural tissues. Note that for amino-acids of the glycine class, the radical yield increases linearly with dose, until doses of approximately $3 \cdot 10^5$ R (possibly even higher) are reached, in contrast to the curve for natural tissues which shows a tendency to saturate at considerably lower doses.[79] In addition to this, irradiated proteins and tissues, unlike the majority of amino-acids, give an E.S.R. signal intensity which decreases rapidly (in the course of hours or days) until the signal completely disappears. The effect of oxygen and humidity affects this process very strongly.

Fig. 9.14 shows a typical singlet spectrum of a γ-irradiated protein.

The fact that in the E.S.R. spectra of irradiated proteins no lines from radicals of the individual amino-acids were observed, led Gordy and his co-workers[39] to the concept that radiation damage to the protein structure wanders to particularly weak positions; e.g. to the S-atom of a leftover cystein. On the basis of the narrowness of the E.S.R. signal, of the lack of an H.F.S., and the reduced radiation yield for many natural proteins, Blumenfeld and Kalmanson[71,72] concluded that in natural protein structure the unpaired electron becomes delocalized to a considerable degree.† This leads to an exchange narrowing, to a disappearance of the H.F.S. and to an increase in the probability of recombination of the free valencies. It was also suggested that the possibility of delocalization was connected with the fact that in natural protein there is a very dense network of peptide-hydrogen-bridge bonds, and that the delocalization of the unpaired electron within this network can be considered as a movement of a charge in the conduction band of a semiconductor.[80]

In fact, if the protein or tissue is denatured before irradiation so that the usual hydrogen-bridge is destroyed, then the radiation yield is increased, and in place of the singlet appears a signal with distinct doublet structure and a splitting of approximately $0 \cdot 6$ mWb m^{-2}.[72] Recently Kajuschin and co-workers[76] suggested that the appearance of the E.S.R. singlets in irradiated natural protein was connected in some way with the action of oxygen. The doublet signal appears as a direct result of the irradiation. In natural protein this signal is transformed by the action of O_2 into a singlet, whilst in denatured protein the doublet remains. It would be very interesting to apply the analytical methods given in Chapter 5 to these results. The possibility is also not excluded that the 'wandering of the radiation damage' is connected not only with a possible delocalization of the unpaired electron but

† This is naturally a 'low frequency' delocalization ($10^8 - 10^9$ s^{-1}) of the type considered earlier.

also with the transfer of the excitation energy which leads to the primary disturbance of a bond (see above, §9.2).

An even clearer characteristic of the E.S.R. spectra of irradiated polymers was observed by Schen Pai-gen *et al.*[74,75] in the case of nucleic acids

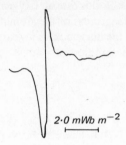

2·0 mWb m^{-2}

Fig. 9.14. E.S.R. spectrum of γ-irradiated egg protein.

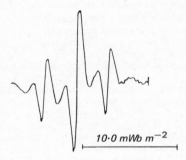

10·0 mWb m^{-2}

Fig. 9.15. E.S.R. spectrum of γ-irradiated guanyl acid.

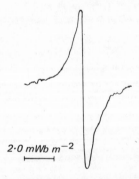

2·0 mWb m^{-2}

Fig. 9.16. E.S.R. spectrum of γ-irradiated desoxyribonucleic acid.

and nucleotides. The nucleotides (the monomers from which the high-molecular nucleic acids are built) give, after irradiation, a wide E.S.R. signal with a characteristic H.F.S. (see, e.g. Fig. 9.15). The nuclear acids after irradiation always give symmetrical singlets with considerably smaller intensity (see Fig. 9.16).† In this case an oxygen effect is not observed. Evidently the normal arrangement of the aromatic purine and pyrimidine bases in the structure of the nucleic acids favours delocalization and the exchange of unpaired electrons.

References

1. Fessenden, R., Schuler, R. J.: *J. Chem. Phys.*, **33** (1960), 935.
2. Molin, Ju. N., Tschcheide, I. I., Buben, N. Ja., Voevodski, V. V.: *Kinetika i Kataliz*, **2** (1961), 192.
3. Szwarc, H., Marx, R.: *J. Chem. Phys.*, **57** (1960), 683.
4. Jermolajew, W. K., Molin, Ju. N., Buben, N. Ja.: *Kinetika i Kataliz*, **3** (1962), 58.
5. Ayscough, P., Ivin, K., O'Donnell, J. M., Thompson, C.: *V. International Symposium on Free Radicals*. Uppsala 1961, paper 4.
6. Maga, M.: *Doklad v IChF AN SSSR Moskau* 1961.
7. Chochran, E. L.: *IV. International Symposium on Stabilizea Free Radicals*. Washington, 1959.
8. Zvetkov, Ju. D., Buben, N. Ja., Makulski, M. A., Lasurkin, Ju. S., Voevodski, V. V.: *C.C.R. Acad. Sci. U.R.S.S.*, **122** (1958), 1053.
9. Rexroad, H., Gordy, W.: *J. Chem. Phys.*, **30** (1959), 399.
10. Lebelev, Ja. S., Zvetkov, Ju. D., Voevodski, V. V.: *Optika i Spektroskopija*, **8** (1960), 84.
11. Heller, C., McConnell, H.: *J. Chem. Phys.*, **32** (1960), 1535.
12. Ghosh, D., Whiffen, D.: *Mol. Phys.*, **2** (1959), 285.
13. Kisseljov, A. G., Makulski, M. A., Lasurkin, Ju. S.: *Vysokomelekuljarnye soedinenija*, **2** (1960), 1678; Molin, Ju. N., Korizki, A. T., Schamschew, W. N., Buben, N. Ja., (Molin, Ju. N., Korickij, A. T., Samsev, V. N., Buben, N. Ja.): *Vysokomolekuljarnye soedinenija*.
14. Lebedev, Ja. S., Zvetkov, Ju. D: *Z. strukt. Chimii*, **2** (1961), 607, Fischer, H., Hellwege, K.: *V. International Symposium on Free Radicals*. Uppsala 1961, paper 23.
15. Lebedev, Ja. S., Zvetkov, Ju. D., Shidomirow, C. M.: *Z. strukt. Chimii*, **3** (1962), 21.
16. Talrose, W. L., Frankevich, E. L.: *IV. International Symposium on Stabilized Free Radicals*. Washington 1959.
17. Tschernjak, N. Ja., Bubnow, N. N., Poljak, L. S., Zvetkow, Ju. D., Voevodski, V. V.: *Optika i Spektroskopija*, **6** (1959), 564.
18. Shidomirov, G. M., Bubnov, N. N.: *Optika i Spektroskopija*, **12** (1962), 445.
19. Smaller, B., Matheson, M. S.: *J. Chem. Phys.*, **28** (1958), 1169.
20. Tschcheidse, I. I., Molin, Ju. N., Buben, N. Ja., Voevodski, V. V.: *C.C.R. Acad. Sci. U.R.S.S.*, **130** (1960), 1291.

† The yield of free radicals increases noticeably when the irradiation and measurement are carried out at low temperatures.

21. Tolkatschew, W. A., Molin, Ju. N., Tschcheidse, I. I., Buben, N. Ja., Voevodski, V. V.: *C.C.R. Acad. Sci. U.R.S.S.*, 141 (1961), 4, 911.
22. Manion, J. P., Barton, M.: *J. Chem. Phys.*, 56 (1952), 560.
23. Frank, J., Rabinowitsch, E.: *Trans. Far. Soc.*, 70 (1934), 120.
24. Molin, Ju. N., Tschcheidse, I. I., Buben, N. Ja., Voevodski, V. V.: *Z. strukt. Chimii*, 2 (1961), 293.
25. Abraham, R., Melville, H., Ovenall, D., Whiffen, D.: *Trans. Far. Soc.*, 54 (1958), 1138; Abraham, R., Whiffen, D.: *Trans. Far. Soc.*, 54 (1958), 1291.
26. Molin, Ju. N., Tschcheidse, I. I., Petrow, Al. A., Buben, N. Ja., Voevodski, V. V.: *C.C.R. Acad. Sci. U.R.S.S.*, 131 (1960), 125.
27. Molin, Ju. N., Tschcheidse, I. I., Buben, N. Ja., Voevodski, V. V.: Doklad na 2 *Vsesojusnoj konferenzii po radiazionnoj chimii, Moskau* 1960; Molin, Ju. N., Tschcheidse, I. I., Buben, N. Ja., Voevodski, V. V.: *Kinetika i Kataliz*, 2 (1961), 192.
28. Lamborn, J., Swallow, A.: *J. Phys. Chem.*, 65 (1961), 920.
29. Alexander, F., Charlesby, A.: *Nature*, 173 (1954), 578.
30. Chilton, H. T. J., Porter, G.: *J. Phys. Chem.*, 63 (1959), 904.
31. Hammill, W. H.: *Ann. Rev. Phys. Chem.*, 11 (1960), 101.
32. Molin, Ju. N.: *Dissertat. IChKiG SO AN SSSR*, Nowosibirsk 1961.
33. Terenin, A. N.: *Acta Physicochem. URSS*, 18 (1943), 210.
34. Kasha, A.: *Disc. Far. Soc.*, 9 (1950), 14.
35. Dewhurst, H. A.: *J. Phys. Chem.*, 62 (1958), 15.
36. Molin, Ju. N.: *Kinetika i Kataliz*, 2 (1961), 490.
37. Combrisson, J., Uebersfeld, J.: *Compt. Rend. Acad. Sci. (Paris)*, 238 (1954), 1397.
38. Whiffen, D. H.: *Symp. Free Radicals in Biological Systems*. Academic Press, New York–London (1960), 227.
39. Gordy, W., Ard, W. B., Shields, H.: *Proc. Nat. Acad. Sci. USA*, 41 (1955), 983.
40. Gordy, W., Ard, W. B., Shields, H.: *ibid*, 41 (1955), 996.
41. Gordy, W.: *Radiation Res.*, 1 (1950), 491.
42. Gordy, W., Shields, H.: *Bull. Am. Phys. Soc., ser 11*, 1 (1956), 199.
43. Gordy, W., Shields, H.: *Bull. Am. Phys. Soc. ser. 11*, 1 (1956), 267.
44. Gordy, W., Shields, H.: *Radiation Res.*, 9 (1958), 611.
45. Gordy, W., Miyagawa, I.: *Radiation Res.*, 12 (1960), 211.
46. Gordy, W., Shields, H.: *Proc. Nat. Acad. Sci. USA*, 46 (1960), 1124.
47. Shields, H., Ard, W. B., Gordy, W.: *Bull. Am. Phys. Soc.*, ser 11, 1 (1956), 200.
48. Shields, H., Gordy, W.: *Proc. Nat. Acad. Sci. USA*, 45 (1959), 269.
49. Shields, H., Gordy, W.: *J. Phys. Chem.*, 62 (1958), 789.
50. Berffet, G.: *Ann. Phys. (Paris)*, ser. 13; 3 (1958), 629.
51. Boag, J. W., Müller, A.: *Nature*, 18 (1959), 831.
52. Couger, A. O., Raudolf, M. L.: *Radiation Res.*, 11 (1954), 54.
53. Ehrenberg, A., Ehrenberg, L.: *Arkiv for Fysic*, 14 (1950), 133.
54. Ehrenberg, A., Ehrenberg, L., Zimmer, G. G.: *Acta Chem. Scand.*, 11 (1957), 199.
55. Fairbanks, A. J.: *Radiation Res.*, 7 (1957), 314.
56. Ghosh, D. K., Whiffen, D. H.: *Mol. Phys.*, 2 (1959), 285.
57. Ghosh, D. K., Whiffen, D. H.: *J. Chem. Soc.*, (1960), 1869.
58. Katayama, M., Gordy, W.: *Bull. Am. Phys. Soc.*, ser. 11, 5 (1960), 253.
59. Kurita, Y., Gordy, W.: *ibid.*, 5 (1960), 253.
60. McCormick, G., Gordy, W.: *J. Phys. Chem.*, 62 (1958), 783.
61. Miyagawa, J., Gordy, W.: *J. Chem. Phys.*, 32 (1960), 255.
62. Miyagawa, J., Kurita, Y., Gordy, W.: *J. Chem. Phys.*, 33 (1960), 1599.
63. Patten, F., Gordy, W.: *Proc. Nat. Acad. Sci. USA*, 46 (1960), 1137.

64. Randolph, M. L., Parrish, D. L.: *Radiation Res.,* 9 (1958), 170.
65. Rexroad, H. N., Gordy, W.: *Proc. Nat. Acad. Sci. USA,* 45 (1959), 256.
66. Servant, R., Augoyard, C., Chau, N. N.: *Compt. Rend. Acad. Sci. (Paris),* 249 (1959), 75.
67. Servant, R., Augoyard, C., Chau, N. N.: *Phys. Radium,* 21 (1960), 70.
68. Windle, J.: *J. Chem. Phys.,* 31 (1959), 859.
69. Henricsen, T.: Symp. *Free Radicals in Biological Systems.* Academic Press, New York–London (1960), 279.
70. Powers, E. L., Ehret, C. F., Smaller, B.: *ibid.,* (1960), 351.
71. Blumenfeld, L. A., Kalmanson, A. E.: *Biofizika,* 2 (1957), 552.
72. Blumenfeld, L. A., Kalmanson, A. E.: *Biofizika,* 3 (1958), 87.
73. Kalmanson, A. E., Blumenfeld, L. A.: *Biofizika,* 3 (1958), 735.
74. Schen Pei-gen, Blumenfeld, L. A., Kalmanson, A. E., Passynski, A. G.: *Biofizika,* 4 (1959), 263.
75. Schen Pei-gen, Blumenfeld, L. A., Kalmanson, A. E., Passynski, A. G.: *Biofizika,* 6 (1961), 534.
76. Pulatowa, M. K., Paguminowa, W. N., Kajuschin, L. P.: *Biofizika,* 6 (1961), 548.
77. Van Roggen, van Roggen, A. L., Gordy, W.: *Bull. Am. Phys. Soc.,* 1 (1956), 266.
78. Randolph, M. L.: Symp. *Free Radicals in Biological Systems.* Academic Press, New York–London (1960), 249.
79. Zimmer, K. G., Ehrenberg, L., Ehrenberg, A.: *Strahlentherapie,* 103 (1957), 3.
80. Evans, M. G., Gergely, J.: *Biochim. biophys. Acta,* 3 (1949), 188.
81. Fischer, H.: *Koll. Zs.,* 180 (1962), 64.

Chapter 10

The Kinetics of Radical Reactions in the Solid Phase

From the last chapter it will be clear that the application of E.S.R. to the study of irradiated solids opens up many possibilities for the quantitative study of the reaction rate of free radicals in the condensed phase. Such investigations allow us to determine, with an accuracy previously unattainable, the connection between the structure of the radicals and their chemical activity. Secondly, in the course of such measurements, we may come to very important conclusions as to the influence of the surrounding medium on the rate of the radical reactions. From this we will know to what extent the radical reactions in the solid phase are determined by the specific chemistry of the primary reaction, and to what extent by the characteristics of the matrix in which the reaction occurs.

§10.1

DETERMINATION OF THE REACTION RATES OF FREE RADICALS IN IRRADIATED POLYMERS

The most detailed of the kinetic measurements have been carried out on irradiated polymers. This may be explained on the one hand by the large practical value of irradiated polymer studies, and on the other hand by the fact that in polymers, the temperature range within which the radicals have a reasonably long lifetime coincides with the temperatures at which the radical reactions occur with normal values of the activation energy and with measurable reaction rates.

Between the years 1958 to 1961 detailed kinetic studies of this kind were carried out at ICP on the radicals formed by the irradiation of polytetrafluorethylene (Teflon). The melting point of this polymer lies at 300°C, and radicals formed within the sample by irradiation recombine at a noticeable rate only at temperatures above 150 to 200°C. The spectra of the radicals [$\sim CF_2-\dot{C}F-CF_2\sim (\dot{R})$], shown in Fig. 6.4, were submitted to a detailed interpretation,[1] and concentration measurements could therefore be performed with great accuracy. For the reasons given above these materials were very suitable for detailed kinetic measurements.[2,3] As these experiments were, so far as we know, the first detailed studies of the reaction kinetics of free radicals in the solid phase, and since they were performed using a series of special techniques which could be very useful for the solution of analogous problems, we would like to deal with them in somewhat more detail.

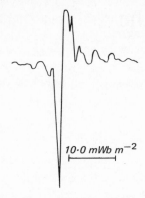

Fig. 10.1. Change in the spectrum of fluoralkyl radicals in the presence of air. The asymmetric singlet at the centre is a radical of the peroxide type.

First it was shown[1] that in the absence of oxygen the E.S.R. spectrum of the radical (R) (see Fig. 6.4) at temperatures of $25-100°C$ goes over into an asymmetric single line (Fig. 10.1) which is caused by a peroxide radical:

$$\underset{\sim CF_2-CF-CF_2\sim}{\overset{O-\dot{O}}{|}} \qquad (\dot{R}O_2)$$

The very clear differences between the spectra of the radicals $\dot{R}$ and $\dot{R}O_2$ makes E.S.R. ideally suitable for the study of the kinetics of the reversible reaction

$$\dot{R} + O_2 \rightleftharpoons \dot{R}O_2$$

A preliminary study of the equilibrium showed[3] that with increasing temperature the equilibrium is shifted to the left, i.e. that the bonding of the oxygen results from the production of heat. On the basis of these experiments the value $[\dot{R}O_2]/[\dot{R}] . P_{O_2}$, which is equal to the product of the equilibrium constant K and the solubility constant K_L, was determined at different temperatures. From these data, it followed that the sum of the reaction heat Q and the solubility heat ΔH_L was 20 kcal/mol and that the product of the factors before the exponential function was approximately

10^{-10} torr^{-1}. In order to obtain the true equilibrium constant and its temperature-dependence, the solubility of oxygen in Teflon and its temperature-dependence had to be measured independently. These data were obtained by special kinetic measurements.

Owing to the exothermic character of the direct reaction it was to be expected that at moderate temperatures, at which the reaction could be considered as irreversible, a limitation would be set by the diffusion.

Whilst carrying out the reaction directly in the cavity of the E.S.R. spectrometer with a sufficiently large sample (a cylinder of 2–3 mm diameter and 15 mm length), it was expected that the radical concentration averaged over the whole sample, $[\overline{\dot{R}O_2}]$, would increase according to the following law:

$$[\overline{\dot{R}O_2}]_t = \frac{r_0^2 - r^2}{r_0^2} [\dot{R}]_0 \tag{10.1}$$

where $[\dot{R}]_0$ is the initial concentration of the radicals $\dot{R}$, r_0 the radius of the sample and $r = r_0 - x$ (x being the width of the zone into which oxygen diffuses in a time t).

For small penetration depths of the oxygen, we can put with reasonable accuracy $x = \sqrt{(2Dt)}$,[4] and we easily obtain an expression for the dependence of the concentration $[\dot{R}O_2]$ on time, in the form

$$[\overline{\dot{R}O_2}]_t = \frac{3}{r_0} [\dot{R}]_0 \sqrt{(Dt)} \tag{10.2}$$

The curves shown in Fig. 10.2 show that this equation is fulfilled with very good accuracy. The curves also show how the average concentration of the primary radicals changes with time, for which the following relationship holds:

$$[\overline{\dot{R}}] = \left(1 - \frac{3}{r_0} \sqrt{(Dt)}\right) [\dot{R}]_0 \tag{10.3}$$

From these data the diffusion coefficient of oxygen in Teflon was calculated to be

$$D \approx 6 \cdot 10^{-4} \exp\left[\frac{-4600}{RT}\right] \text{cm}^2 \text{ s}^{-1}$$

The factor before the exponential function, and the activation energy of the diffusion, have very reasonable values.

The next group of experiments were concerned with the decomposition of the peroxide radical $\dot{R}O_2$. These experiments were carried out on cylindrical samples and on thin films with a thickness $d = 0.25$ mm. A previously irradiated sample was put into a tube and placed in the spectrometer cavity. This sample was then saturated with oxygen until a complete transformation of $\dot{R}$ into $\dot{R}O_2$ took place. The reaction was investigated at different temperatures whilst the oxygen was continually pumped out. The kinetic curves of the dependence of log $[\dot{R}O_2]$ on t proved to be quite complicated (Fig. 10.3). They are apparently made up of two connected linear sections.

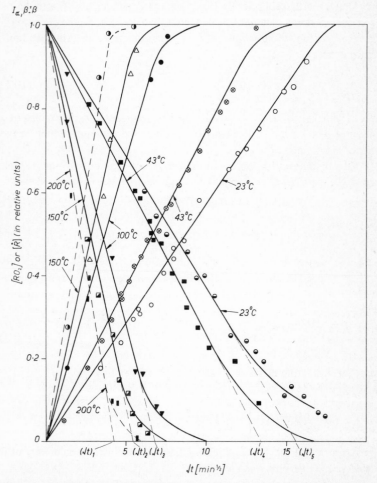

Fig. 10.2. Kinetic curves of the diffusion of oxygen in Teflon at different temperatures. (The concentrations of $\dot{R}$ and $\dot{R}O_2$ are measured in the same relative units.)

The figure below shows all three processes occurring in the sample, the dissociation of $\dot{R}O_2$ into $\dot{R}$ and O_2 the reverse reaction of the interaction of $\dot{R}$ with O_2 and the diffusion of the absorbed oxygen to the sample surface from where it is pumped out.

$$\dot{R}O_2 \xrightarrow{k_1} \dot{R} + O_2$$

$$\dot{R} + O_2 \xrightarrow{k_2} \dot{R}O_2$$

$$O_2 \xrightarrow{k_D} \text{pump}$$

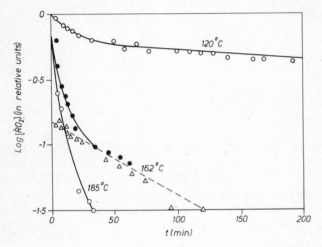

Fig. 10.3. Logarithmic plot of the decomposition kinetics of the radical $\dot{R}O_2$ on a surface.

The constant k_D is calculated for a planar sample according to the following known formula:[5]

$$k_D \approx 12 \frac{D}{d^2}$$

and when the expressions for D and d are introduced,

$$k_D \approx 10 \exp\left(-\frac{4600}{RT}\right) \quad \text{s}^{-1}$$

assuming that because of the small value of $[O_2]_L$ the semi-stationery concentration method of N. M. Semenov may be applied, i.e. with

$$\frac{d[O_2]}{dt} \approx 0$$

the authors obtained the following expression for the rate with which the average concentration $[\dot{R}O_2]$ is reduced:

$$-\frac{d[\dot{R}O_2]}{dt} = k_1[\dot{R}O_2]\frac{k_D}{k_D + k_2[\dot{R}]}$$

$$= k_1[\dot{R}O_2]\frac{k_D}{k_D + k_2([\dot{R}O_2]_0 - [\dot{R}O_2])} \tag{10.4}$$

Initially, when $[\dot{R}] \ll [\dot{R}O_2]_0$ the following is valid.

$$-\frac{d[\dot{R}O_2]}{dt} = k_1[\dot{R}O_2] \tag{10.5}$$

As the reaction becomes well advanced ($[\dot{R}O_2] \ll [\dot{R}O_2]_0$), we get

$$-\frac{d[\dot{R}O_2]}{dt} = \frac{k_1 k_D}{k_D + k_2[\dot{R}O_2]_0}[\dot{R}O_2] \tag{10.6}$$

From the equations (10.5) and (10.6), it follows that the curve $\log[\dot{R}O_2] = f(t)$ approximates to a straight line for large and small t. This corresponds to the results shown in Fig. 10.3.† From the slope of the linear region we can determine k_1 and $k_1 k_D/(k_D + k_2[\dot{R}O_2]_0)$. Since k_D and $[\dot{R}O_2]_0$ are known, we can calculate k_2 and the ratio $k_2/k_1 = K$, and since we have previously determined the product $K \cdot K_L$ we can also find K_L.

The measurement and calculations give the following results:

$$\dot{R}O_2 \rightarrow \dot{R} + O_2 \qquad k_1 = 10^8 \exp\left(-\frac{20000}{RT}\right) \text{s}^{-1}$$

$$\dot{R} + O_2 \rightarrow \dot{R}O_2 \qquad k_2 = 10^{-15} \exp\left(-\frac{6000}{RT}\right) \text{cm}^3 \text{ s}^{-1}$$

$$\dot{R}O_2 \rightleftarrows \dot{R} + O_2 \qquad K = 10^{-23} \exp\left(\frac{14000}{RT}\right) \text{cm}^3$$

$$(O_2) \rightleftarrows (O_2)_{sol} \qquad K_L = 10^{-3} \exp\left(-\frac{6000}{RT}\right)\frac{\text{cm}^3 O_2}{\text{cm}^3 . \text{torr}(O_2)}.$$

† If in equation (10.4) the term $k_2[\dot{R}O_2]_0$ is not neglected, then we obtain a more complicated expression, which can however be represented as a linear plot $f([\dot{R}O_2]) = A - Bt$ for $t \neq 0$. If the data measured at 162°C are processed in this manner, we actually get a straight line (see dotted line and triangles), which serves as further proof of the validity of the assumed mechanism.

E.S.R. in Chemistry

In order to verify the graphs and calculations, the solubility of O_2 in Teflon at 20°C was determined by a simple manometrical method, and the result compared with the results of the calculations on the basis or the expression for K_L deduced above. The values obtained by the two methods agreed within an accuracy of approximately 10 per cent.

Another series of quantitative measurements on the radicals $\dot{R}$ and $\dot{R}O_2$ in Teflon was devoted to the systematic study of the quadratic recombination process of these radicals.[6,7] In the course of this work it was established that the recombination processes for the amorphous and crystalline phases occur in different temperature intervals. Some difficulties arose in the investigation of the recombination of $\dot{R}O_2$ at higher temperatures, through the simultaneous decomposition into $\dot{R}$ and O_2. However, success was achieved with the help of a method of calculation analogous to the one above in determining the values of the reaction-rate constant for the recombination of $\dot{R}O_2$. In Table 10.1 are shown the compiled results for the values of k_0^{eff} and E_{eff} for the radical recombination in Teflon.

Table 10.1

Phase	Degree of crystallization (%)	Recombination temperature (°C)	k_0^{eff} (cm^3/s)	E_{eff} (kcal/mol)
		radical $\dot{R}$		
crystalline	74	220–270	10^{+6}	65 ± 5
	46	200–220	10^{-3}	40 ± 4
amorphous	46	100–220	10^{-7}	30 ± 3
		radical $\dot{R}O_2$		
crystalline	74	160–200	10^{-10}	26 ± 3
	46	140–180	10^{-8}	26 ± 3
amorphous	74	120–200	10^{-16}	10 ± 2
	40	110–180	10^{-15}	12 ± 2

The values of k_0^{eff} and E_{eff} not only differ from each other in the crystalline and amorphous phases, but also depend on the degree of crystallization of the sample studied. This evidently agrees well with current ideas on the structure of polymers, according to which different parts of a polymer chain can belong to the amorphous phase as well as to the crystalline phase.

But to what can we now attribute the large differences in the values of E_{eff} and k_0^{eff}? If we retain the usual chemical concepts, we would have to assume that in Teflon we are dealing with several different mechanisms for the recombination processes. However, the fact that k_0^{eff} changes in such a way that the increase in the activation energy is compensated for in a particular range, attracts our attention. This fact is illustrated particularly well in Fig. 10.4, from which it follows that these two values depend linearly on each other:

$$\log k_0^{\text{eff}} = A + B E_{\text{eff}} \tag{10.7}$$

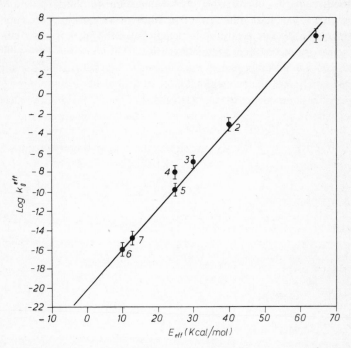

Fig. 10.4. Dependence of the logarithm of the factor before the exponential function on the activation energy, for the radical recombination reaction in Teflon.

Such a dependence, called a *compensation effect*, is observed in a whole series of physico-chemical phenomena in the condensed phase. The present one is the Meier-Neldel effect, which was already observed in 1927 in the study of the electrical conductivity of unipolar semiconductors,[8] the results of conductivity measurements on organic semiconductors,[9] the change of heterogeneous catalysts,[10] the change in catalytic activity of homogenous catalysts,[11] etc. Although until now a convincing interpretation of the compensation effect is still missing, we may evidently assume that in this case the different values of E_{eff} in the various series of experiments should not be considered as a proof of different mechanisms, but as an expression of a single mechanism, to which however the normal kinetics do not apply.

The data given above on the radical recombination in Teflon, which represent the results of very accurate kinetic measurements, allow us to analyse the problem somewhat more deeply. The basis of this analysis is the hypothesis that in the temperature range in which the compensation effect is observed, a change in the activation energy results from some reversible change of the type and character of lattice movements.[7] Such changes can be produced by a phase transition or by approach to the melting point. In the case of Teflon this hypothesis is completely justified, as in the amorphous phase at 170°C a phase transition takes place, and the recombination in the crystalline phase was studied close to the melting point of approximately 300°C (see Table 10.1). If, however, the activation energy is temperature-dependent, then the Arrhenius law, $k = k_0 \exp(-E/RT)$, is no longer valid.

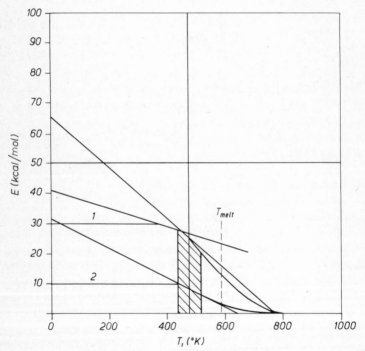

Fig. 10.5. Assumed dependence of the activation energy of the recombination in Teflon on temperature
   (1) crystalline phase
   (2) amorphous phase
The temperature range in which the recombination was observed is shaded.

If we plot these values in the coordinates $\log k$ and $1/T$ then, provided that E does not change rapidly, we obtain approximately a straight line, where naturally the values determined for k_0^{eff} and E_{eff} depend on dE/dT:

$$E_{\text{eff}} = E - T \frac{dE}{dT} \tag{10.8}$$

$$k_0^{\text{eff}} = k_0 \exp\left(-\frac{1}{R}\frac{dE}{dT}\right) \tag{10.9}$$

From Fig. 10.5, we see that E_{eff} can be considerably larger than E. But since k_0 was assumed to be temperature-dependent, and k is increasing faster than is indicated by the law $\exp(-E/RT)$, then the increase in E_{eff} must be compensated for by a very large increase in k_0^{eff}. From (10.8) and (10.9) we get

$$\log k_0^{\text{eff}} \approx \log k_0 - \frac{E}{R\bar{T}} + \frac{E_{\text{eff}}}{R\bar{T}} \tag{10.10}$$

which is in complete agreement with (10.7). Here $\bar{T}$ is the average temperature of the interval in which the measurements were performed.

By using this equation we were successful in determining the true activation energy for the recombination process in Teflon. Firstly, it should be noted that these values for the radicals $\dot{R}$ and $\dot{R}O_2$ are of the same magnitude. This means that the recombination is limited by the relative movement of the chain segments and not by the specific chemical features of the recombining groups. Furthermore, it was seen that k_0 in the crystalline phase has the usual value for bimolecular reactions of 10^{-10} cm^3 s^{-1}, but in the amorphous phase a lower value of approximately 10^{-15} cm^3 s^{-1}. The activation energies are 26 and 10 kcal/mol respectively.

It is interesting that an analogous analysis of experimental data by different authors on the recombination kinetics of radicals in polymers with hydrocarbon chains (polyethylene, polypropylene,[12] polyvinyl chloride,[13] polymethylmethacrylate[14]) for which E changes from approximately 20 to 40 kcal/mol, also gave a straight line in the coordinates $\log k_0 = \psi(E)$. This straight line does not coincide with that for Teflon, since the freezing-in of the internal motion follows a different law from that in Teflon.

We have not attempted to give a universal explanation of the compensation effect—there can be no single explanation of it. It may be connected with quite different causes, which result in a temperature-dependence of the activation energy of the process under investigation. The basic final conclusions from the work we have considered are the following:

1. One cannot take the anomalous large values of k_0^{eff} and E_{eff}, obtained by application of the Arrhenius formula to the results of recombination rates in the condensed phase, as the true reaction constants.

2. The presence of the compensation effect proves that the change of the true activation energy with increasing temperature is not accompanied by an increase of the true value of k_0, since if the opposite were true, the linear relationship (10.7) would not hold.

§10.2

ON SOME PERCULIARITIES OF THE REACTION KINETICS OF RADICAL RECOMBINATION IN THE SOLID PHASE

In the previous section we have shown, with the help of E.S.R., that for the recombination of free radicals in irradiated Teflon, the rate of the recombination process is not determined by the specific chemical features of these radicals, but by the characteristics of the matrix. We saw that changes in the characteristics of the matrix in a particular temperature range led to large deviations from the classical kinetic laws. It should be noted that this temperature range lies lower for the amorphous phase than for the crystalline phase.

In polymers, particularly in Teflon, the above-mentioned deviations can be caused by movement of large parts of the macro-molecule. In order to obtain some direct conclusions as to the role of the surrounding medium, it is interesting to investigate the recombination laws of free radicals in irradiated solids of simpler structure. Naturally these studies were also carried out using E.S.R., which permits an identification of the radicals formed by the irradiation, and the determination of the changes in concentration at different temperatures.

In the work of Ermolaev *et al.*[15] the radical recombination was investigated in a series of frozen organic substances after irradiation by high velocity electrons with an energy of 1·6 keV. The experiments were carried out in the following way. The frozen sample was irradiated at a constant temperature $T_0 \approx 100°$K, at which there was virtually no recombination. After this, the sample was rapidly heated (in the spectrometer cavity) to a temperature T_1, where it remained for two minutes, and then it was cooled again to T_0 for the measurement of $[\dot{R}]$. Thereafter, the same procedure was repeated at correspondingly higher temperatures T_2, T_3, ..., up to the temperature at which the time of two minutes was sufficient for the recombination of all radicals. The 'thaw curves' obtained in this way are reproduced in Fig. 10.6 in the coordinates $[\dot{R}]/[\dot{R}_0] = f(T/T_{melt})$. The curves shown fall into two classes. In methyl alcohol, benzene and *n*-octyl alcohol, which solidify into crystalline form, there resulted a large decrease in the radical concentration in the vicinity of the melting point. In the amorphous samples, glycerine, *n*-butyl alcohol and *n*-nonyl alcohol, however, the radicals already start to recombine rapidly in the vicinity of the so-called glassy-point, which usually lies at $T_g \approx 0.6-0.7\ T_{melt}$. One of the

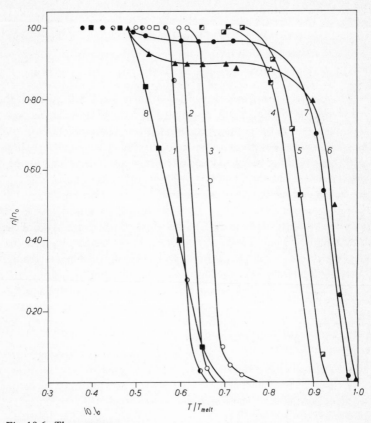

Fig. 10.6. Thaw curves,
1. *n*-butyl alcohol (193°K)
2. *n*-nonyl alcohol (268°K)
3. glycerine (292°K)
4. methyl alcohol (175°K)
5. benzene (278°K)
6. *n*-octyl alcohol (256°K)
7. crystalline 1,1-dicyclohexyldodecane (300°K)
8. amorphous 1,1-dicyclohexyldodecane (300°K).

The figures in brackets refer to the melting point of the material.

samples studied, 1,1-dicyclohexyldodecane, could solidify in the crystalline as well as the amorphous state. Fig. 10.6 shows, accordingly, that the recombination curve belongs either to the first or to the second class. In the case of n-octyl alcohol the curve shows a spread-out step at approximately $0 \cdot 6$ T_{melt}, which clearly indicates the joint presence of the amorphous and crystalline phases.

These studies resulted in the need for an explanation as to which types of motion, other than the diffusion appearing at the melting point and above T_g, could still lead to an intensive recombination in the solid phase. Particularly interesting were the materials for which the freezing-in of the motion at low temperatures was shown by means of nuclear magnetic resonance (N.M.R.).

In Fig. 10.7 are shown the 'thaw curves' for cyclohexane and cyclopentane, which solidify into crystalline form. The temperatures at which the molecular rotation is frozen in, as determined by N.M.R.,[16] are shown by arrows on the abscissa. In addition to this it has been shown that at these points a change occurs in the crystal lattice, accompanied by a freezing-in not only of the rotation but also of the self-diffusion.[17] This posed the question as to which of these two types of motion is responsible for the recombination. To answer this, Schamschew[18] recorded the thaw-curve for the radicals in irradiated hexamethylbenzene, since it was known that in $C_6(CH_3)_6$ at $T \approx 150°-220°K$ the rotation thaws, without the appearance of self-diffusion.[19]

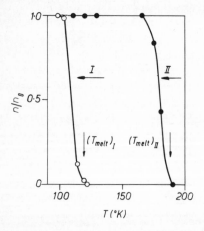

Fig. 10.7. Thaw curves of cyclopentane ($T_{\text{melt}} = 180°K$) and cyclohexane ($T_{\text{melt}} = 280°K$). The arrows show the points of the polymorphous transition, which is accompanied by the thawing of the rotation of the molecule about all three axes.

The experiments showed (Fig. 10.8) that in this temperature range only approximately 40 per cent of the radicals recombine. This evidently proves that the rotation makes the recombination easier only for those radicals which lie relatively close to each other. For the recombination of more separated radicals, a self-diffusion is required.

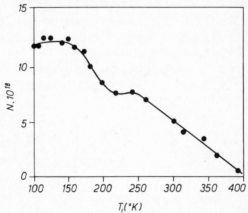

Fig. 10.8.   Thaw curve of hexamethylbenzene (T_{melt} = 439°K).

Although the results obtained with the help of the thaw curves are extremely interesting, naturally one should not believe that they can give a complete picture of the recombination. Nor should it be forgotten that the recording time of each experiment was arbitrarily limited to two minutes. To obtain a complete picture, more accurate measurements were carried out in the temperature range in which the thaw curves fall rapidly.

With amorphous materials the usual kinetic curves of the second order are observed. Here, the recombination process is evidently influenced by simple diffusion. With crystalline materials, however, a 'step-like' recombination curve is seen: at each temperature, the concentration falls to a certain value $R(T)$ which is dependent on this temperature and on the initial concentration (see p. 233, Fig. 9.1). Such results were obtained with cyclohexane and n-octyl alcohol irradiated with high-velocity electrons[20] and with U.V.-irradiated frozen aqueous solutions of H_2O_2.[21] In order to explain this peculiarity, the assumption was made (in reference 20) that this was caused by an inhomogeneous structure of the polycrystalline samples. These are assumed to consist of more or less large regions characterized by different values of the phase transition temperature. Different conditions of solidification of the sample can naturally lead to a method of distinguishing between the distributions of such regions, which cause such large differences in the radiation yield as the values given above (see p. 232) of $G_R = 1.6$ and 4·0 for cyclohexane, and also create corresponding differences in the recombination kinetics (see Fig. 10.9). Semenov also assumed that the irradiation itself could influence the character of the inhomogeneities.[22]

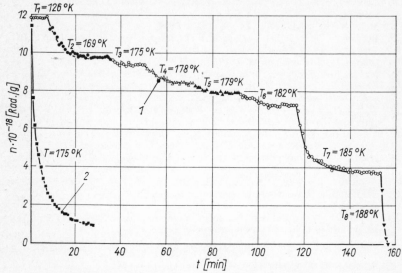

Fig. 10.9. Recombination kinetics of radicals in cyclohexane
1. rapidly frozen sample, irradiated at 126°K, $D = 30$ Mrd
2. tempered sample, irradiated at 126°K, $D = 40$ Mrd

One sees that we are still far from an explanation of the recombination mechanism of radicals in the solid phase. We can say, however, that the study of the recombination process has evidently led to the creation of a very fine method for the analysis of the lattice characteristics of solids, which reflects the features of the crystalline and amorphous state on a more microscope scale than ever before possible.

Further work in this direction can lead to the clarification of the actual kinetic processes in the solid state, as well as to a deeper understanding of the structure of the solids investigated.

References

1. Zvetkov, Ju. D., Buben, N. Ja., Makulski, M. A., Lasurkin, Ju. S., Voevodski, V. V.: *C.C.R. Acad. Sci. U.R.S.S.*, **122** (1958), 1053 .
2. Zvetkov, Ju. D., Lebedev, Ja. S., Voevodski, V. V.: *Vysokomolekuljarnye soedinenija*, **1** (1959), 1519.

3. Zvetkov, Ju. D., Lebedev, Ja. S., Voevodski, V. V.: *Vysokomolekuljarnye soedinenija,* 1 (1959), 1634.
4. Zvetkov, Ju. D.: *Dissertat. IChKiG SO AN SSSR,* Nowosibirsk 1961.
5. Semenov, N. N.: *Acta Physicochim. URSS,* 18 (1943), 93.
6. Zvetkov, Ju. D., Lebedev, Ja. S., Voevodski, V. V.: *Vysokomolekuljarnye soedinenija ,* 3, (1961), 882.
7. Lebedev, Ja. S., Zvetkov, Ju. D., Voevodski, V. V.: *Kinetika i Kataliz,* 1 (1960), 496.
8. Meier, W., Neldel, H.: *Phys. Zs.,* 38 (1937), 1014.
9. Balabanow, Je. I., Berlin, A. A., Parin, W. P., Talrose, W. L., Frankewitsch, E. D., Tscherkaschin, M. I.: *C.C.R. Acad. Sci. U.R.S.S.,* 134 (1960), 1123.
10. Cremer, E.: *Adv. in Catalysis,* 7 (1955), 75.
11. Marcus, R. J., Zwalinsky, B. J., Eyring, H.: *J. Phys. Chem.,* 58 (1954), 432.
12. Ohnishi, S., Kashiwagi, M., Ikeda, I., Nitta, I.: *Conference on Application of Large Radiation Sources in Industry and Chemical Processes.* Warsaw 1959.
13. Kuri, Z., Ueda, H., Shida, S.: *J. Chem. Phys.,* 32 (1960), 371.
14. Ohnishi, S., Nitta, I.: *J. Polymer Sci.,* 38 (1959), 451.
15. Ermolaev, V. K., Molin, Ju. N., Buben, N. Ja.: *Doklad na II vsesojusnom sovescanii po radiacionnoj chimii.* Moskau 1960; see also reference 20.
16. Andrew, E. R.: *Nuclear Magnetic Resonance,* Cambridge 1955; Rushworth, F. A.: *Proc. Roy. Soc.,* A 222 (1954), 526.
17. Andrew, E. R.: *Phys. Chem. Solids,* 18 (1961), 9.
18. Schamschew, N. W.: See N. N. Semenov, reference 22.
19. Andrew, E. R.: *J. Chem. Phys.,* 18 (1950), 607.
20. Jermolajew, W. K., Molin, Ju. N., Buben, N. Ja.: *Kinetika i Kataliz,* 3 (1962), 58.
21. Sergejew, G. B., Gurman, W. S., Papissowa, W. I., Jakowenko, E. I.: *V. International Symposium on Free Radicals.* Uppsala (1961), 63.
22. Semenov, N. N.: XVIII Congress of JUPAC, Montreal 1961.

Chapter 11

The Application of E.S.R. in the Study of Catalysts and in Primary Reactions on Surfaces

It is well known that chemists in various specialist fields are very interested in explaining the mechanism of heterogeneous catalysis. There are however no direct methods at the researcher's disposal for the investigation of the structure and characteristics of the active intermediary bonds formed in the course of the catalytic process. It is not surprising, then, that the intensive use of E.S.R. for the solution of very diverse chemical problems, has also led to experimental use of E.S.R. in the study of the catalysis mechanism. This work can be divided into two main groups.

Firstly, starting from the idea that heterogeneous catalytic processes can follow a radical—or radical chain—mechanism, a series of E.S.R. investigations was devoted to working out methods by which free radicals can be detached from solid surfaces and their reaction kinetics studied. Since one of the most effective ways of forming free radicals on surfaces is the action of ionizing radiation, this group of studies is closely connected with tentative results on the correlation of the change in catalytic activity under the action of radiation, and the corresponding changes in the E.S.R. spectra.

The second important division is the study of the E.S.R. spectra of catalysts containing some kind of paramagnetic ion. By an analysis of the E.S.R. spectra, as we shall see below, interesting results are obtained on the change of the electronic structure of these ions as a function of the method of formation, the method of activation, the intensity of the catalytic process, etc. In other words, we have the possibility of determining a connection between the activity of the catalyst and the electronic characteristics of the ions contained within it.

§11.1

FREE RADICALS WHICH ARE ADSORBED
ON SOLID SURFACES

The idea of the possible existence of free radicals in the adsorbed state has been put forward several times within the last 40 years in attempts to explain the action of heterogeneous chain-breaking of the first order. The general concept of heterogeneous recombination,

$$\dot{R} + \text{surface} \underset{k_2}{\overset{k_1}{\rightleftharpoons}} (\dot{R})_{ads}, \qquad \left\{ \begin{matrix} (1) \\ (2) \end{matrix} \right\}$$

$$\dot{R} + (\dot{R})_{ads} \overset{k_3}{\rightleftharpoons} R_2 \qquad\qquad (3)$$

proved to be applicable in most cases,[1] under the condition that the adsorbed radical $(\dot{R})_{ads}$ is sufficiently active for reaction (3) to occur without a larger activation energy, and that at the same time the bond on the surface is strong enough for reaction (2) to occur sufficiently slowly. Until recently no methods for the study of adsorbed radicals have been available, so the research worker has had to be satisfied with these obvious, but as yet unproven, hypotheses.

The existence of free radicals adsorbed on a solid surface was first demonstrated by Livingston, Zeldes and Taylor[2] by the γ-irradiation of quartz at 77°K. The possibility of stabilizing hydrogen atoms on a solid surface was proved by the appearance of a clear doublet spectrum with a splitting of approximately 50 mWb m^{-2}. According to the authors, the source of the hydrogen atoms was adsorbed hydrogen molecules and hydroxyl groups on the surface. Following the action of heavy water on the surface, i.e. after partial substitution of the hydrogen by deuterium, the spectrum of the irradiated sample showed, in addition to the hydrogen doublet, the triplet of deuterium with a splitting $\Delta B_{HFS} \approx 7 \cdot 8$ mWb m^{-2}. This result is again strong evidence in favour of the hypothesis that hydrogen atoms are in fact formed under these conditions.

E.S.R. spectra of H-atoms have been obtained by Bubnov, Poljak *et al.*,[3] by the γ-irradiation of quartz, silica gel and ordinary sodium glass. In all cases ΔB_{HFS} was approximately equal to 50 mWb m^{-2}, although the width of the H.F.S. components depended very strongly on the structure of the lattice: for quartz $\Delta B_i = 0 \cdot 8$ mWb m^{-2}, for silica gel $\Delta B_i = 0 \cdot 24$ mWb m^{-2}, and for glass $\Delta B_i = 0 \cdot 45$ mWb m^{-2}.

In the last two cases, the variation can be attributed to the presence of paramagnetic impurities and nuclei with magnetic moments. It is essential that ΔB_{HFS} should agree with the value obtained for the free hydrogen atom[4]. This agreement shows that the electronic structure of the hydrogen atom is to all practical purposes unchanged by the adsorption. In the light of these results, however, the high stability of the hydrogen atoms is very difficult to understand. We have already seen that the hydrogen atoms on a hydrocarbon lattice at these temperatures have a sufficiently high mobility to guarantee a high recombination rate. There has been no success in detecting hydrogen atoms even in water irradiated at 77°K.[5] The hydrogen atoms formed by the irradiation of silica gel and quartz, however, do not recombine at all at 77°K. A possible explanation of this is as follows. The hydrogen atoms being formed by the dissociation of the surface OH groups or by the adsorbed water molecules diffuse into the inside of the solid, and there they are stabilized by some of the symmetrical lattice points, as in the radiolysis or photolysis of frozen acid solutions (see §8.6). If such an interpretation were correct, then the idea of adsorbed atoms and radicals would be completely invalidated.

With the object of clarifying this problem, Kasanski and Pariski[6,7] undertook a systematic study of the behaviour of hydrogen atoms formed by the irradiation of silica gel. First of all they studied the conditions of recombination by heating the sample in a vacuum. It was shown that the recombination becomes observable between 120 and 130°K. The kinetic recombination curve at 143°K is shown in Fig. 11.1 (curve 1). It can easily be shown to satisfy an equation of the first order.

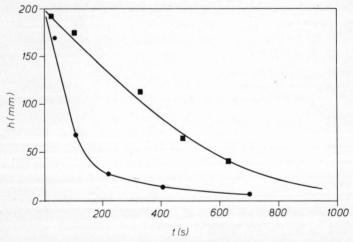

Fig. 11.1 Kinetic curves of the adsorption of hydrogen atoms in irradiated silica gel in vacuum (■) and in an atmosphere of oxygen (●) at 143°K

By measurement at different temperatures, the authors found an expression for the rate constant of the monomolecular recombination process:

$$k \approx 10^{+1} \exp\left(-\frac{2000}{RT}\right) s^{-1}$$

The small value of the activation energy tends to confirm the assumption that the chemical bond of the hydrogen atoms is very weak, a conclusion which was obtained on the basis of $\Delta B_{HFS} \approx 50$ mWb m^{-2}. One should also take into account the unusually small value of the factor before the exponential term, which will ensure a slowing down of the recombination at liquid nitrogen temperatures.

Kasanski and Pariski also showed[8] that the adsorption rate of hydrogen atoms increases if the heating is carried out in oxygen or ethylene. As can be seen from Fig. 11.1 (curve 2), the adsorption rate of hydrogen atoms at $T = 143°K$ is three times larger in the presence of oxygen than it is in vacuum. In the presence of ethylene at $120°K$ the rate is 30 times larger than in vacuum.

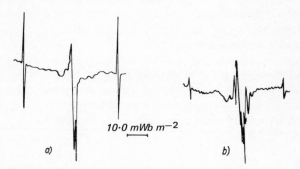

10·0 mWb m^{-2}

a)

b)

Fig. 11.2. Reaction of hydrogen atoms with ethylene,
(a) spectrum of irradiated silica gel
(b) spectrum of the same sample after heating it for 30 s in an ethylene atmosphere at $-120°C$.
The gain is the same in both cases.

In the last case the disappearance of the hydrogen atoms is accompanied by the appearance of some additional lines at the centre of the spectrum of the irradiated silica gel, which are strongly reminiscent of the spectra of the alkyl radicals (see Fig. 11.2). The strong action of gases on the hydrogen atoms makes it appear probable that these atoms are nevertheless stabilized either at the surface or somewhere very close to the surface.

In another paper by the same authors with the participation of Burschtein,[9] this question was subject to further scrutiny. It was demonstrated that in the presence of molecular oxygen at 77°K a broadening of the H.F.S. components of the hydrogen atoms was observed (from 0·10 to 0·15 mWb m^{-2}), and that the saturation effect of the signal on increasing the microwave power almost completely disappeared (Fig. 11.3).

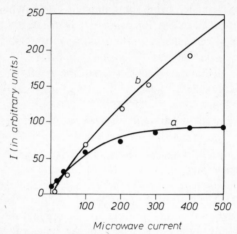

Fig. 11.3. Saturation curves of the signal of hydrogen atoms in (*a*) vacuum, and (*b*) oxygen, at liquid nitrogen temperatures.

Since both effects can only be explained by an interaction between the magnetic moments of the hydrogen atoms and the adsorbed oxygen molecules, this fact alone strengthens the above assumption as to the localization of the atoms near the surface. The authors adapted Bloembergen's theoretical equations, for the magnetic interaction between the electron and the nucleus,[10] to the case of an interaction of two electron spins, in order to calculate the average separation between the adsorbed oxygen molecule and the hydrogen atom. This separation was approximately 1·0 to 1·2 nm. From this they concluded that the hydrogen atoms formed during the primary reaction are localized in small cavities on the surfaces of the solid SiO_2 and are separated from the oxygen molecules adsorbed on the surface by 1·0 to 1·2 nm (Fig. 11.4). Although these atoms are energetically very weakly bound to the base, the probability that they will come out from the cavities to the surface is so remote that the recombination rate at low temperatures in vacuum is extremely small.

The adsorbed oxygen or ethylene molecules, which can react easily with the hydrogen atoms, can thus help the trapped atoms to escape from the cavities within which they are stabilized (see Fig. 11.4). No success was achieved in detecting the radical HO_2 which is formed by this reaction. In ethylene however, as we have already stated, the products of the reaction of the hydrogen atoms with the ethylene gave a detectable E.S.R. spectrum.

A comparison of this spectrum (see Fig. 11.2*b*) with the known spectrum of the ethyl radical (see Fig. 9.2) shows that in the case we are considering the total splitting is smaller, being approximately 10·5 mWb m^{-2} instead of

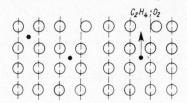

Fig. 11.4. Sketch of the adsorption of hydrogen on the surface of silica gel; the influence of adsorbed gases

12·2 mWb m^{-2}. On the basis of the considerable width of the edge components and the size of the total splitting, we can say that the spectrum obtained corresponds to the E.S.R. spectra of the radicals R–$\dot{C}H_2$ which would be formed if the primary reaction

$$(\dot{H})_{ads} + C_2H_4 \rightarrow (\dot{C}_2H_5)_{ads}$$

were followed by a polymerization:

$$(\dot{C}_2H_5)_{ads} \xrightarrow{C_2H_4} (\dot{C}_4H_9)_{ads} \xrightarrow{C_2H_4} (\dot{C}_6H_{13})_{ads} \text{ etc.}$$

On the basis of the results obtained, we can prove that in each case the hydrogen atoms are actually capable of reaching the ethylene molecules on the surface of the solid. The radicals R–$\dot{C}H_2$ are also chemically active enough for this. It was demonstrated in the same paper that with the addition of oxygen, the R–$\dot{C}H_2$ goes over into the peroxide radical R–CH_2–O–$\dot{O}$.

The results do not of course prove conclusively that the heterogeneous hydration and oxidation reactions actually take place according to a radical mechanism. However, the possibility in principle of such a mechanism may be considered as proven.

The results obtained also completely validate the generally accepted picture of the heterogeneous recombination of atoms and radicals during chain reactions. Hydrogen atoms in the gaseous phase are adsorbed on the surface, they fall into the cavities described above, and so the constant k_2 (see p. 279) becomes very small. At the same time the bond of the atom with the surface is so weak that it reacts very easily with other atoms in the gas phase. As we have seen, it is precisely these two conditions which were postulated in the earlier studies of the chain theory.

It now becomes clear why the numerous attempts to obtain a large concentration of atoms on the surfaces of solids by freezing out from the gaseous phase have not been successful. When highly porous adsorbants, for which the atomic heat of adsorption is low (as in the case of silica gel), are used for this purpose the recombination process is always localized in the vicinity of the mouths of the pores, and the atoms cannot reach the main part of the surface. This problem may be by-passed by slowing down the process (3) by using materials which interact more strongly with the atoms as acceptors to olefins, aromatic compounds, etc. It has proved to be extremely difficult however to produce materials with large surface areas. This has been successful in the case of specially-produced polystyrols.[11] The research workers here did not, of course, observe any adsorbed atoms, but a radical produced by the action of the hydrogen atoms with the polystyrol.

The concept of the localization of free atoms in cracks on solid surfaces can also prove useful in another field. From the results obtain by Pariski and Kasanski it follows that by application of this effect radicals of any structure can be obtained in the adsorbing layer.

It should be noted that these authors[12] obtained adsorbed ethyl radicals by γ-irradiation of a monomolecular layer (or less) of adsorbed ethane† at $77°$K. The spectrum of $(C_2H_5)_{ads}$ is identical, with regard to number of components and total splitting, to the E.S.R. spectra of the ethyl radicals in liquid ethane and in a fixed matrix (see Figs. 11.5 and 9.2).‡ This agreement in the values of ΔB_{HFS} proves that the unpaired electron in the adsorbed radical is in the same state as in the C_2H_5 radical in liquid ethane, i.e. that the chemical activity and the activation energy of the subsequent reactions are in principle not influenced by the adsorption.

Particularly interesting is the fact that the ethyl radical adsorbed on the silica gel is still completely stable up to temperatures of $-60°$C, and that even at $-10°$C its lifetime is of the order of a few minutes. These experiments have thus revealed, for the first time, the persistence of active radicals of the alkyl type at or near room temperature.

† The work of Kolbanowski *et al.*[13] demonstrated for the first time the possibility of the formation of free radicals by the irradiation of adsorbed hydrocarbons (without giving any explanation of the structure of the radicals so formed).

‡ In determining the number and intensity of the components one should take into account that overlapping occurs in the central part of the spectrum of silica gel (see e.g. Fig. 11.2).

Another effective method for the production of adsorbed radicals of a given structure is the photolysis of frozen adsorbed halides of the general type RX. Under normal conditions (in pure materials or in solid matrices of inert materials) the following process occurs:

$$RX \xrightarrow{h\nu} \dot{R} + \dot{X} \tag{A}$$

as a result of the shielding effect with unusually low yields, since here the overriding majority of the radicals formed by (A) recombine again with the corresponding X atoms. If the same materials are irradiated in an adsorbing monomolecular layer, then the halogen atoms can be effectively stabilized in surface cracks, which considerably reduces the recombination probability and consequently strongly increases the quantum yield. On a sufficiently expanded surface, one can count on obtaining sufficiently high radical concentrations.

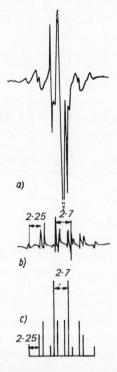

Fig. 11.5
(*a*) Spectrum of the ethyl radical adsorbed on the surface of silica gel;
(*b*) Spectrum of the ethyl radical in liquid ethane;[14]
(*c*) Structure of the spectrum (*b*).

As an example of this we can consider the E.S.R. spectrum obtained by Pariski and Kasanski[15] by the U.V. irradiation (λ = 253·7 nm) at 77°K of CH_3I adsorbed on a monomolecular layer of silica gel (Fig. 11.6).

We see that the spectrum consists of four components with approximately the same splitting as in the case of the $\dot{C}H_3$ radical in irradiated polymethylsiloxane (see Fig. 6.3). The difference between these spectra is that the components of the E.S.R. spectrum of $(\dot{C}H_3)_{ads}$ have differing widths. This stems from the fact that because of the impossibility, in this case, of a rotation about arbitrary axes, considerable differences can be observed in the anisotropic broadening of the components, which correspond to different values of the total nuclear magnetic moment of the three methyl protons. Thus by a quantitative analysis of the spectra of adsorbed radicals, one may in addition come to certain conclusions about the possible states of motion of these particles.

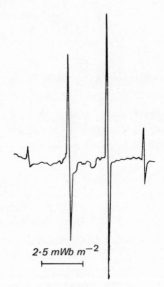

2·5 mWb m^{-2}

Fig. 11.6. Spectrum of the methyl radical adsorbed on the surface of silica gel.

Unfortunately there are very few results on the direct use of E.S.R. for a clarification of the action of ionizing radiation on catalytic activity. It has been shown by Kasanski and Petscherskaya[16] that one of the components of the complex E.S.R. spectrum of γ-Al_2O_3 irradiated at 77°K disappears simultaneously with, and at the same temperature as, the onset of catalytic activity in the irradiated sample for the reaction $H_2 + D_2 \rightleftharpoons 2HD$. The authors believe that the increased activity of the irradiated γ-Al_2O_3 and the unstable E.S.R. signal are caused by the same carrier. Taylor and Kohn[17] also observed an increase in the catalytic activity for the same reaction H_2 + $D_2 \rightleftarrows 2HD$ in the hydration of ethylene by the irradiation of silica gel which was carefully pumped down at 500 to 600°C.

By E.S.R., Kasanski and Pariski[8] observed the formation of a small concentration of surface radicals in samples which had previously been heated at 200 to 300°C for 8 hours, and then irradiated at room temperature. The radicals formed by the irradiation were transformed into peroxide radicals by the action of oxygen, the final concentration being several times larger than the initial concentration of the primary radicals. This evidently suggests that, by irradiation in vacuum, several different types of radicals are formed, and some have such wide lines that they cannot be identified before the reaction with molecular oxygen.

Even though very few data are available as yet, on the basis of what is known, we can say that the change in catalytic activity produced by irradiation is not connected with the formation of hydrogen atoms, since in no case has a correlation been observed between the activity and the hydrogen atom concentration.

In concluding this short section, the work of Mistschenko, Boreskow *et al.*[18] should be mentioned. They observed a change in the catalytic activity of γ-irradiated titanium dioxide, and recorded the E.S.R. spectrum in parallel. The isotopic exchange reaction of the hydrogen after irradiation was speeded up by three or four orders of magnitude (the irradiation dose was about 17 Mrd carried out at 77°K). On heating to room temperature the rate constant rapidly fell, and at 0°C, within one hour had decreased to about one-hundredth part of its original value. The E.S.R. signal produced by irradiation remained unchanged at 77°K, but at 0°C its intensity decreased over a period of one hour. Thereafter there were no further noticeable changes in the intensity or signal shape. Thus in TiO_2, as also in Al_2O_3 and SiO_2, a certain correlation is to be observed between the changes in the E.S.R. spectra and the catalytic activity induced by ionizing radiation. However, the question of how the E.S.R. spectra produced by the paramagnetic centres are related to the increase in catalytic activity, remains to this day unanswered.

§11.2

THE STUDY OF CATALYTIC AGENTS WHICH CONTAIN PARAMAGNETIC IONS

The large range of catalytic agents based on metals with variable valency, Fe, Cr, Mn, Mo, Co, Ni, V, etc., has attracted the attention of research workers for many years. The high activity and selective action of these catalysts has often been related to the rather special features of the *d*-electrons of the corresponding ions. A direct study of these materials is, of course, best carried out by examining the magnetic properties of the corresponding systems. However, despite the large number of such studies, most of which were carried out in the U.S.A. by Salwood,[19] success was not achieved until now in detecting any direct correlation between the magnetic properties and the catalytic properties. These failures may perhaps be attributed to the fact that the magnetic susceptibility is too small a characteristic function of the electronic structure of the paramagnetic ion. The shortcomings of this method become abundantly clear in the investigation of complex molecules and materials with multi-electron bond systems.

The development of the techniques and theory of E.S.R. opened up new approaches with very good prospects for solving this problem. It is clear from earlier chapters that the application of E.S.R. enables us to study processes which often otherwise could not have been studied, and from these processes we may deduce details of the electron structure of paramagnetic ions. Now these ions are components of various different bonds, particularly those of catalysts. This opens up many new possibilities for laying the groundwork of a relationship between the electronic structure of the individual ions and the catalytic activity.

In addition to this, E.S.R. allows us to investigate complex systems in which there exist many different types of paramagnetic centres, and to single out just some of these centres even in cases where the relative concentration is very small. Clearly these types of measurement are not possible with the usual magnetic methods.

Despite these glowing prospects for success in the application of E.S.R. to problems of heterogeneous catalysis, investigations in this direction were only carried out relatively recently, simultaneously in the U.S.S.R., U.S.A., Holland and Germany. Since this work is relatively new, and no theories have yet been put forward in this field, we will limit ourselves to a short summary of published work.†

The E.S.R. spectra investigated in most detail were those of various chromium catalysts. These catalysts are widely used in the hydration of unsaturated compounds, in the aromatization of paraffins and in the polymerization of olefins. The main component of all these catalysts is chromium oxide. The oxide contains Cr^{3+} ions with three unpaired *d*-electrons, which give a very large spin-lattice relaxation time easily observed

---

† The review article by O'Reilly[20] published in 1960 only deals with the theory of nuclear and electron resonance, and does not cover any experimental work in this field.

by E.S.R. at reasonably high temperatures. Crystalline α-Cr_2O_3 is antiferromagnetic with a Neel temperature of approximately 40°C,[21] and a resonance will only be observed above this temperature. If the chromium oxide is placed in a diamagnetic base (e.g. aluminium oxide, silica gel, etc.) then the exchange interaction in the Cr_2O_3 microcrystals decreases and the Neel temperature drops considerably. In aluminium-chromium catalysts with small chromium oxide content, a resonance is even observed at liquid nitrogen temperatures.

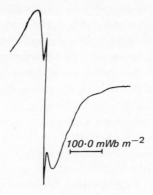

$100 \cdot 0 \ mWb \ m^{-2}$

Fig. 11.7. Spectrum of an aluminium-chromium catalyst with a chromium content 9·2 per cent.

Kasanski and Petscherskaya[22] investigated the E.S.R. spectra of aluminium-chromium catalysts with varying chromium oxide content, and demonstrated that certain conclusions may be drawn as to the structure of these catalysts from the resonance spectra. In samples with a chromium content of about 10 per cent, lines were observed which were characteristic of crystalline chromium oxide, whereas with a chromium content of under 5 per cent the signal was noticeably broadened and became asymmetrical. The authors explained this by noting that the small chromium oxide crystallites are flat scales a few atomic layers thick, growing from the substratum. Such a microcrystallite form leads to an anisotropy of the g-factor, and with it a broadening and asymmetry of the observed signal.

O'Reilly and McIver[23] observed in reduced aluminium-chromium catalysts, in addition to the Cr_2O_3 lines, a signal from the amorphous chromium ions bound to the base. In the same work, oxidized aluminium-chromium catalysts were also studied, and these showed two lines, a wide one ($\approx$ 50–60 mWb m^{-2}) from the Cr_2O_3 microcrystals, and a narrower one, 4·0 mWb m^{-2} wide (Fig. 11.7) which O'Reilly and McIver attributed to

Cr^{5+} ions. These conclusions were drawn from the absence of a fine structure, which would have to be observed if this line had originated from the Cr^{3+} ions.

Kasanski and Petscherskaya claimed that this conclusion was not strictly valid, since a single narrow line can also be observed in Cr^{3+} ions if there is a strong exchange interaction. In order to determine accurately the valency of the chromium ions giving this narrow line, these authors carried out an E.S.R. study of oxidized aluminium-chromium catalysts at two frequencies, 9 and 1·3 GHz. If the narrow line had been caused by Cr^{3+} ions and the fine structure of the spectrum smeared out by exchange interaction, then at a lower frequency, a signal broadening and a change in the g-factor would be expected. Both values, however, remained unchanged, thus giving independent proof that the narrow E.S.R. line was caused by the Cr^{5+} ions. The same conclusion was arrived at by measurements of the magnetic susceptibilities.

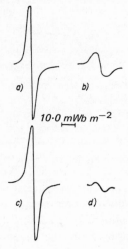

Fig. 11.8. The influence of oxygen on the narrow signal of an aluminium-oxygen catalyst.

Kasanski and Petscherskaya demonstrated that in addition to this, the Cr^{5+} ions are on the surface of the carrier and do not form a solid solution with the bulk of the aluminium oxide. The basis of this result was that the adsorption of paramagnetic oxygen molecules on the surface of a catalyst at room temperature causes a broadening of the signal (Fig. 11.8*a*, *b*). This effect apparently follows from a dipole-dipole broadening of the signal as a result of the magnetic fields formed by the adsorption of paramagnetic oxygen molecules. Since the dipole-dipole interaction decreases very rapidly with the distance between the paramagnetic particles, for this effect to appear the ions must be on the surface of the base material. Kasanski and Petscherskaya also succeeded in observing a change in the spectrum of the Cr^{5+} ions at liquid nitrogen temperatures, as a result of oxygen adsorption (Fig. 11.8c, d). In this case the area under the curve becomes smaller, without the line width changing. The process which occurs can be represented in the following way:

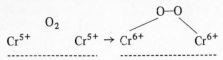

Since at liquid nitrogen temperatures the oxygen molecules cannot penetrate deeply into the lattice base, this result is further evidence that the Cr^{5+} ions lie on the surface.

Cr^{5+} ions have also been observed by E.S.R. in partially saturated chromium oxide in other carriers (alumino-silicates,[25] silica gel[26]). These systems are used as catalysts in ethylene polymerization, and their study is thus of considerable interest.

We have already stated that E.S.R. is well suited to the study of exchange interaction in magnetically dense systems with a strong exchange between the paramagnetic particles. An example of this is given by the work of Petscherskaya and Kasanski,[27] in which the process of thermal activation of Cr_2O_3 gel was investigated, and at the same time the activity of the catalysts for the hydration of ethylene was measured. The results obtained are shown in Fig. 11.9. Chromium oxide gel, precipitated with ammonia from an aqueous nitrate solution and dried at 100°C, contains a considerable quantity of structural water and is completely inactive in the ethylene hydration. If it is heated in a hydrogen atmosphere, then as the temperature increases the water goes out from the lattice; this decreases the separation between the Cr^{3+} ions, and the E.S.R. spectrum widens as a result of the increased dipole-dipole interaction. From about 350°C, the exchange interaction begins to increase considerably, leading initially to a strong narrowing of the E.S.R. signals and then to the appearance of antiferromagnetism. (In samples heated to above + 400°C an E.S.R. signal is observed only above 50°C, i.e. above the Neel temperature; the line width in these samples is equal to that of α-chromium oxide.) It is interesting to note that in the same temperature interval, the catalytic activity

of the chromium oxide gel increases strongly. It could be that antiferromagnetism and high catalytic activity are a common result of the strong
exchange interaction between the Cr^{3+} ions in dehydrated samples, so that
the exchange interaction is also a factor which influences the catalytic
activity.

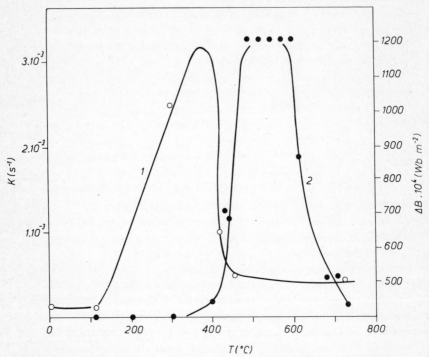

Fig. 11.9. 1. Dependence of the width of the E.S.R. signal of chromium oxide gel
against the temperature at which it had previously been tempered in a hydrogen atmosphere. 2. Dependence of the rate constant for the hydration of ethylene at room
temperature, calculated from a first-order equation, against the temperature at which
the catalyst had previously been tempered in a hydrogen atmosphere.

As another example of the parallel study of catalytic activity and
E.S.R. spectra, we will consider the work of Kasanski *et al.*[28] on mixed
vanadium-molybdenum oxide catalysts. Vanadium pentoxide catalysts are
frequently used in the industrial oxidation of hydrocarbons.[29] Oxides and
salts of other metals are often added to the vanadium pentoxide in order
to increase the activity and selectivity of the reaction. Improved results are
obtained in this way if molybdenum trioxide is added to the vanadium

pentoxide in the oxidation of benzene to malonic acid anhydride. The studies showed that in the mixed vanadium-molybdenum catalyst an E.S.R. spectrum was observed, although pure vanadium pentoxide and molybdenum trioxide are diamagnetic and do not give an E.S.R. signal. In samples with a small molybdenum trioxide content, an H.F.S. was resolved

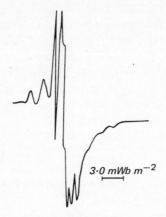

Fig. 11.10. Spectrum of vanadium pentoxide with 0·5 per cent molybdenum trioxide added.

(Fig. 11.10), from which it could be deduced that the E.S.R. signal is related in some way to the appearance of V^{4+} ions in the vanadium pentoxide lattice. By comparison of the E.S.R. data with the results of an X-ray structure analysis, the following model of the catalyst was constructed:

$$V^{5+} \quad V^{5+} \quad V^{5+} \quad V^{5+} \quad V^{5+}$$
$$V^{5+} \quad V^{5+} \quad V^{4+} \quad Mo^{6+} \, V^{5+}$$
$$V^{5+} \quad V^{5+} \quad V^{5+} \quad V^{5+} \quad V^{5+}.$$

The molybdenium ions form a solid solution in the V_2O_5 lattice, where they replace the V^{5+} ions. For the maintenance of electrical neutrality a partial reduction of the V^{5+} ions into V^{4+} ions occurs, and this is the origin of the E.S.R. signal.

From the standpoint of the semiconductor theory of catalysis, the V^{4+} ions in the V_2O_5 lattice create disturbed levels, which influence the electrical and catalytic features of the vanadium pentoxide. In this particular study, a correlation was actually obtained between the intensity of the E.S.R. signal and the catalytic activity of the samples. So we see how useful E.S.R. can be in the study of disturbed levels in oxidic semiconducting catalysts.

The same problem was studied by Nicolau and Thom,[30] who observed weak E.S.R. signals in various oxidic catalysts and attributed them to admixtures. The nature of the admixtures was not however determined, so the results must be considered as very preliminary. In our view, more interesting results come from another investigation of the same authors, in which they observed a resonance of metallic platinum and palladium distributed on carbon.[31] Nicolau and Thom assumed that the platinum atoms were stabilized between the aromatic rings of the graphite lattice rather like a sandwich bond. This model is in agreement with other works in which the structure of carbon has been investigated by E.S.R.

In closing, we would like to mention the work of Hollis and Selwood,[32] who observed a change in the ferromagnetic resonance of nickel when hydrogen was adsorbed on the surface of an aluminium nickel catalyst. This work opens up a new application for E.S.R.–the study of the mechanism of adsorption on ferromagnetic catalysts.

From this short section it is clear that the application of E.S.R. to the problems of heterogeneous catalysis is only in the early stages of its development. Most of the studies are devoted to the structure of the catalysts. From the viewpoint of the general mechanism of catalysis, by far the more interesting works are those on the study of chemisorption on active paramagnetic centres, and the nature of the chemical bonds formed, and the active intermediate products in the course of catalytic processes. Also of great interest is the relationship between the catalytic activity and exchange effects, which can be studied in detail by E.S.R. The relationship was, until now, observed most clearly in the case of chromium oxide gel. If these observations are confirmed in other systems, and if it is shown that such a relationship is really significant in a large number of known catalytic processes, then, considering the distant-action effects in a multi-electron catalytic reagent system, complete new approaches for the clarification of the catalysis are opened up. These ideas can hardly be developed any further without new experimental data. One may be sure, however, that systematic E.S.R. studies of how the production and activation processes, the adsorption of different gases, and finally the catalytic process itself, influence the characteristics of the electron shell of the atoms of the catalysts, will contribute to the solution of a multitude of problems in this interesting field of modern chemistry.

§11.3

THE STUDY OF THE PROCESSES OF ENZYME CATALYSIS

For many years the mechanism of enzyme catalysis was considered to be one of the most puzzling problems in modern science. The actual reasons for the unusually high acceleration of chemical processes under the influence of specific protein catalysts were not understood, nor were many of the properties of these processes, particularly the high degree of activity in using up energy from exothermic reactions in order to sustain endothermic reactions.

Biochemists paid particular attention to the study of biological oxidation, the most important chemical process in the cell, which supplies the energy for the maintenance of life. Already by the 1930s it was clear that free radicals must be formed as intermediate products in the energy consumption process of the cell, both from the materials oxidized and also from a few active low-molecular compounds of the pigment type which play important roles in biocatalysis. Michaelis[33] put forward the hypothesis of gradual oxidation, according to which the dehydration of materials occurs according to the following mechanism:

$$AH_2 \rightarrow \dot{A}H + \dot{H} \rightarrow A + 2\dot{H}$$

The relatively stable free radicals of the type $\dot{A}H$, which occur as intermediate products during the stages of oxidation, Michaelis called semiquinones. He carried out extensive spectrophotometric and potentiometric studies, which can be considered as providing indirect proof of his hypothesis. The appearance of free radicals during the dehydration of some pigments was proved by Michaelis[34] by means of direct measurement of the magnetic susceptibility. The direct detection of free radicals in active enzyme systems and in cells and tissues in which bio-oxidation processes occur was made possible, however, only by the development of E.S.R. The appearance of intermediate products with an odd number of electrons during the biological oxidation, was directly predictable from the original ideas of the biochemists on the mechanism of this process. According to the results of numerous investigations in the 1940s, the essential stage of the oxidation of substrates in the cell occurred in the following way. The substrate AH_2, in the specific protein-enzyme dehydrogenases, loses two hydrogen atoms and is transformed into the oxidized form A. As an example, succinic acid $COOH . CH_2 . CH_2 . COOH$ during dehydration transforms into fumaric acid $COOH . CH : CH . COOH$. The freed hydrogen

atoms† are used in the reduction of a series of co-enzyme groups and pass
along a redox-reaction chain, with a gradual lowering of the potential. Thus
the first stage of the oxidation of the substate involves the separation and
transfer of two hydrogen atoms. On the other hand, the final stages of
biological oxidation, in which cytochrome enzymes participate, result in a
one-electron transfer between iron-porphyrin complexes, the active centres
of the cytochrome. From this it follows that in the reaction chain of the
biological oxidation, there must be elements in which free radicals of the
semiquinone type appear. As we shall now see, the application of E.S.R. to
biological catalysis is not limited to a direct experimental proof of
Michaelis' hypothesis, which even without additional proof was never in
doubt. These studies resulted in many new possibilities for the solution of
the problem of the principal mechanism of biocatalytic processes.

Commoner, Townsend and Pake[35] were the first to obtain E.S.R. signals
from animal and plant tissue. This study, as well as the majority of later
works,[36-39] was carried out on lyophilized tissue.‡ It is assumed that if the
preparation of the lyophilized tissue is carried out sufficiently rapidly and
carefully (without melting the sample in the drying process), then there will
be no noticeable change in the radical content. Although this assumption
lacks a sound basis, recent studies by Commoner and co-workers on natural
biological materials containing water, have led to the same dependence of
the concentration of unpaired electrons on the intensity of the enzyme
process, as have the studies on lyophilized materials. The first studies of
Commoner and co-workers, as well as similar studies carried out at ICP,
led to the following conclusions.

1. All biological samples lyophilized in enzyme reactions give an asym-
metric E.S.R. singlet with a half-width of $0 \cdot 6 - 0 \cdot 8$ mWb m^{-2}, the g-factor of
which differs very little from that of the free electron. The radical concentration here is $10^{-6} - 10^{-8}$ mol per gram of dry material. A typical E.S.R.
signal from lyophilized tissue is shown in Fig. 11.11. The intensity of the
signal in different tissues changes in a similar way to the exchange activity
of the material.

2. The signal intensity decreases if the sample is stored in air. Any
previous denaturation of the tissue by heating (before drying) leads to a
strong decrease in the signal intensity, or even to its complete disappearance. In dried preparations a considerable quantity of the radicals respon-

† We reproduce here only the general features of the reaction scheme.
‡ Lyophilization is described as the sublimation in vacuum of ice from frozen tissue.

sible for the E.S.R. signal disappear on heating to 100°C. In some preparations, some of the paramagnetic centres survive even after a longer period of heating at 100°C. This is caused by the presence of condensed aromatic systems, similar to melanin pigment, in such tissue.† It has been shown by fractionation experiments that the part of the signal which disappears on heating is concerned with the protein component of the preparation.

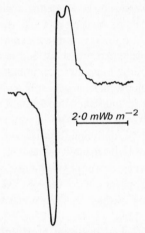

$2 \cdot 0 \ mWb \ m^{-2}$

Fig. 11.11.   E.S.R. signal from lyophilized rat liver (after reference 37).

With the increase in detection sensitivity of E.S.R. spectrometers, it has been possible to examine biological samples which have not previously been dried. Materials which have been investigated are redox-enzyme systems with isolated enzymes and free radicals, which are all formed by the non-enzyme gradual oxidation of biochemical substrates and of co-enzyme groups. In the case of non-enzyme oxidation of biological substrates and of co-enzymes like flavin mononucleotides, an E.S.R. spectrum was formed with $\Delta B_{1/2} \approx 3$ mWb m^{-2} and with a proton H.F.S.[41] In redox-enzyme processes with flavin enzymes, a narrow signal ($\Delta B_{1/2} = 1 \cdot 3$ mWb m^{-2}) without H.F.S. is observed. It has been shown in many kinetic experiments[42-44] that the E.S.R. signal originates from the formation of a complex of the enzyme with the substrate. The shape and width of the E.S.R. signal proves the low-molecular free radicals adsorbed on the enzyme-protein are indeed the source of the unpaired electrons; the unpaired elec-

† More details on the magnetic properties of systems with conjugated bonds are given in Chapter 12.

tron density, however, is distributed over a somewhat larger volume. In fact, the signals observed in the enzyme reaction are characterized not only by the disappearance of the H.F.S. (which could also be explained by a broadening of the individual H.F.S. components through a reduced mobility of the protein molecule), but also by a reduction in the total width, which can only be understood in terms of delocalization or exchange effects (see Chapter 3).

Recently, in a very interesting study of enzyme systems, Beinert and Sands[45] discovered E.S.R. signals with $g \approx 4.3$, which clearly came from iron ions. It was shown that a direct or indirect electron transfer was possible between the paramagnetic centres responsible for this signal and the enzyme-substrate complexes, which gives a normal signal with $g \approx 2.004$.

Extremely interesting results were obtained by Kalmanson, Liptschina and Tschetverikov,[46,47] who investigated the E.S.R. spectra of various semiquinone radicals adsorbed on protein structures in normal and cancerous tissue. They showed that in all cases, after the adsorption on the protein structure, the semiquinone radicals gave identical 'enzyme' signals.

In 1957 the idea was put forward[37] that E.S.R. signals observed in naturally occurring enzyme systems were caused by unpaired electrons which originated from the gradual oxidation of low-molecular substrates. The narrow line width and the absence of an H.F.S. indicated that these unpaired electrons were to a considerable extent delocalized around the protein structure of the enzyme. From this viewpoint, one can consider the protein components of the enzyme system as sorts of 'locally disturbed' semiconductors in which the low molecular substrate plays the role of the local disturbance. In fact, it had already been assumed many years ago that the arrangement of the lattice of hydrogen bridge bonds in natural protein structures can lead to the formation of a conduction band in the energy spectrum of the system. But since this band lies approximately 3 eV above the valence band, in pure protein at normal temperatures it is empty, and so the protein itself does not show any semiconducting properties. The unpaired electron formed in the course of the reaction, by satisfying certain geometric and energetic conditions (in the neighbourhood of the corresponding levels of the substrate and protein), can get into the conduction band of the protein by a complex formation with the substrate and by a gradual oxidation or reduction.† The unpaired electron here is delocalized about the hydrogen bridge system and peptide bonds of the protein molecule, and wanders through the structure until it meets an acceptor,

---

† Note that a similar description was given above in the case of the E.S.R. spectra of irradiated proteins (see §9.4).

which causes a redox-reaction between the two low molecular bonds spatially distant from each other.

It is clear that such a mechanism must lead to a very large activity cross-section for the enzyme reaction, as has long been recognized in bio-chemistry.[44] In addition, it follows that in this mechanism, an excess of unpaired electrons may accumulate within the conduction band of the protein. It was fairly recently discovered[48] that the E.S.R. signal originating from the interaction of adenosintriphosphoric acid (ATP) with the protein actomyosin complex, has a line shape analogous to the signal shape of lyophilized enzyme preparations. The individual components of the system do not by themselves give a signal. One can assume that the mechanism of the signal formation is analogous to that described above.

Naturally the unpaired electrons can in some cases be localized on radical centres or ions with a changeable valency. On the other hand, an electron transfer can result from processes analogous to the formation of charge transfer complexes.[49]

From what we have said, it is clear that the application of E.S.R. to the investigation of enzyme catalysis is only just beginning. At the present time, quantitative kinetic studies are the most needed. Since E.S.R. allows us, in principle, to measure not only the concentration of the unpaired electrons, but also the transfer between their individual active centres, and their delocalization, it can be an extremely helpful tool in finding solutions to such important present-day problems as enzyme catalysis.

References

1. Buben, N. Ja., Schechter, A. B.: *Acta Fhysicochimica URSS,* **10** (1939), 371; Laidler, K., Schuler, K.: *J. Chem. Phys.,* **17** (1949), 1212; Lawrowskaja, G. K., Voevodski, V. V.: *J. phys. Chem., Moscow,* **26** (1952), 1165.
2. Livingston, R., Zeldes, H., Taylor, E. H.: *Disc. Far. Soc.,* **19** (1955), 166.
3. Bubnow, N. N., Voevodski, V. V., Poljak, L. S., Zwetkow, Ju. D.: *Optika i Spektroskopija,* **6** (1959), 565.
4. Beringer, R., Heard, M. A.: *Phys. Rev.,* **95** (1954), 1474.
5. Siegel, S., Flournoy, J. M., Baum, L. H.: *J. Chem. Phys.,* **34** (1961), 1782.
6. Kasanski, W. B., Pariski, G. B., Voevodski, V. V.: *Kinetika i Kataliz,* **1** (1960), 539.
7. Kazansky, V. B.: *II Congrès International de Catalyse.* Paris Technip (1961), 615.
8. Kasanski, V. B., Parijsky, G., Voevodski, V. V.: *Disc. Far. Soc.,* **31** (1961), 203.
9. Kasanski, W. B., Pariski, G. B., Burschtein, A. I.: *Optika i Spektroskopija,* **31** (1962), 45.
10. Bloembergen, N.: *Physica,* **15** (1949), 386.
11. Ingall, R. B., Wall, L. A.: *V. International Symposium on Free Radicals,* Uppsala (1961), 25.
12. Kasanski, W. B., Pariski, G. B.: *Kinetika i Kataliz,* **2** (1961), 507.
13. Kolbanowski, Ju. A., Kustanowitsch, I. M., Polak, L. S., Stscherbakowa, A. S.: *C.C.R. Acad. Sci. U.R.S.S.,* **129** (1959), 145.

14. Fessenden, R., Schuler, R.: *J. Chem. Phys.,* 33 (1960), 935.
15. Kasanski, W. B., Pariski, G. B.: *Kinetika i Kataliz,* 2 (1961), 507.
16. Kasanski, W. B., Petscherskaja, Ju. I.: 34 (1960), 477.
17. Kohn, H. W., Taylor, E. H.: *J. Chem. Phys.,* 63 (1959), 966.
18. Mistschenko, Ju. A., Boreskow, G. K., Kasanski, W. B., Pariski, G. B.: *Kinetika i Kataliz,* 2 (1961), 296.
19. Salwood, P.: *Advances in Catalysis,* 9 (1957), 93.
20. O'Reilly, D.: *Advances in Catalysis,* 12 (1960), 31.
21. Maxwell, R., McGuire, T. R.: *Rev. Mod. Phys.,* 25 (1953), 279.
22. Kasanski, W. B., Petscherskaya, Ju. I., Voevodski, V. V.: *Kinetika i Kataliz,* 1 (1960), 257.
23. O'Reilly, D. E., McIver, D. S.: *Am. Chem. Soc.,* Div. Petrol. Chem., Gen. Papers, 4 (1959) 2; *Advances in Catalysis,* 12 (1960), 100.
24. Kasanski, W. B., Petscherskaya, Ju. I., (Kazanskij, V. B., Pegerskaja, Ju. I.): *Kinetika i Kataliz,* 2 (1961), 454.
25. Cossee, L. L., van Reijen: *II Congrès International de Catalyse.* Paris, Technip (1961), 1679.
26. Petcherskaja, Ju. I., Kazansky, V. B., Voevodsky, V. V.: *II Congrès International de Catalyse.* Paris, Technip (1961), 2121; Petscherskaya, Ju. I., Kasanski, W. B.: *J. phys. Chem., Moscow,* 34 (1960), 2617.
27. Petscherskaya, Ju. I., Kasanski, W. B., Voevodski, V. V.: *Kinetika i Kataliz,* 3 (1962), 111.
28. Kasanski, W. B., Jeshkowa, S. I., Ljubarski, A. G., Voevodski, V. V., Ioffe, I. I.: *Kinetika i Kataliz,* 2 (1961), 862.
29. Ioffe, I. I., Jeshkowa, S. I., Ljubarski, A. G.: *J. phys. Chem., Moscow,* (1961), 2343.
30. Nicolau, C., Thom, H. G.: *II Congrès International de Catalyse.* Paris, Technip (1961), 1326.
31. Nicolau, C., Thom, H. G., Pobitshak, E.: *Trans. Far. Soc.,* 55 (1959), 1430.
32. Hollis, D. P., Selwood, P. W.: *J. Chem. Phys.,* 35 (1961), 378.
33. Michaelis, L.: *J. Biol. Chem.,* 96 (1932), 703.
34. Michaelis, L., *et al.: JACS,* 59 (1937), 2460.
35. Commoner, B., Townsend, J., Pake, G.: *Nature,* 174 (1954), 689.
36. Commoner, B.: *Progress Report on Physical Mechanisms of Biological Electron Transport.* Washington Univ., St. Jonis (1960).
37. Blumenfeld, L. A.: *Bull. Acad. Sci. U.R.S.S., ser. biol.,* 3 (1957), 285.
38. Blumenfeld, L. A., Kalmanson, A. E.: *Biofizika,* 3 (1958), 1.
39. Morosowa, G. K., Blumenfeld, L. A.: *Biofizika,* 5 (1960), 235.
40. Szent-Gyorgyi, A.: *Nature,* 148 (1941), 157.
41. Commoner, B., Lippincott, B. B.: *Proc. Nat. Acad. Sci. USA,* 46 (1960), 405.
42. Hollocher, G., Commoner, B.: *Proc. Nat. Acad. Sci. USA,* 46 (1960), 416.
43. Commoner, B., Lippincott, B. B.: *ibid.,* 44 (1958), 1110.
44. Commoner, B., Lippincott, B. B., Passonnenau, J. K.: *ibid.,* 44 (1958), 1099.
45. Beinert, H., Sands, R. H.: *Free Radicals in Biological Systems.* Academic Press, New York (1961), 17.
46. Kalmanson, A. E., Liptschina, L. P., Tschetwerikow, A. G.: *Biofizika,* 6 (1961), 410.
47. Kalmanson, A. E., Liptschina, L. P., Tschetwerikow, A. G.: *C.C.R. Acad. Sci. U.R.S.S.,* 141 (1961), 230.
48. Kajuschin, L. P., Kofman, Je. B., Golubev, I. N., Lvov, N. M., Pularowa, M. K.: *Biofizika,* 6 (1961), 20.
49. Szent-Gyorgyi, A.: *Introduction to Submolecular Biology.* Academic Press, New York 1960.

Chapter 12

The Application of E.S.R. to the Investigation of Organic Structures

As one can see from the title, our twelfth and last chapter is devoted to a consideration of some of the new problems in structural chemistry and chemical kinetics which have only arisen since the wide application of E.S.R. to chemical studies. The major role in this new field is played by the structure of E.S.R. signals in materials which should be diamagnetic according to current concepts in chemistry. In recent years there have been an increasing number of publications on the observation of E.S.R. signals in systems in which there was no apparent reason for the presence of the unpaired electrons causing the paramagnetism. Since in the majority of these studies it was shown that the E.S.R. signals could not be ascribed to any normal paramagnetic or ferromagnetic impurities, and as the systems in which these anomalies were observed contained a large number of similar materials with so-called ordered structures, which are very important in chemistry and biology (pigments, polymers, biopolymers etc.), so the problem resolves into a question of the nature of the paramagnetic carriers.

We would also like to point out that, up to the present time, there are no completely satisfactory theories to explain these effects, and so we have been forced to limit ourselves to clarifying the more likely theories and making a few general comments.

Because of the great confusion caused by contradictory data, it is first of all necessary to classify accurately the observed facts, to determine the common features of the materials investigated, to look for differences resulting from structural peculiarities of the individual systems, and to weed out the cases in which the contradictory results are attributable to insufficient reproducibility or unreliable experimentation.

In presenting this material, we will begin by describing experiments which at first sight do not appear to be at all relevant to the question in

hand. By this, we mean E.S.R. studies of coal and other carbonaceous
products of organic substances. It has already been shown, by Juza and
co-workers,[1] through precise measurements of the magnetic susceptibility
of activated sugar carbons, that the diamagnetism of the materials is so small
that to explain it the existence of some paramagnetic centres had to be
assumed. It is clear, however, that at that time, no definite statements on
the nature of the paramagnetic carriers could be made.

After the discovery of E.S.R. it was found, quite independently of the
earlier experiments of Juza, that very diverse samples of mineral coal give
E.S.R. signals,[2] in some cases (e.g. anthracite) with a signal intensity corresponding to a concentration of over 10^{20} unpaired electrons per gram. The
symmetric narrow E.S.R. line observed ($\Delta B \approx 0.2$–0.4 mWb m^{-2}), with
$g \approx g_{el}$, proved so popular that in some laboratories, besides DPPH, carbon
was used as a calibrating sample for g-factor measurements and for the
determination of the relative concentration of paramagnetic particles. In the
course of these studies, the influence of oxygen on the paramagnetism of
carbon was discovered. The E.S.R. signal is sometimes considerably
broadened in the presence of oxygen, and sometimes it disappears completely.† If one begins to pump down the oxygen immediately after the
adsorption, then in most cases, the intensity and shape of the E.S.R. signal
is completely restored, even if the oxygen was acting for several minutes at
room temperature. If however one pumps down only after a few days, then
there is no change in the signal; this is a result of the formation of stable
peroxide forms, as is shown by the chemical studies of the surface oxidation
of carbon.[3]

Natural mineral carbons are very complex structures and contain many
different admixtures. The structure and admixture content of coal varies a
great deal from deposit to deposit, from shaft to shaft and even from sample
to sample. Although it is possible to use coal samples pumped down and
sealed in a tube as calibrating samples, the problem of free valencies in
carbons cannot be solved by a study of natural coals.

Recently, several laboratories have devoted effort to the study of the
carbonization products of organic materials, in most cases sugar carbon: the
sugar was carbonized in air, in vacuum or in an inert atmosphere at 400 to
700°C.

The number of papers published on this subject is unusually large.[4] One
can say without exaggeration that almost every laboratory which concerned
itself with E.S.R. in the years 1952 to 1957 chose as one of the first
materials to study one or other of the many coke or coal samples, and the

† In some natural carbons the oxygen does not influence the E.S.R. signal.

research workers generally found something new and sufficiently interesting to publish. We have been mainly concerned with the influence of tempera- ture and duration of the heat treatment on the intensity, shape and width of the E.S.R. signals. This work originated in our assumption that the source of the paramagnetism in carbons is usually free radicals, in localized side chains connected together by the condensed aromatic lattice, or in corners and broken bonds within the lattice itself. The influence of oxygen on the E.S.R. spectra of coke was considered to be the result of the interaction of oxygen with these valencies according to the reaction $\dot{R} + O_2 \rightarrow R\dot{O}_2$; the regeneration of the signal on pumping down was considered to be a result of the attendant dissociation of the bond $R{-}\dot{O}_2$, and the irreversible adsorp- tion a result of the formation of peroxides, in agreement with the above- mentioned chemical data on carbons.

It is generally accepted in most laboratories outside of the Soviet Union, that there exists a large concentration of free radicals in natural and artifi- cial carbons (calculated for the gaseous phase corresponding to a partial pressure of the radicals of approximately 10 atm!).

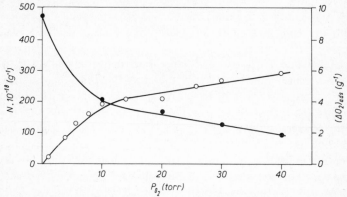

Fig. 12.1. Dependence of the number of paramagnetic centres in coke (●) and the number of adsorbed oxygen molecules (○) on the oxygen pressure

A series of experiments[5] carried out at ICP did show, however, that this assumption is in contradiction with experimental results. In fact, the E.S.R. signals were caused by known free radicals (or even by delocalized electrons), so that the change in the integrated intensity of the E.S.R. signals through the action of adsorbed gases resulted from the maintenance of a certain stoichiometric ratio between the number of radicals reacting and the number of adsorbed molecules. In order to verify this conclusion, comparisons were made between the change in the number of paramagnetic carries ΔN brought about by the action of the oxygen, and the number of adsorbed oxygen molecules $(\Delta O_2)_{ads}$. These experiments were repeated several times, and led beyond any doubt to the conclusion that at the adsorption of one oxygen molecule, the intensity of the E.S.R. signal decreases by a value which corresponds to some ten paramagnetic centres. As examples of this, Fig. 12.1 and Table 12.1 gives values for the adsorption of oxygen on sugar carbon (obtained by burning sugar in air at 600°C).†

As can be seen from these data, the ratio $N/(O_2)_{ads} \approx 70$ remains constant at this temperature until the build-up of a complete monomolecular layer.

It should be stressed here that, as we have already shown,[5] the E.S.R. line width undergoes large changes only until the monolayer is complete (Fig. 12.2). The linear increase in ΔB at higher oxygen pressures is caused by the broadening due to the impacts of the paramagnetic oxygen molecules in the gaseous phase.

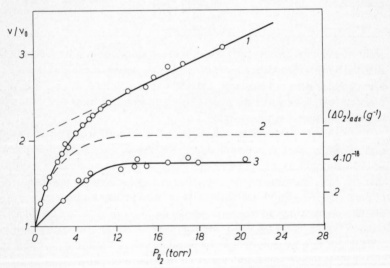

Fig. 12.2. Dependence of the relative width of the E.S.R. line of coke on oxygen pressure (1). Curve (2) was obtained by calculation of the line broadening due to impacts of the oxygen atoms in the gaseous phase. Curve (3) shows the quantity of adsorbed oxygen.

† The values of ΔN were obtained with the help of the method of calculation given in Chapter 9, from the values $(I_0')G$, ΔB_{max}^G, $(I_0')L$, B_{max}^L, obtained by linear anamorphosis. It should be noted that the magnitude of the effect considerably exceeds the possible errors due to inaccuracies in the determination of ΔN or $(\Delta O_2)_{ads}$.

The investigation of the dependence of ΔB_G, ΔB_L and ΔB_e on the amount of oxygen adsorbed showed that the line broadening due to oxygen adsorption is not caused by a decrease in the exchange, as was thought previously, but by a simultaneous increase of ΔB_G and ΔB_e. The effective width is well described by the equation (4.43):

$$\Delta B_L = \frac{\Delta B_G^2}{\Delta B_e}$$

In the experiments shown in Table 12.1, the exchange frequency obtained from the E.S.R. line width is $\nu_e = 10^7$ and 2.10^7 Hz at $P_{O_2} = 0$ and 40 torr respectively.

Table 12.1

P_{O_2} [torr]	$N[g^{-1}]$	$\Delta N[g^{-1}]$	$(\Delta O_2)_{ads}$ [g^{-1}]	$\Delta N/(\Delta O_2)_{ads}$
0	458.10^{18}	–	–	–
10	200.10^{18}	258.10^{18}	$3.8.10^{18}$	68
20	152.10^{18}	306.10^{18}	$4.1.10^{18}$	74
30	116.10^{18}	342.10^{18}	$5.2.10^{18}$	66
40	76.10^{18}	382.10^{18}	$5.7.10^{18}$	67

In special experiments carried out in many laboratories it has been shown that the temperature-dependence of the E.S.R. signals of carbon (the structure of which does not change at reduced temperatures) obeys a $1/T$ law precisely, which excludes the possibility of interpreting these signals as due to the excitation of a triplet state.

From the parallel investigation of the E.S.R. of carbon and of the adsorption of oxygen, we can conclude that the magnetic centres in carbon cannot be ordinary radicals, since in that case $\Delta N/(\Delta O_2)_{ads}$ would not be greater than two. For the same reason, the effect cannot be ascribed to the action of paramagnetic admixtures, since it is not possible to formulate a mechanism by which an oxygen molecule interacts with 50 to 60 admixed atoms.

If in this way we can exclude the possibility of interpreting the effect by free radicals or even by random isolated paramagnetic particles, we arrive at the conclusion that the paramagnetism of the carbon must be connected in some way with the specific features of this complicated system, which is now seen as consisting of planar aromatic 'nets' or lattices of varying sizes which to a certain extent are assembled in 'packets' and connected by aliphatic chains. From the data given it follows that the exchange frequency of the unpaired electrons between the individual 'nets' or 'packets' (10^{17} Hz) cannot noticeably influence the energy levels of the system.

Despite this, one can see that it is just this weak interaction of the strongly coordinated system which causes the paramagnetism in the ground state of some structures, without which free valencies, in the full meaning of the word, would be formed. The action of the oxygen can then be explained in the following way. The adsorbed O_2 molecule influences the ordered system of conjugated bonds in such a way as to change the character of the electron exchange interaction, and consequently the number of 'effective' spins measured by E.S.R. If one assumes, according to the hypothesis of Frumkin,[6] that the oxygen can penetrate between individual 'nets', then it is reasonable to assume that while it causes $N\Delta B_G$ to decrease (through the build-up of local fields), it increases B_e by making exchanges between neighbouring 'nets' much easier.

The explanation which we have put forward for the E.S.R. effect in carbons cannot be regarded as a theory, but only as an attempt to understand the experimental results given above. It might appear, however, that these concepts may have a more general importance in connection with the increased interest in the 'narrow' E.S.R. signals observed within the last few years in very varying saturated molecular structures. If it transpires that the nature of both effects is the same, then the explanations of the effects must be the same.

In the year 1959, Berlin *et al.*,[7] discovered that 'narrow' E.S.R. signals were observed from polymers with conjugated double bonds like the polyphenylacetylenes:

$$\sim CH=C-CH=C-CH=C\sim$$
$$\quad\;\; | \qquad\quad | \qquad\quad |$$
$$\quad C_6H_5 \quad\; C_6H_5 \quad\; C_6H_5$$

Following this discovery, analogous effects were observed in a large number of other polymers with extended nets of conjugated bonds, in pure carbon chains as well as in chains of hetero-atoms (polyphenylene, polyaminoquinone, polytertiaryethylene, etc.)[8-11] In these cases the E.S.R. signals originated in (one-dimensional) chain systems, as well as in polymers, which form a two- or three-dimensional system of conjugated bonds.

The essential characteristics of these E.S.R. signals may be listed as follows:

1. 'Narrow' E.S.R. signals always originate in polymers with conjugated bonds and are never observed in polymers without conjugation chains.

2. The signals are symmetrical singlet lines of Lorentzian shape with $g = 2 \cdot 003 - 2 \cdot 006$ and $\Delta B \approx 0 \cdot 4 - 0 \cdot 8$ mWb m^{-2}.

3. The signal intensity increases with increasing molecular weight (or more correctly, with an increase in the expansion of the system of conjugated bonds) and can reach a figure of $10^{15}-5 \cdot 10^{19}$ spins per gram. For soluble polymers this corresponds on the average to a concentration of from one spin per 10^4 molecules to one spin per 10 molecules of the polymer. (polymers with an unusually high spin concentration are generally not soluble). The signal intensity for a polymer with a given degree of conjugation does not depend on the preparation procedure.

4. The temperature dependence of the E.S.R. signals, within the limits of experimental accuracy, corresponds to the Curie law. This means that the number of 'paramagnetic particles' is temperature-dependent.

5. The 'narrow' E.S.R. lines remain after the polymers are dissolved, and their intensity is independent of the dilution (see Fig. 12.3).

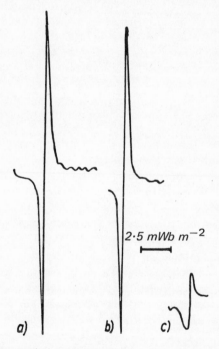

Fig. 12.3. E.S.R. spectrum of polyphenylacetylene

   (*a*) In the solid state;
   (*b*) preparation (*a*) dissolved in benzene;
   (*c*) preparation (*b*) diluted five-fold, with the same volume as for preparation (*b*).

6. In some cases polymers with conjugated bonds which contain built-in free radicals have been obtained. In these cases, in addition to the usual 'narrow' E.S.R. line, broader signals are also formed. On further polymerization or dilution, the additional signals disappear, but the 'narrow' signals remain.

The sum total of the experimental facts given above led the research workers to the conclusion that the observed 'narrow' E.S.R. signals in the cases considered do not come from the usual free radicals which originate during the polymerization process, but are caused by peculiarities of the intra- and inter-molecular interactions in polymers with conjugated bonds. In fact, it is a question, for example, of the normal molecular radicals $\dot{R}$ formed during polymerization, so a continuation of the polymerization could not lead to an increase in the concentration of unpaired electrons per polymer weight. We might try to explain the effect in terms of biradicals formed in the system when there is a strong decrease in the activation energy of a triplet-state, but this also contradicts the experimental results. The temperature-independence of the measured number of unpaired electrons proves that the magnetic state is either a ground state, or lies in the immediate vicinity of the ground state ($\Delta E \ll kT$). For this supposition the number of unpaired electrons would have to be comparable with the number of molecules, whereas in the experiment it is found to be much smaller.

One might imagine that in polydispersed polymer preparations there is an anomalous distribution of molecular weights which will always lead to the presence of a high molecular fraction in the sample, for which the excitation energy in the triplet state (ΔE) lies close to zero, and a low molecular fraction, with $\Delta E \gg kT$. Thus the molecular fraction from the central region is completely missing, and this is the fraction which would give the temperature-dependence of the number of magnetic centres. This idea, very improbable in itself, is contradicted by the appearance of anomalous effects in a series of organic low-molecular monodispersed systems. Exactly the same E.S.R. signals are obtained from many pigments, which exhibit an elongated system of conjugated bonds,[12,13] from non-metallic phthalocyanine and its complexes with diamagnetic metals,[14,15] and from many other compounds. Here, as in the case of polymers with conjugated double bonds, narrow symmetric singlet signals ($\Delta B \approx 1$ mWb m^{-2}) are observed, the g-factor of which is very close to the free spin value, and with an intensity which corresponds to a concentration of one unpaired spin per 100 to 5000 molecules. The signal completely disappears in solution, but reappears at the formation of the solid phase. This proves that the formation of the signal depends, not only on the characteristics of the single molecule, but also on its position in the lattice. As measurements over a wide temperature range have shown, the small concentrations of unpaired electrons observed experimentally are temperature-independent. This is evidence that the ground state of the paramagnetic region is magnetic. The signals are preserved during recrystallization and distillation under high vacuum.[15] It should be mentioned, however, that signals have not been obtained from single crystals of phthalocyanine.[14] Through the recrystallization or distillation whereby polycrystalline preparations are formed, the E.S.R. spectrum reappears.†

A study of the compounds exhibiting the above effects shows that they are all characterized by a reduced ionization potential I and an increased electron-affinity A. This led Benderski and Blumenfeld[16] to the idea that in all these cases, the appearance of unpaired electrons is connected with the formation of charge transfer complexes (see also Chapter 8). Mulliken[17,18] carried out a theoretical study of the charge transfer process, and showed that complex formation is accompanied by an electron transition from the highest filled molecular orbit of the donor to the lowest empty orbit of the acceptor. Since both the donor and acceptor are saturated molecules with an even number of electrons, formation of the charge transfer complex coincides with the formation of two unpaired electrons. In fact, Bijl *et al.*,[19] in a study of charge transfer complexes formed from aromatic amines (donor) and aromatic quinones (acceptor), have shown that these complexes give narrow E.S.R. signals of the type considered above. The signal intensity for different donor-acceptor pairs increases with a decrease in the value of $I - A$, where I is the ionization potential of the donor and A the electron affinity of the acceptor. In the cases studied,[19] the measured concentration of the unpaired electrons was between 0·4 and 80 per cent of the number of pairs. This figure was independent of temperature in all cases. In reference 16 the assumption was made that in all the cases considered above, the paramagnetism is caused by regions in the solid phase in which the state of the charge transfer complex is made energetically more favourable by changes in the lattice (such regions can grow dislocations, for example). Any destruction of the conjugation in whatever form, leads to an increase in the value of $I - A$, and thus to a large reduction in the number of charge transfers complexes in the ground state of the system.

† It has since been shown that only one of the two possible crystalline forms of the phthalocyanine (α-form) is paramagnetic.[33] In addition to the paramagnetism, the α-form is characterized by an electrical conductivity which is six orders of magnitude greater than the diamagnetic β-form.

A water-tight theory of these effects is still missing. Without doubt, one cannot consider the explanation suggested in reference 16 the only one possible. There are reasons to assume that the anomalous magnetic characteristics of organic systems with an extended net of conjugated bonds, which show themselves in the E.S.R. spectra, are connected in some way with the increase in electrical conductivity of these systems. Further experimental and theoretical studies of these extremely interesting effects are needed.

Recently, results have appeared which show evidence of the existence of large magnetic effects like ferromagnetism and antiferromagnetism in highly ordered organic structures, and which are caused by collective spin interactions. In magnetic resonance spectra this leads to the appearance of extremely wide lines ($10-100$ mWb m^2) with a very large integrated intensity. These effects were first observed on biopolymers—nucleic acids and nucleotides[20,21]—and later in synthetic polymers with conjugated bonds.[22,23] The appearance of 'wide' lines is accompanied by the appearance of a positive magnetic susceptibility, which is saturated in relatively weak magnetic fields. There are cases in which the resonance line is so strongly broadened that it can no longer be observed. The anomalous magnetic properties can only be judged on the basis of static magnetic measurements.[33] The information collected[24,25] has led to the conclusion that the effect is connected somehow with structural irregularities in the materials studied. Changes in the magnetic properties of biological structures have been observed and identified in some important biological processes.[26] The results obtained were later confirmed by other laboratories (see e.g. references 27, 28).

Considering all the available data, it is very difficult to decide between the two possible explanations of these effects:

(*a*) a purely structural explanation, in which the appearance of unpaired spins and their collective interaction is a property of the organic structure,

(*b*) by the presence of microscopic ferromagnetic enclosures, stablized by the structure.[29,30]†

The problem requires further careful study.

Research has been carried out to give a theoretical interpretation of the observed effects on the basis of the first of the two explanations.[31,32] One of these research programmes involved the charge transfer complexes men-

---

† Later studies[34] have shown that evidently this is the case for the formation of mixed metallo-organic ferrites, the formation and properties of which are determined by the organic structure.

tioned above.[31] One assumes here that the transition into the complex state does not result in isolated pairs in such systems, but occurs throughout the whole region of the polymer structure.

In this chapter we have shown many examples of how the application of E.S.R. has allowed us to discover unknown properties of organic compounds. We are still far from a complete understanding of these effects. However, there is no doubt that further studies will eventually clarify the physical mechanism and the meaning of the rather surprising properties discovered in highly ordered organic structures. Magnetic radiospectroscopy will without doubt play an important role in the solution of these problems.

References

1. Juza, R., Lübbe, H., Heilbein, L.: *Naturwiss.*, **25** (1937), 522; *Zs. Angew. Chemie*, **51** (1938), 354.
2. Uebersfeld, J., Etienne, A., Combrisson, J.: *Nature*, **174** (1954), 614; Garifjanow, N. S., Kosyrew, B. M.: *J. exp. theor. Phys.*, **30** (1956), 272; de Ruiter, E., Ischamberg, H.: *Brennstoff-Chemie*, **40** (1959), 2, 41.
3. Dubinin, M. M.: *Uspechi Chimii*, **24** (1955), 513.
4. Ingram, D. J. E., Tarrley, J. G., Jackson, R., Bond, D. L.: *Nature*, **174** (1954), 797; Austin, D. E., Tarrley, J. G.: *Trans. Far. Soc.*, **54** (1958), 400; Castle, J. S.: *Phys. Rev.*, **95** (1954), 846; Pastor, R. C., Were, J. A., Brown, T. H., Turkevitch: *J. Phys. Rev.*, **102** (1956), 918; Uebersfeld, J., Erb, E.: *J. Phys. et Radium*, **16** (1955), 340; Wobshall, D., Akamatu, U., Mrosowski, S.: *Bull. Am. Phys. Soc.*, **3** (1958), N 2; 4 (1959), 3.
5. Tichomirowa, N. N., Markin, M. I., Nikolajewa, I. W., Voevodski, V. V.: *Problemy Kinetika i Kataliza*. T. 10, Izd-vo AN SSSR (1960), 426; Tichomirowa, N. N., Nikolaewa, I. W., Voevodski, V. V.: *Ž. strukt. Chimii*, **1** (1960), 99.
6. Levina, S., Frumkin, A., Lunew, A.: *Acta Physicochim.*, **3** (1935), 397.
7. Berlin, A. A., Blumenfeld, L. A., Tscherkaschin, M. I., Kalmanson, A. E., Selskaja, O. G.: *Vysokomolekuljarnye soedinenija*, **1** (1959), 1361.
8. Toptschijew, A. W., Geiderich, M. A., Dawydow, B. E., Kargin, W. A., Krenzel, B. A., Kustanowitsch, I. M., Poljak, L. S.: *C.C.R. Acad. Sci. U.R.S.S.*, **128** (1959), 312.
9. Blumenfeld, L. A., Berlin, A. A., Matwejewa, N. G., Kalmanson, A. E.: *Vysoko-molekuljarnye soedinenija*, **1** (1959), 1647.
10. Blumenfeld, L. A., Berlin, A. A., Slinkin, A. A., Kalmanson, A. E.: *Ž. strukt. Chimii*, **1** (1960), 103.
11. Liogonki, B. I., Ljubtschenko, L. S., Berlin, A. A., Blumenfeld, L. A., Parin, W. P.: *Vysokomolekuljarnye soedinenija*, **2** (1960), 1494.
12. Moschowski, Ju. Sch.: *C. C. R. Acad. Sci. U.R.S.S.*, **130** (1960), 1277.
13. Tschernjakowski, F. P., Kalmanson, A. E., Blumenfeld, L. A.: *Optika i Spektroskopija*, **9** (1960), 796.
14. Ingram, D. J. E., Bennett, J. E.: *J. Chem. Phys.*, **22** (1954), 1136.
15. Neiman, R., Kivelson, D.: *J. Chem. Phys.*, **95** (1961), 162.
16. Benderski, W. A., Blumenfeld, L. A.: *C.C.R. Acad. Sci. U.R.S.S.*,
17. Mulliken, R. S.: *JACS*, **72** (1960), 600.
18. Mulliken, R. S.: *J. Phys. Chem.*, **56** (1952), 801.

19. Bijl, D., Kainer, H., Rose-Innes, A. C.: *J. Chem. Phys.*, 80 (1959), 756.
20. Blumenfeld, L. A., Kalmanson, A. E., Schen Pei-gen: *C.C.R. Acad. Sci. U.R.S.S.*, 124 (1959), 1147.
21. Blumenfeld, L. A.: *Biofizika*, 4 (1959), 515.
22. Blumenfeld, L. A., Berlin, A. A., Matwejewa, N. G., Kalmanson, A. E.: *Vysokomolekuljarnye soedinenija*, 1 (1959), 1647.
23. Blumenfeld, L. A., Berlin, A. A., Slinkin, A. A., Kalmanson, A. E.: Ž. *strukt. Chimii*, 1 (1960), 103.
24. Woswyschajewa, L. W., Blumenfeld, L. A.: *Biofizika*, 5 (1960), 579.
25. Schen Pei-gen, Blumenfeld, L. A., Kalmanson, A. E.: *Biofizika*, 5 (1960), 645.
26. Samoilowa, O. P., Blumenfeld, L. A.: *Biofizika*, 6 (1961), 15.
27. Müller, L. A., Hotz, G., Zimmer, K. G.: *Biochem. and Biophys. Res. Comm.*, 4 (1961), 214.
28. Blois, M. S., Maling, J. E.: *Biochem. and Biophys. Res. Comm.*, 4 (1961), 252.
29. Lasurkin, Ju. S.: *Lecture on the V International Biochemical Congress*, Moscow, 1961.
30. Shulman, R. G., Walsn, W. M., Williams, H. J., Wright, J. P.: *Biochem. and Biophys. Res. Comm.*, 5 (1961), 52.
31. Blumenfeld, L. A., Benderski, W. A.: *C.C.R. Acad. Sci. U.R.S.S.*, 133 (1960), 1451.
32. Ginsburg, W. L., Dain, W. M.: *C.C.R. Acad. Sci. U.R.S.S.*, 131 (1960), 785.
33. Wihkse, K., Newkirk, A. E.: *J. Chem. Phys.*, 34 (1961), 2184.
34. Blumenfeld, L. A.: *C.C.R. Acad. Sci. U.R.S.S.*,

Appendix 1

TABLES OF THE CHARACTERS OF THE IRREDUCIBLE REPRESENTATIONS OF SOME SYMMETRY GROUPS

Note: R is the element of the group, Γ the representation.

1. C_1

Γ \ R	E
A	1

2. C_2

	E	C_2
A	1	1
B	1	-1

3. C_3

	E	C_3	C_3^2
A	1	1	1
E $\big\{$	1	α	α^2
	1	α^2	α

$\alpha = e^{2\pi i/3}$

4. C_4

	E	C_2	C_4	C_4^3
A	1	1	1	1
B	1	1	-1	-1
E $\big\{$	1	-1	i	$-i$
	1	-1	$-i$	i

5. C_5

	E	C_5	C_5^2	C_5^3	C_5^4
A	1	1	1	1	1
E' $\big\{$	1	α_4	α^2	α^3	α^4
	1	α_4	α^3	α^2	α
E'' $\big\{$	1	α^2	α^4	α	α^3
	1	α^3	α	α^4	α^2

$\alpha = e^{2\pi i/5}$

6. C_6

	E	C_6	C_3	C_2	C_3^2	C_6^5
A	1	1	1	1	1	1
B	1	-1	1	-1	1	-1
E' $\big\{$	1	α	α^2	α^3	α^4	α^5
	1	α^5	α^4	α^3	α^2	α
E'' $\big\{$	1	α^2	α^4	1	α^2	α^4
	1	α^4	α^2	1	α^4	α^2

$\alpha = e^{\pi i/3}$

7. C_{2v}

	E	C_2	σ_v	σ_v'
A_1	1	1	1	1
A_2	1	1	-1	-1
B_1	1	-1	-1	1
B_2	1	-1	1	-1

8. C_{3v}

	E	$2C_3$	$3\sigma_v$
A_1	1	1	1
A_2	1	1	-1
E	2	-1	0

9. C_{4v}

	E	C_2	$2C_4$	$3\sigma_v$	$2\sigma_d$
A_1	1	1	1	1	1
A_2	1	1	1	-1	-1
B_1	1	1	-1	1	-1
B_2	1	1	-1	-1	1
E	2	-2	0	0	0

313

10. C_{5v}

	E	$2C_5$	$2C_5^2$	$5\sigma_v$
A_1	1	1	1	1
A_2	1	1	1	-1
E_1	2	$2\cos\beta$	$2\cos 2\beta$	0
E_2	2	$2\cos 2\beta$	$2\cos 4\beta$	0

$$\beta = \frac{2\pi}{5}$$

11. C_{6v}

	E	C_2	$2C_3$	$2C_6$	$3\sigma_d$	$3\sigma_v$
A_1	1	1	1	1	1	1
A_2	1	1	1	1	-1	-1
B_1	1	-1	1	-1	-1	1
B_2	1	-1	1	-1	1	-1
E_1	2	-2	-1	1	0	0
E_2	2	2	-1	-1	0	0

12. C_{1h}

	E	σ_h
A_1	1	1
A_2	1	-1

13. C_{2h}

	E	C_2	σ_h	i
A_g	1	1	1	1
A_u	1	1	-1	-1
B_g	1	-1	-1	1
B_u	1	-1	1	-1

14. $C_{3h} = C_3\sigma_h$

	E	C_3	C_3^2	σ_h	S_3	$(\sigma_h C_3^2)$
A	1	1	1	1	1	1
B	1	1	1	-1	-1	-1
$E_1\{$	1	α	α^2	1	α	α^2
	1	α^2	α	1	α^2	α
$E_2\{$	1	α	α^2	-1	$-\alpha$	$-\alpha^2$
	1	α^2	α	-1	$-\alpha^2$	$-\alpha$

$$\alpha = e^{2\pi i/3}$$

15. $C_{4h} = C_4 . i.$ 16. $C_{5h} = C_5\sigma_h.$ 17. $C_{6h} = C_6 . i.$

18. D_2

	E	C_2^z	C_2^y	C_2^x
A_1	1	1	1	1
B_1	1	1	-1	-1
B_2	1	-1	1	-1
B_3	1	-1	-1	1

19. D_3

	E	$2C_3$	$3C_2$
A_1	1	1	1
A_2	1	1	-1
E	2	-1	0

20. D_4

	E	C_2	$2C_4$	$2C_2'$	$2C_2''$
A_1	1	1	1	1	1
A_2	1	1	1	-1	-1
B_1	1	1	-1	1	-1
B_2	1	1	-1	-1	1
E	2	-2	0	0	0

21. D_5

	E	$2C_5$	$2C_5^2$	$5C_2'$
A_1	1	1	1	1
A_2	1	1	1	-1
E_1	2	$2\cos\beta$	$2\cos 2\beta$	0
E_2	2	$2\cos 2\beta$	$2\cos 4\beta$	0

$$\beta = \frac{2\pi}{5}$$

22. D_6

	E	C_2	$2C_3$	$2C_6$	$3C_2'$	$3C_2''$
A_1	1	1	1	1	1	1
A_2	1	1	1	1	-1	-1
B_1	1	-1	1	-1	1	-1
B_2	1	-1	1	-1	-1	1
E_1	2	-2	-1	1	0	0
E_2	2	2	-1	-1	0	0

23. D_{2d}

	E	C_2	$2S_4$	$2C_2'$	$2\sigma_d$
A_1	1	1	1	1	1
A_2	1	1	1	-1	-1
B_1	1	1	-1	1	-1
B_2	1	1	-1	-1	1
E	2	-2	0	0	0

24. $D_{3d} = D_3 . i$ 25. $D_{2h} = D_2 . i$ 26. $D_{3h} = D_3 . \sigma_h$

27. $D_{4h} = D_4 . i$ 28. $D_{5h} = D_5 . \sigma_h$ 29. $D_{6h} = D_6 . i$

30. T 31. $T_h = T \cdot i$

	E	$3C_2$	$4C_3$	$4C_3'$
A	1	1	1	1
E $\Big\{$	1	1	α	α^2
	1	1	α^2	α
T	3	-1	0	0

$\alpha = e^{2\pi i/3}$

32. O 33. $O_h = O \cdot i$

	E	$8C_3$	$3C_2$	$6C_2$	$6C_4$
A_1	1	1	1	1	1
A_2	1	1	1	-1	-1
E	2	-1	2	0	0
T_1	3	0	-1	-1	1
T_2	3	0	-1	1	-1

34. T_d 35. $C_{\infty v}$

	E	$8C_3$	$3C_2$	$6\sigma_d$	$6S_4$
A_1	1	1	1	1	1
A_2	1	1	1	-1	-1
E	2	-1	2	0	0
T_1	3	0	-1	-1	1
T_2	3	0	-1	1	-1

	E	$2C_\varphi$	σ_v
A_1	1	1	1
A_2	1	1	-1
E_1	2	$2\cos\varphi$	0
E_2	2	$2\cos 2\varphi$	0
$\ldots$			

36. $D_{\infty h}$

	E	$2C_\varphi$	C_2'	i	$2iC_\varphi$	iC_2'
A_{1g}	1	1	1	1	1	1
A_{1u}	1	1	1	-1	-1	-1
A_{2g}	1	1	-1	1	1	-1
A_{2u}	1	1	-1	-1	-1	1
E_{1g}	2	$2\cos\varphi$	0	2	$2\cos\varphi$	0
E_{1u}	2	$2\cos\varphi$	0	-2	$-2\cos\varphi$	0
$\ldots$						

Appendix 2

SPIN FUNCTIONS AND PAULI MATRICES

Let $\psi(x, y, z, \sigma)$ be the complete wavefunction of a particle, where σ is the z-component of the spin and assumes values between $-S$ and $+S$. At $S = \frac{1}{2}$, σ can assume two values ($\pm \frac{1}{2}$). In matrix form this may be written

$$\psi \left(\tfrac{1}{2}\right) = \begin{pmatrix} 1 \\ 0 \end{pmatrix}$$

$$\psi \left(-\tfrac{1}{2}\right) = \begin{pmatrix} 0 \\ 1 \end{pmatrix} \tag{1}$$

Pauli introduced spin operators in the form of matrices with two rows:

$$\hat{S}_z = \tfrac{1}{2}\begin{pmatrix} 1 & 0 \\ 0 & -1 \end{pmatrix} \qquad \hat{S}_x = \tfrac{1}{2}\begin{pmatrix} 0 & 1 \\ 1 & 0 \end{pmatrix} \qquad \hat{S}_y = \tfrac{1}{2}\begin{pmatrix} 0 & -i \\ i & 0 \end{pmatrix} \tag{2}$$

From this representation we can see that the functions $\psi(\tfrac{1}{2})$ and $\psi(-\tfrac{1}{2})$ are eigenfunctions of the operator $\hat{S}_z$. In fact the following relationships hold:

$$\hat{S}_z \psi(\tfrac{1}{2}) = \tfrac{1}{2}\begin{pmatrix} 1 & 0 \\ 0 & -1 \end{pmatrix}\begin{pmatrix} 1 \\ 0 \end{pmatrix} = \tfrac{1}{2}\begin{pmatrix} 1 \\ 0 \end{pmatrix} = \tfrac{1}{2}\psi(\tfrac{1}{2})$$

and

$$\hat{S}_z \psi(-\tfrac{1}{2}) = \tfrac{1}{2}\begin{pmatrix} 1 & 0 \\ 0 & -1 \end{pmatrix}\begin{pmatrix} 0 \\ 1 \end{pmatrix} = -\tfrac{1}{2}\begin{pmatrix} 0 \\ 1 \end{pmatrix} = -\tfrac{1}{2}\psi(-\tfrac{1}{2})$$

We can thus build up the following 'multiplication' table for the operator:

$$\hat{S}_x \psi(\tfrac{1}{2}) = \tfrac{1}{2}\psi(-\tfrac{1}{2}) \qquad \hat{S}_z \psi(\tfrac{1}{2}) = \tfrac{1}{2}\psi(\tfrac{1}{2})$$

$$\hat{S}_x \psi(-\tfrac{1}{2}) = \tfrac{1}{2}\psi(\tfrac{1}{2})$$

$$\hat{S}_y \psi(\tfrac{1}{2}) = \tfrac{i}{2}\psi(-\tfrac{1}{2}) \qquad \hat{S}_z \psi(-\tfrac{1}{2}) = -\tfrac{1}{2}\psi(-\tfrac{1}{2}) \tag{3}$$

$$\hat{S}_y \psi(-\tfrac{1}{2}) = -\tfrac{i}{2}\psi(\tfrac{1}{2})$$

Appendix 3

INTENSITY DISTRIBUTION IN AN H.F.S. SPECTRUM FOR *n* EQUIVALENT NUCLEI WITH $I = \frac{1}{2}$, 1 AND $\frac{3}{2}$

Table 1.   Intensity distribution in an H.F.S. spectrum for *n* equivalent nuclei with $I = \frac{1}{2}$ $(n \leqslant 20)$

n	Relative intensity
1	1 1
2	1 2 1
3	1 **3** **3** 1
4	1 4 **6** 4 1
5	1 5 **10** **10** 5 1
6	1 6 15 **20** 15 6 1
7	1 7 21 **35** **35** 21 7 1
8	1 8 28 56 **70** 56 28 8 1
9	1 9 36 84 **126** **126** 84 36 9 1
10	1 10 45 120 210 **252** 210 120 45 10 1
11	1 11 55 165 330 **462** **462** 330 165 55 11 1
12	1 12 66 220 495 792 **924** 792 495 220 66 12 1
13	1 13 78 286 715 1287 **1716** **1716** 1287 715 286 78 13 1
14	1 14 91 364 1001 2002 3003 **3432** 3003 2002 1001 364 ...
15	1 15 105 455 1365 3003 5005 **6435** **6435** 5005 3003 1365 ...
16	1 16 120 560 1820 4368 8008 11440 **12870** 11440 8008 4368 ...
17	1 17 136 680 2380 6188 12376 19448 **24310** **24310** 19448 12376 ...
18	1 18 153 816 3060 8568 18564 31824 43758 **48620** 43758 31824 ...
19	1 19 171 969 3876 11628 27132 50388 75582 **92378** **92378** 75582 ...
20	1 20 190 1140 4845 15504 38760 77520 125970 167960 **184756** 167960 ...

Table 2.   Intensity distribution in an H.F.S. spectrum for *n* equivalent nuclei with $I = 1$ $(n \leqslant 8)$

n	Relative intensity
1	**1 1 1**
2	1 2 **3** 2 1
3	1 3 6 **7** 6 3 1
4	1 4 10 16 **19** 16 10 4 1
5	1 5 15 30 45 **51** 45 30 15 5 1
6	1 6 21 50 90 126 **141** 126 90 ...
7	1 7 28 77 161 266 357 **393** 357 ...
8	1 8 36 112 266 504 784 1016 **1107** 1016 ...

Table 3.   Intensity distribution in an H.F.S. spectrum for n equivalent nuclei with $I = \frac{3}{2}$ $(n \leqslant 8)$

n	Relative intensity
1	**1** **1** **1** **1**
2	1 2 3 **4** 3 2 1
3	1 3 6 10 **12** **12** 10 6 3 1
4	1 4 10 20 31 40 **44** 40 31 20 10 . . .
5	1 5 15 35 65 101 135 **155** **155** 135 101 . . .
6	1 6 21 56 120 216 336 456 546 **580** 546 . . .
7	1 7 28 84 203 413 728 1128 1554 1918 **2128** **2128** . . .
8	1 8 36 120 322 728 1428 2472 3823 5328 6728 7728 **8092** 7728 . . .

INDEX

(The principal references to a subject are indicated by the use of bold type.)

Allyl radical, 93
Aminoacids, 253
Aprotic solvents, 192, 226
Aromatic anion radicals, 182, 203
Aromatic free radicals, 89

Benzonitrile, 226
Benzonitrile ion, 226
Biological oxidation, 295

Carbon, 302
Catalysts, 218, **278**, 287
Catalyst, chromium, 288
Catalysis, enzyme, 295
Chain molecule, 138
Characters, 59, 66
Character tables, 61
Charge transfer complexes, 216, 309, 310
Chromium, catalysts, 288
Chromium, oxide, 288
Compensation effect, 269
Conjugated bonds, 188, 192, 306, 308, 310
Conjugated double bonds, 196, 211
Contact interaction, 86
Coupling coefficients, 12
Crystal field, 48, 64
Crystal field, medium, 65
Crystal field, strong, 64
Crystal field, weak, 65

Deficiency structure, 197
Dibenzolchrome, 197
Dicarbonic acid, 243
Dipole–dipole interaction, 86
Direct product, **62**
Double modulation method, 33
DPPH, 42, 111, 151, 189

Effective volume, 11, 42
Electron transfer, 299
Ethane, irradiated, 233
Ethyl radicals, 283, 284
Excess noise, 16
Exchange narrowing, **102**

Fine structure, 81, 84

Ferrocene, 197
Free radicals, 231, **279**, 295, 308
Free radicals, aromatic, 89
Free radicals, reaction kinetics, 263
Frequency modulation model, **102**
Frequency mixing, 20

g-factor, 46, **72**
g-factor, anisotropy, **81, 84**, 127
Gaussian line, 101, 117, 127
Gaussian model, **100**
Group theory, 49

Hamiltonian operator, 62
Heterodyne spectrometer, 21, 24, 29
Hydrogen atom, 180, 221, 224, 279
Hydrogen atom, hot, **248**
Hydrogen, atomic, 145
Hyperfine structure, 7, 85, **143**

Integral intensity, 108
Ion radicals, 225
Ion pairs, 215, 224
Irreducible representation, 58, 61
Irreducible representation of the rotational group, 66

Jahn–Teller theorem, 74

Kramer's theorem, 72, 83

Lattice, 48, 95, 97
Line width, 94, **134**
Line shape, 115
Lorentzian line, 117
Lorentzian model, 99
Lorentzian shape, 100
Lyophilized tissue, 296

Magnetic field modulation, **31**
Molybdenum trioxide, 292

Naphthalene ion, 214
Natural tissue, 257
Nickel, ferromagnetic resonance, 294
Nuclear moment, 85, 145
Nucleic acid, 258, 310

321

Orbital moment, quenching, 75
Oxidation, biological, 295

Paramagnetic particles, minimum
    detectable number, 41
Perinaphthene, 92, 194
Phthalocyanine, 308
Polarography, 226
Polycrystal, 125
Polymers, 211
Polyphenylacetylene, 306
Proteins, 256, 298
Protic solvent, 192

Quenching, 75

Radiation yield, 230
Radicals, 283
Radicals, allyl, 93
Radicals, aromatic anion, 203
Radicals, aromatic free, 89
Radicals, ethyl, 283, 284
Radicals, free, 231, 279, 295, 308
Radicals, free, reaction kinetics, 262
Radical recombination, 232
Radiolysis, 230, 236
Radiolysis, biological materials, 252
Raman scattering of lattice phonons, 97
Reaction kinetics, 213
Reaction kinetics, free radical, 262
Recombination, 280
Recombination kinetics of triphenyl-
    methyl radicals, 183
Representation theory, 52
Representation, double-valued, 70
Resolution, 8
Rotational group, 65
Rotational group, irreducible
    representation of, 66

Sandwich complexes, 197
Sandwich compounds, 294
Saturation, 8, 40, 98, 282
Semiconductor diodes, 15
Semiquinones, 182, 191, 228, 295
Sensitivity, limiting, 40
Solvent, aprotic, 192, 226
Solvent, protic, 192
Spectral lines, distortion of shape, 39
Spin density, negative, 92, 197, 200
Spin-Hamiltonian operator, 81
Spin-lattice interaction, 94
Spin-lattice relaxation time, 96
Spin-orbit coupling, 96
Spin-orbit interaction, 76
Spin-spin interaction, 98
Spin temperature, 95
Stark effect, 64, 70
Stilbene, 207
Structure, fine, 81, 84
Structure, hyperfine, 7, 85, 143
Sugar carbon, 302
Susceptibility, minimum detectable, 40
Sweep, 32, 33
Symmetry groups, 52
Symmetry operations, 52

Teflon, 139, 234, 262
Tissue, lyophilized, 296
Tissue, natural, 257
Transition probability, 95
Triphenylmethyl, 92, 182
Triphenylmethyl radicals, recombination
    kinetics, 182

U.V. light, 221

Vanadium pentoxide, 292
Video spectrometer, 32